Professionalizing
Medicine

Professionalizing Medicine

*James Reeves and the Choices
That Shaped American Health Care*

JOHN M. HARRIS, JR.

McFarland & Company, Inc., Publishers
Jefferson, North Carolina

Library of Congress Cataloguing-in-Publication Data

Names: Harris, John M. (John Malcolm), 1948– author.
Title: Professionalizing medicine : James Reeves and the choices
that shaped American health care / John M. Harris Jr.
Description: Jefferson, North Carolina : McFarland & Company, Inc.,
Publishers, 2019. | Includes bibliographical references and index.
Identifiers: LCCN 2019007709 | ISBN 9781476676364
(paperback : acid free paper) ∞
Subjects: LCSH: Reeves, James E. (James Edmund),
1829–1896—Health. | Medicine—United States—Biography. |
Medicine—United States—History—Biography.
Classification: LCC R133 .H375 2019 | DDC 610.92 [B] —dc23
LC record available at https://lccn.loc.gov/2019007709

British Library cataloguing data are available

ISBN (print) 978-1-4766-7636-4
ISBN (ebook) 978-1-4766-3622-1

Front cover: James Reeves (National Library of Medicine)

Printed in the United States of America

*McFarland & Company, Inc., Publishers
Box 611, Jefferson, North Carolina 28640
www.mcfarlandpub.com*

To Dr. Robin B. Harris, my wife
and companion in medical history

Table of Contents

Preface

An ailing James Reeves traveled from his home in Chattanooga for a consultation with Baltimore's William Osler in October 1895. The two physicians were prominent American pathologists and knew each other well. Reeves hoped his diagnosis was a benign liver tumor, but Osler found untreatable cancer. Reeves sent Osler three collectible medical books to thank him for his courtesy. Each was dedicated "To Dr. Wm Osler with Love. James E. Reeves, Chattanooga, Tenn. October 17th '95."

Osler gave one of Reeves' books to Maryland's state medical society and bequeathed the other two, and eight thousand more, to McGill University in Montreal. The medical society eventually purged its holdings and a Philadelphia dealer sold the first book to a young physician in 1976. It was an 1824 edition of A.P.W. Philip's *Treatise on Indigestion*. Much later, this book prompted the question "Who was James Reeves?"

Reeves was an apostle of nineteenth-century medical science and a founder of the American public health movement. He was nationally recognized in his time, but is now mostly remembered as the physician brother of Ann Reeves Jarvis, the West Virginia Sunday school teacher who inspired Mother's Day.

Reeves' story is worth knowing because it personalizes the hectic fifty-year period when medical science transformed the American health care landscape. Today's medical science may seem breathtakingly advanced, but no more so than Koch's discovery of the tubercle bacillus was to those alive in 1882. The era has been amply described by medical sociologists and historians, each with their interpretations of the big issues, but there are few serious biographies of the players, men like Nathan Davis who founded the American Medical Association, Stephen Smith who founded the American Public Health Association, and James Reeves, who was a leader in both. Reeves' life puts a human lens on the issues and times that shaped our own while offering a deeper perspective into their nature.

Reeves' story is appropriate for health care practitioners and educators because he was a relatively unique blend of practicing physician, scientist, moralist, and community activist. He organized medical societies, but he did not see them as many physicians did, professional fraternities demanding loyalty. He saw them as open temples to nature that had to earn their place in society by humility and devotion to science. He confronted a hard moral question that is still with us—to whom did medical science belong? For Reeves the answer was medical science belonged to everyone, which meant that his profession was in partnership with society, not distinct from it. But his response was in the minority.

Most nineteenth-century American physicians saw themselves as inhabitants of a besieged professional citadel where medical science was their crown jewel. Their professional citadel metaphor led them to another metaphor that underlies today's vision of medical professionalism, that health care delivery is part of a social bargain in which practitioners use their science for good and society reciprocates with status and professional autonomy. This image guides health care's vision of itself and how it trains tomorrow's physicians. It encourages right behavior, but it also fosters a disturbing sense of entitlement. I argue that health care's social contract metaphor is incomplete, destructive, and historically inaccurate. Reeves' story offers a way to re-examine the relationship's origins and explore an alternative connection between those who deliver health care and society.

My five-year effort to discover James Reeves and pull his story together was often solitary, but never unaccompanied. I owe debts to many folks for their encouragement, criticism, and fact-finding. In particular, to the late Kate Quinn who kept Reeves' name alive in her community and graciously introduced my wife and me to Wheeling and its health officer, Dr. William Mercer.

I am grateful to Reeves' great-great granddaughters, Joan Webb and Barbara Boren, for sharing their family mementos and for their kind support over these past years. Professors Ken Fones-Wolf and Connie Rice in the University of West Virginia History Department and the staff at the West Virginia and Regional History Center took care of me and offered helpful guidance on my trips to Morgantown.

Eva Grimsley at the Rappahannock Historical Society found census records on the Reeves family that I could have never located. Barbara Smith in Philippi graciously, and purely for the fun of it, tracked down deeds, lawsuits, and facts that made sense of Reeves' early life. Allison Piazza and Arlene Shaner at the New York Academy of Medicine did a wonderful job of locating obscure hard-copy references in their files, as did David Clapp and Suzette Raney in Chattanooga. Caroline Hoag and Sue Hersman, descendants of John Hupp and Frank Dent, kindly supplied materials to the cause. There were many more who answered email requests, phone calls, and the occasional drop-in with kind professionalism. Thanks to all.

From the perspective of a twenty-first century historian, I must give a shout-out to Google co-founder Larry Page and the many academic partners that make Google Books and similar projects possible. My story fell into a bibliographic sweet spot where key written resources were easily understood, out of copyright, and often digitized. I could not have constructed Reeves' life or his medicine without these resources. As one example, my book contains 319 references from newspaper articles, 95 percent of which are digitized and searchable. From the pain of visually scanning the 5 percent that now exist only on microfilm, I can confidently say that this story could not have been written before Google Books.

I owe thanks to the wonderful people who slogged through the many versions of this manuscript with me. In particular, Cris Campbell and Tim DeWolf, genuine bibliophiles, offered good suggestions and kind words, as did Drs. Thomas and Barbara Elliott, Dr. Jacalyn Duffin, and Dr. Herbert Swick. I extend a special thank you to recently retired University of Oregon history professor James Mohr, who patiently gave me hours of helpful advice. His grad students were lucky to have him. Jim often reminds me that, to this point, he and I are the only members of the James Reeves fan club.

And lastly, I thank my wife, Robin Harris—for a lot, but in this case for joining me on trips to Virginia and West Virginia, for encouraging me and listening to my ideas as I found yet another shiny nugget of nineteenth-century medicine to explore, and for reading and critiquing the whole thing, more than once.

Prologue
One of the Best and Truest Men in the Profession

His funeral was a civic event. The Chattanooga *Times* devoted a page to his accomplishments and the doctor's national stature: "He was esteemed by great men in the profession—Chattanooga loses a good friend." The memorial service was packed with Chattanooga's leading citizens. The local medical society called a special meeting to issue a resolution acknowledging his many contributions to the city and the medical profession, naming him one of the foremost physicians of his age.[1]

That evening, January 5, 1896, a train transported Dr. James Reeves' body from Tennessee to Wheeling, West Virginia, where he had spent most of his professional life. On January 7 there was a second funeral service and the scene was again notable for the large number of physicians. Mayor Caldwell was one of pallbearers who carried the famous doctor's remains to Greenwood Cemetery.[2]

Three months before his death Reeves travelled to Baltimore, Maryland, where William Osler, the country's best-known physician, diagnosed Reeves with untreatable liver cancer. Soon afterwards Chattanooga's mayor, George Ochs, sent a grim letter to Wheeling's mayor Benjamin Caldwell, telling him that Reeves was wasting away and could die soon. Both men knew Reeves well and admired his integrity and his fortitude. They also appreciated his scientific work. Ochs wrote, "I regard Dr. Reeves as one of the most eminent specialists of this country, and his discoveries and achievements in microscopy will, as years roll by, place him among the foremost of American specialists."[3]

Reeves was a renowned microscopist, but to his longtime friends he was also a founder of the country's public health movement and a champion of his profession. Reeves wrote and enforced West Virginia's Board of Health Act, and, when the Act's licensing provisions were upheld by the U.S. Supreme Court in 1889, Reeves' law provided Constitutional justification for the state regulation of all professions. After making the fatal diagnosis, Osler shared the sad news with mutual friends George Gould, editor of Philadelphia's *Medical News*, and James Baldwin, a prominent Ohio surgeon. Gould, who supported Reeves in one of his last battles against quackery, wrote to Baldwin, "He is one of the best and truest men in the profession, as you say, and has done noble work for us all and for humanity."[4]

4

Reeves labored at the nexus of medical science, clinical practice, and public health during the half century when American medicine emerged from a disjointed trade to the respected profession and government-sanctioned industry it now is. He frequently described medicine as his "true church"; however, his deeds and his values did not always align with other physicians' professional goals. Instead, they exposed difficult choices that still trouble American health care. Once the funeral ceremonies were done, his profession preferred to forget Reeves, much as a congregation loses interest in a demanding and recently departed itinerant preacher.

⑈ 1 ⑈

The Age of Jackson Begins

Wednesday, March 4, 1829, was the nicest day for a presidential inauguration in the young nation's history and Old Hickory walked comfortably to his swearing-in without a hat. After the ceremony President Andrew Jackson rode his horse down Pennsylvania Avenue to the White House where pandemonium quickly followed. Twenty thousand people pressed the building, from which Jackson barely escaped. An observer recorded the scene: "Ladies fainted, men were seen with bloody noses, and such a scene of confusion took place as is impossible to describe—those who got in could not get out by the door again, but had to scramble out of windows." It was a prophetic beginning for the turbulent period between 1829 and Jackson's death in 1845, a time later known as "the Age of Jackson."[1]

In neighboring Amissville, Virginia, Josiah and Nancy Reeves celebrated the birth of their first child, James Edmund, on April 5, a month after Jackson's inauguration. Josiah was a nineteen-year-old tailor who had moved to Virginia from Maryland. Nancy Kemper Reeves was a year older, descended from Germans who had immigrated to Virginia in 1714. Many of Nancy's German relatives lived in nearby Fauquier County; however, Nancy's mother, Elizabeth Bayse, was from Amissville and belonged to one of the two original English families in town, the other family having given the town its name. Josiah and Nancy lived near Nancy's sister, Elizabeth Kemper.[2]

Today Amissville is a pastoral village and Washington, D.C., bedroom community, located in rural Rappahannock County. It was in Culpeper County in 1829 and even less pretentious than now, with only a store, schoolhouse, and blacksmith shop. Three members of the Amiss family bought land that year for a Methodist church to be built opposite the schoolhouse.[3] This was positive news for Josiah because the young tailor had goals of becoming a Methodist preacher.

Josiah raised his family in a strict Methodist household and his son was a product of early nineteenth-century American Methodism. Reeves' father was formally ordained as a deacon in 1859, but probably from his time in Amissville, he was one of the many tradesmen who served as Methodist lay preachers.[4]

The Methodism that inspired Josiah and shaped his son was different from the twentieth century's liberal United Methodist Church. It was a young, evangelical, Protestant sect, founded in Oxford (England) by Anglican priest, John Wesley. Wesley's zealous preaching, his methodical daily approach to Christian perfection, and the religious clubs formed by his friends gave rise to epithets, one of which was "Sacramentarians," another was "Oxford Methodists."[5]

American Methodists followed Wesley's doctrines after the Revolutionary War, but they developed their own branch of his church. The American Methodist Church was flexible and community-focused. By encouraging tradesmen like Josiah to minister, the Church became a haven for ordinary people seeking the meaning of the Gospel.

James' life path, as set down by his church, was one of personal industry, moral correctness, and genuine humility. He regularly saw itinerant preachers, modeled on Wesley's own peripatetic ministry, who personified nineteenth-century American Methodist virtues. Methodist itinerants visited each community in their two hundred to five hundred-mile circuits every two to six weeks and were often one of the few outsiders many rural villages saw. When the preacher arrived on horseback he would stay with a local family, offer a sermon, and examine the local classes. Unless there was a quarterly assembly or a camp meeting, he was off the following day.

The Methodist Church of Jackson's age was America's largest and fastest-growing denomination, and Methodist teachings amplified and shaped Reeves' professional life. Wesley sermonized that Methodists must be slow to judge, but when encountering false prophets they should judge firmly. Wesley admonished Methodists to call out to their brothers and sisters who had erred, not to keep quiet or to ignore their transgressions. Reeves followed these principles, often creating friction with physicians who preferred fraternal harmony. Reeves adopted the humanistic metaphor of a "true church" to portray medicine's dedication to science, but, in the spirit of his Methodism, he saw professional boasting as more than unscientific hubris or unethical professionalism; it was sinful.[6]

Wesley wrote his own medical book and popularized the phrase "cleanliness is next to Godliness."[7] As nineteenth-century regular physicians moved away from the flawed theories of heroic medicine and rediscovered the healing powers of nature, Reeves found a professional home in Wesley's doctrines of sanitation and preventive medicine.

Nearby events altered the Reeves family's future. Visitors to the Capitol rotunda during Jackson's inauguration in 1829 could see a suspended half pound weight affixed with sewing cotton move a 1,760 pound load along a set of rails. An observer summed up the implications: "From the results of those experiments and the information which has been received, who will doubt the great superiority of railroads to that of canals?"[8]

A railroad was a bed of rails over which horse-drawn carriages travelled when Reeves was born, and there were less than forty miles of railroads in the entire country. In neighboring Baltimore the city's merchants and bankers were spurred by the success of New York's Erie Canal to invest in a railroad connecting their Atlantic port with the Ohio River; they planned to use animal power. However, on October 10, 1829, Robert Stephenson's Rocket won a contest in Merseyside, England to develop a practical steam locomotive. The directors of the Baltimore and Ohio Railroad Company challenged Peter Cooper's Baltimore iron works to develop a locomotive based on Stephenson's model that could navigate the tight turns across the mountains to the Ohio River. Despite losing a race to a horse in 1830, Cooper's Tom Thumb demonstrated that a nimble, coal-powered, American-built locomotive was feasible.[9, 10]

One nineteenth-century historian called the rail line that eventually connected Baltimore and the Ohio River port of Wheeling, Virginia: "the world's first really important railroad." Within a generation the B&O disrupted centuries of established communication and transportation patterns. The railroad determined where the Reeves family lived and brought the Civil War to Josiah's home town. It fostered the state's near religious devotion to development as Reeves began his public health career in West Virginia.[11]

Railroads made mobility and geographic expansion synonymous with progress. The 1845 inaugural issue of *Scientific American* featured a railroad car on its first page as an exemplar of the country's scientific accomplishments. Railroads allowed physicians to develop their national organizations while providing an omnipresent image of the power of modern science.[12]

Another local event that occurred the year he was born also shaped Reeves' future. The Virginia state legislature called a constitutional convention on October 5, 1829, to address discord between the eastern and western parts of the state. The country watched to see how the Old Dominion would handle its difficulties.

The key constitutional problems were legislative representation and suffrage, growing pains that troubled many states. The population was 39 percent slaves and had more than doubled since the American Revolution. Most of Virginia's inhabitants and 90 percent of its slaves lived in the eastern tidewater area. The eastern landowners, descended from English immigrants, ran the state, but the growth was in the west.

Western delegates wanted representation based on white population, while eastern representatives favored a combination of white population and property value. In terms of suffrage, westerners wanted the vote for all free men, as did many Jacksonians, while easterners wanted to restrict the vote to free men of property. For easterners, property included their "peculiar institution" of slavery.

The Convention's debates degenerated into attacks over loyalty, honor, tyranny, and treason, diatribes that often overwhelmed thoughtful presentations of economics and politics. William Gordon of Albemarle said of his fellow Virginians, "a more gallant people is not on the earth; the only fear they know, is the dread of a dishonorable action."[13] Moral causes, not voting rights, were what people killed and died for. In the end, the delegates handed their problems to the next generation. The new state constitution allowed for reapportionment, but it could not occur until 1841 and then only if most of the eastern counties agreed. The eastern slaveholding counties continued with business as usual.

Affronted westerners wanted satisfaction, by secession from Virginia if necessary, even though the U.S. Constitution prohibited the creation of a new state from an existing one without the original state's agreement and Congressional approval. A writer in the Wheeling *Gazette* of April 1830 demanded that a convention in the West be called to appoint commissioners: "To treat with the eastern nabobs for a division of the state— peaceably if we can, forcibly if we must."[14] Secession would become the answer, but peace and cooler heads prevailed in 1829.

Josiah and Nancy had another son, Joseph Henry Clay, in 1830. The census showed them living in Amissville that year with two young sons and three slaves: a mother and two daughters. Tax records from 1834 and 1835 also placed Josiah and his family in Amissville, but, by 1839, the Reeves family had moved across the Blue Ridge, to New Market, Virginia. Unlike rural Amissville, New Market was an active mercantile center, located on the axis of the Shenandoah Valley, with a population of seven hundred, three churches (Lutheran, Baptist, Methodist), a large brick academy, five stores, three taverns, one lawyer, and four doctors. A good situation for a young tailor.[15]

New Market was also a seat of learning that could inspire a curious boy. Industrious Germans from Pennsylvania had entered the fertile valley more than one hundred years before Josiah's arrival. Ambrose Henkel set up a German press in New Market in 1806 and several generations of English-speaking Henkels continued his printing legacy. One historian noted, "It is not an accident that an academy was chartered at New Market in 1817; that a theological seminary was launched there in 1821; that Shenandale College was projected in 1849."[16]

Several of New Market's German residents had an interest in medicine and one of them would later tutor an aspiring Reeves. By the time of Josiah's arrival, Dr. Jacob Neff, son of Dr. David Neff, was well-established in New Market.[17] Several years later, Jacob Neff provided Reeves with his first real training in medicine.

In contrast to the English settlers east of the Blue Ridge, Valley Germans did not usually own slaves. About three quarters of Shenandoah County's white population was of German heritage in 1840 and 9 percent of the County's 11,600 inhabitants were slaves, compared to almost 50 percent of Virginia's eastern population. Germans tended to have large families, whose members worked in their fields and shops. In addition, the German Mennonites and Dunkers (German Baptists), like the English Methodists, were religiously opposed to slavery.[18]

However, as in Amissville, Josiah Reeves was at least a part-time slaveholder during his New Market years. He reported two slaves in 1840 and 1843, whereas in 1839, 1841, and 1842, he had none.[19] The 1840 federal census showed the family owning one slave, a female age thirty-six to fifty-five, probably a domestic servant.[20] The most likely reason that Josiah reported slaves in some years but not others was that he hired or loaned them out during the years they were not counted as his property. Josiah's practical Methodist morality could have accepted the ownership of a slave or two as a domestic servant, so long as the servant was well-treated.

Reeves attended school in New Market, but Josiah made him help the family as a part-time tailor's apprentice. The son resented this work from the beginning. Reeves' sister, Ann, wrote almost 60 years later, "My father resolved that James must learn some kind of a trade, and to this end decided upon that of tailoring. Nothing could have been more distasteful to him, as he preferred an intellectual pursuit."[21]

A lingering economic depression began 1837 and word arrived of new opportunities along the railroad. Virginia's agricultural economy suffered and the state's sons and daughters crossed the mountains. Josiah sold his house and property in New Market in 1842. This sale may have included his slaves because there is no record of Josiah owning slaves once he left New Market. The following year, 1843, he purchased a one-quarter acre lot from William Wilson in Barbour County's recently platted county seat.[22]

Barbour County was one hundred fifty miles west of New Market, over the formidable Allegheny Mountains. The newly-formed Virginia county was named for Philip Pendleton Barbour, president of the Constitutional Convention of 1829, Speaker of the U.S. House of Representatives, and a U.S. Supreme Court Justice. Barbour County's seat, mostly empty bottom land adjoining a ferry crossing, was first called "Phillippa," possibly to honor Philip Barbour or his daughter, Philippa, but by 1844 the emerging settlement was known as Philippi.[23]

Historians disagree on the number of children, the year that Reeves' sister Ann was born, and when the family moved to Philippi.[24] The family Bible listed five children, four of whom were likely born in Amissville: James Edmund, the eldest (born in 1829), Joseph Henry Clay (1830), Ann Maria (1832), and George Washington (1834). The fifth child, Emily Hersey (1839) was likely born in New Market.[25] The 1840 U.S. census listed six children, including another baby girl, but did not give names.[26] The family had a seventh child, Thomas Asbury Reeves, who was seven years old in the 1850 census and born about the time of their move to Philippi. However, the 1850 census only recorded four children living with Josiah and Nancy: Joseph, Ann, Emily, and Thomas. By then James had left home and, presumably, George and the young girl from the 1840 census were no longer alive.[27] Josiah's granddaughter, Anna Jarvis, only recorded five children: James, Joseph, Ann, Emily, and Thomas.[28]

According to Josiah's 1882 obituary, most likely written by Reeves, Josiah moved his family to Philippi in 1843, after the sale of his New Market property and at the time of his first land purchase in Philippi. Josiah rented space near Philippi's new courthouse for his tailoring shop and went into business with bootmaker Edmund Compton.[29] That year, when Reeves was fourteen, Josiah made him leave school and begin working as a full-time tailor's apprentice.[30]

Philippi sat alongside a shallow river in the Tygart Valley. The river was usually too wide to cross on foot or horseback, but too rocky for barges and commercial flatboats. There was no bridge before 1852, so travelers typically crossed by ferry. The river provided Philippi with a source of water and power for mills, while the location offered a convenient transit point for the road connecting Beverly in the southeast with Clarksburg to the west and, after 1852, Fairmont to the northwest. Philippi's location permitted the growth of services such as tailoring, inn keeping, and local transportation.

Most of Barbour County's residents were immigrant subsistence farmers who did not live in town. The hilly land around Philippi probably reminded the Irish and Scot settlers of their ancestral homes, but it was not particularly bountiful. The major crop was corn and the principal livestock

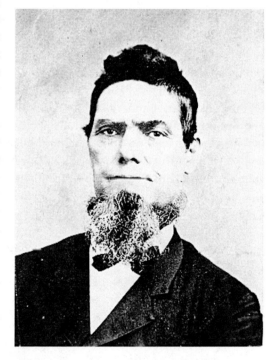

Josiah Washington Reeves (1810–1882), father of James Edmund and Ann Maria Reeves, date unknown. Ann described her father as a stern Methodist minister, but he worked as a tailor and most likely served as a lay preacher during James' early life. He was ordained as a Methodist deacon in 1859. Josiah insisted that James learn tailoring and discouraged his son's interest in medicine (courtesy Joan Webb).

was hogs, although some farmers grew wheat and rye and others raised cattle or sheep. If a settler did not use his grains domestically, he often converted them to whiskey, not only easier to sell, but a staple for house raising, log rollings, and shooting matches.

Philippi was only slightly more civilized than the countryside and a long way from the educated settlement of New Market. A flood deposited water nineteen inches deep in front of the court house in 1846. In 1850 there were only twenty-seven families in Philippi. Animals roamed unchecked, causing property damage and adding to sanitation problems. When the town was finally incorporated in 1871 the first ordinance the council passed authorized the restraint of loose hogs and horses. The council passed a similar ordinance four years later concerning geese.[31]

The Reeves tailoring business was modestly successful in this rough environment, at least by local standards. According to Ann Reeves, "We were always surrounded by comforts equal to, if not superior to those around us." The family home was on a large town lot, consisting of one and one quarter acres of bottomland and three acres of steep hillside.[32]

Barbour County's dominant religion was Methodism. The first two ministers licensed to perform marriages in 1843 were Methodists. After the courthouse and jail, one of the earliest public buildings in Philippi was the Methodist church, completed in 1851, two years before the schoolhouse.[33] As Josiah was settling into Philippi and reconciling his own relationship with slavery, his faith entered a crossroads that forced its adherents to make a difficult choice.

Northern Methodists increasingly viewed Southern resistance to Wesley's antislavery doctrines as heresy and Southern Methodists saw Yankee self-righteousness as external opposition to their mission to spread God's Word, the theological equivalent of treason versus tyranny. Long-simmering issues reached full boil at the 1844 Methodist General Conference in New York City. Northern delegates were adamant that slaveholding, particularly by the clergy, was immoral and incompatible with the Church's purpose. Southerners argued that slavery was not governed by the Methodist Church.

Southern delegates convinced themselves that their Church's founder, Wesley, "never deemed it proper to have any rule, law, or regulation on the subject of slavery, either in the United States, the West Indies, or elsewhere."[34] However, Wesley bitterly and eloquently objected to slavery in any form, anywhere. In his 1774 *Thoughts upon Slavery*, he wrote,

> The grand plea is "They [slaves] are authorized by Law." But can Law, Human Law, change the nature of things? Can it turn Darkness into Light or evil into good? By no means. Notwithstanding ten thousand laws, right is right and wrong is wrong, still.[35]

Subsequent events foreshadowed the cataclysm that followed. Hoping to ensure denominational peace, the Methodist General Conference divided its house, adopting a resolution allowing for a separation into Northern and Southern Churches.

Southern preachers saw themselves as good men who, if they followed the Northern lead, would lose their congregations and their ability to bring Christ's message to enslaved Negroes. Albeit, their message was that masters should treat their slaves kindly and slaves should obey their masters. To them, this message had allowed the Church to prosper in the South, which meant that God endorsed it.

The Southern clergy met on May 1, 1845, in Louisville, Kentucky to formalize the separation. After sixteen days of deliberation, the delegates took the intended step of creating a separate church. During the same month, a group of Southern Baptists met in Augusta, Georgia and declared a separate ministry for the South.

Thoughtful Christians grasped the implications of these rifts in the major Protestant denominations. The Presbyterian *Watchman of the South* (in Richmond) editorialized, "The churches once divided, North and South, Demagogues will have but little [more] to do to dissolve the Union of the States. That done, then we shall see war and horrible contests. Brother will slay brother." A Presbyterian paper in Philadelphia agonized, "If a union cemented by all the finer influences of the gospel could not last, what can?"[36]

The Methodist schism hardened the family's moral commitments. Reeves' sister Ann welcomed a prominent Southern preacher into her house during the Civil War and when the minister tried to persuade her to form a new Southern Methodist church, she suggested he take the next train home. She told him, "her church should not be split over Civil War issues if it was in her power to prevent it."[37] Reeves remained with the Northern Church as he cared for his Confederate neighbors during the Civil War, a difficult choice that many of his closest friends avoided.

⚕ 2 ⚕

Medicine in the Age of Jackson

American physicians struggled with their identity and their science during the Jacksonian Age and Reeves spent his professional life dealing with these issues. Since colonial times, the small number of elite American physicians had copied British educational and organizational models and set themselves up as learned professionals—men of science. But by 1829 they competed in a growing, disorganized medical marketplace with self-help, alternative healers, medical swindlers, and an increasing supply of poorly-trained fellow physicians.

William Shippen, Jr., and John Morgan founded the English colonies' first medical school in 1765 at the College of Philadelphia, later the University of Pennsylvania. Shippen and Morgan's graduates called themselves regularly educated physicians, or "regulars." The few American medical colleges that followed Philadelphia adopted a similar curriculum. These colleges required students to study Latin, mathematics, anatomy, botany, chemistry, medicine, surgery, and *materia medica*. Students had to complete two sets of identical courses, typically four months each, write a dissertation, and apprentice with a seasoned regular physician for at least three years before receiving a diploma.

European physicians and their American counterparts argued that medicine had moved beyond its mystical heritage. It was now a learned profession, based on science. They pointed to the prevention of smallpox with inoculation and vaccination, the prevention and cure of sea scurvy with lemon juice, the treatment of chlorosis (anemia) with iron salts, and the anatomical and surgical advances of John and William Hunter. They claimed a better understanding of human anatomy than their competitors, an understanding garnered from cadavers obtained by grave-robbing, which, in turn, served as a macabre professional initiation rite. For well-trained regulars, surgery was no longer a marginal craft, but an acceptable and scientific medical art. The public agreed. Without the benefits of anesthesia and antisepsis, surgery was still a useful and evolving therapy in the early nineteenth century.[1]

Regular physicians also argued that their emerging profession deserved protection. America's regular physicians adapted England's market-controlling College of Physicians of London to their colonial world. The College was a royal society, chartered in 1518, that functioned as a medieval craft guild and its American equivalent was medical licensure laws. New York City passed a law in 1760 requiring examination and licensure to practice medicine. New Jersey issued a law in 1772 mandating that anyone wishing to practice medicine in New Jersey undergo examination by a licensing panel. Colonial licensing laws supported physicians' claim to social status, but afforded little competitive security beyond the ability to sue for non-payment of fees.

Regular physicians achieved modest guild powers after the American Revolution. New York State's 1806 licensing law required county medical societies to examine and license anyone who sought to practice medicine in the county, which encouraged the formation of local societies. By 1808, nearly every New York county had a medical society with a board of censors and a library. When Reeves was born all but three states required state approval, a medical diploma, or local medical society endorsement to practice medicine.[2]

Later American physicians saw the early nineteenth century as a golden age, when their profession was venerated and protected because of its antiquity and its science. But the age was more chaotic than golden. The U.S. population almost doubled by 1810, from 2.8 million in 1780 to 5.3 million. The handful of staid American medical colleges only produced one hundred graduates in 1810, not nearly enough. The small number of "golden age" medical men with respectable diplomas formed societies and mingled in cities, but most physicians did not attend regular medical colleges and cobbled together lonely rural practices. Many of these doctors had only apprenticed with another physician, one who had not attended a medical college either.[3]

Until physicians like Reeves made their mark, nineteenth-century licensure laws accepted all medical diplomas as evidence of fitness for practice and entrepreneurial medical educators rushed to the opportunity. New medical colleges arose, as one contemporary observer put it, "like mushrooms after a night of rain." The number of American medical colleges tripled from six in 1810 to nineteen in 1830 and the number of graduates increased from one hundred to six hundred per year.[4]

Antebellum medical colleges set their own standards and depended on student fees, thus most entered a race to the bottom. Many new schools only required that the prospective student be acceptable to a preceptor. Some had no admission requirements except the willingness of a student to matriculate. Bending the rules for graduation became a fact of life. An easily-obtained medical diploma became the ticket to state licensure and public acceptance. One in four new licenses in New York was based on a medical diploma in 1820. The proportion was roughly one in three in 1830 and by 1846 it was more than nine in ten.[5]

The burgeoning supply of poorly-trained, diploma-certified physicians threatened the medical profession's claims to privileged status; but this claim was also undermined by larger social forces. America's politicians were well-acquainted with Adam Smith's denunciation of the guild system. Smith's philosophical arguments and Jacksonian frontier egalitarianism opposed elitism and privilege across the board.[6]

New states did not create licensure laws and others began to repeal theirs. Some states, including Reeves' Virginia, never had one. State legislatures in the Jacksonian age did not want to interfere with root doctors, Indian doctors, midwives, or anyone else who provided medical services to the public. By 1849 only New Jersey and the District of Columbia maintained control of medical licensure. Elite regular physicians despaired of their educational institutions, along with any hope of public support in maintaining professional stability and quality. Many families, including Reeves', did not want their sons to become doctors.[7]

Confronted with deteriorating quality in their ranks and loss of legislative protection, regular physicians faced still another problem. The public could see the fruits of mechanical science as locomotives began crossing the countryside, but when it looked at regular medicine, even in the best of hands, it saw flawed theories and harsh treatments: the consequences of regulars' chosen position as men of science. Natural philosophers like Newton and Priestley had made discoveries that changed lives. Wanting to be seen as learned philosophers, regulars often adopted the rhetoric of Sir Francis Bacon (1561–1626), but not his practices. This led them down the path of grand theories.

According to Bacon, data should be used to derive axioms or theories, and theories should be tested with more data. Bacon wrote that the road to truth rises and falls "uphill to axioms and downhill to effects." Unlike Bacon, physicians created competing theoretical systems around small numbers of observations, supported their theories with still more theories until they had a grand "system," and pushed their systems into the world untested. Bacon had witnessed this process and criticized it.[8]

American Founding Father Benjamin Rush exemplified the age's theory-driven, system-building model and set the pattern for early nineteenth-century American regular medicine. Rush theorized in 1790 that inflammation and congestion of the blood vessels caused or complicated not just some, but virtually all diseases. This being the case, his explanatory system dictated that inflammation and congestion must be relieved by antiphlogistic (anti-inflammatory) therapies, specifically ones such as bleeding and purging that caused systemic depletion and reduced the visible signs of inflammation.[9]

Rush's easily-grasped approach guided American practice until it was briefly superseded in 1820 by that of French physician Francois Broussais, who claimed that all diseases were due to inflammation of the gastrointestinal tract rather than the blood vessels.[10] Rush and Broussais arrived at the same point, both advocating bleeding and other depletive measures. Indeed, the more ominous the disease, the more drastically aggressive and "heroic" must be the treatment because nature alone could not cure the problem. Regular physicians presented themselves as heroes coming to rescue nature, but patients knew they had to act heroically to withstand such treatment.

Observant physicians and laymen grasped the underlying problem—that medicine had very few real facts with which to work. Physician to the English King, Sir Gilbert Blane, facetiously noted in 1821 that a few apparent truths based on actual experience could lead to tortuously different, but eventually convergent theoretical systems: "It is also very remarkable, that theories, though widely different, do often wonderfully coincide in matters of practice with each other, and with well-established empirical usages, each bending and conforming, in order to do homage to truth and experience."[11]

Rush's friend, Thomas Jefferson, wrote, "I wish to see a reform, an abandonment of hypothesis for sober facts, the first degree of value set on clinical observation, and the lowest on visionary theories.... The only sure foundations of medicine are an intimate knowledge of the human body and observations of the effects of medical substances on that."[12]

Regular physicians had disavowed the heroic therapies and theory-based medical systems that guided their professional fathers by 1876, but the reasons for their use remain a source of debate. Missing the logical implications, medical leaders of the nation's centennial described their "golden age" predecessors as misguided and blind.[13]

Medical historians often followed this lead. Haller (1981) described physicians of the time (and their patients) as delusional. Rothstein (1992) dismissed the medical therapeutics of the early part of the century as mostly medically invalid. According to Rosenberg (1977), if heroic therapies worked it was due to their symbolic power: "not in a [medical] sense immediately intelligible to a mid-twentieth century pharmacologist or clinician."[14]

To accept that early nineteenth-century regulars were blind and their practices medically nonsensical, one must ignore evidence that the treatments underlying heroic therapies had been used for centuries, in some cases since antiquity.[15] Dismissing heroic therapy as an icon of nineteenth-century pre-science gives short shrift to the observational powers of its users and ample evidence that their treatments helped or even cured. It undervalues the difficulties later physicians, such as Reeves, faced in combatting them and implies that modern medicine has moved beyond the problems that created heroic medicine.

If the patient's ailment was one of many conditions called congestion or dropsy, but now referred to as malignant hypertension or cardio-renal failure, bleeding and purging would have provided benefit. Bleeding and gastrointestinal purging were accepted, medically intelligible treatments for severe congestive heart failure well into the twentieth century.[16]

Likewise, the staples of the heroic pharmacopeia, metallic salts such as mercury and tartar emetic (antimony potassium tartrate), could effectively treat diarrheal diseases and reduce vascular congestion. These drugs have narrow therapeutic indices, where the toxic dose and the therapeutic dose are similar, but they have genuine antibacterial and antiparasitic properties. They were useful treatments for several gastrointestinal ailments, even if physicians did not understand their modes of action. Calomel (mercurous chloride) is also a diuretic and was helpful for fluid removal. Although their toxicities made them far less acceptable as other drugs became available and disease mechanisms were better understood, calomel and tartar emetic were accepted medical therapies into the 1950s.[17]

The evidence suggests that regular medicine's dependence on broad theories and heroic therapies was not due to "blindness," but rooted in issues that still exist. One was a lack of scientific tools. Another was physician propensity to overuse a successful approach. A third was faulty reasoning.

Under the right conditions, where animal experiments or a few well-defined cases could demonstrate a truth, perceptive physicians used Bacon's methods. Such was the case for Hunter's anatomical and surgical studies, as it was for James Lind who showed the benefits of treating scurvy with oranges and lemons in 1747, and Edward Jenner, who demonstrate the protective benefits of vaccination in 1798. The problem was that physicians needed data from large groups of patients with similar problems to test most of their theories and this capability did not exist in the early nineteenth century.[18]

Nineteenth-century physicians extended and pushed the uses of successful therapies, as physicians always have. Benjamin Rush advised in 1796, "Bleeding should be repeated while the symptoms which at first indicated it continue, should it be until four-fifths of the blood contained in the body are drawn away." Calomel was another favorite and Rush recommended it in gram doses: "in such large doses as to effect a salivation" (i.e., mercury toxicity).[19]

Regulars sometimes reasoned badly, but their logical errors were not unique to the early nineteenth century. They were due to deficits in human cognition that their contemporaries recognized. Blane accused his fellow physicians of ignoring evidence for theory, drawing conclusions from small numbers, and following *post hoc* reasoning in 1821. American physicians reiterated Blane's concerns in 1822, noted their persistence in 1978, and updated them in 2005.[20]

Following the language of Baconian inductive reasoning rather than its methods, regulars disparaged their competitors whose treatments simply worked. Regulars derisively called these healers "empiricists" because they did not provide supporting theories.[21] At the same time they prided themselves on their knowledge of medications that also lacked theories, but which they used anyhow. If a regular physician relied solely on the 1830 U.S. Pharmacopeia, he could recommend more than fifteen hundred agents, preparations, pills, and tinctures, typically in his best Latin.[22]

Americans who distrusted regular physicians, did not have access to one, or wanted another opinion chose from armies of dentists, mesmerists, and folk healers, practitioners who also thought their treatments were effective, and outright frauds, who knew they were not. If sufferers or caregivers were literate, they could use home remedy books. Beginning in the eighteenth century, regular physicians, such as Englishman William Buchan and American Anthony Benezet, sold books that advocated regular orthodoxy. Other authors provided alternatives and attacked the practices of regulars. These included the various editors of Methodist leader John Wesley's *Primitive Physick*, first written in 1747 and reprinted in America until 1858, and Samuel Thomson's 1822 *New Guide to Health*.[23]

Regulars had coexisted with these competitors for centuries; however, Samuel Thomson proved to be more than a folk healer with a printing press. He started out with a powerful message of self-empowerment that evolved to a new medical sect, one that emphasized herbs and botanicals versus bloodletting and metallic salts.

Thomson was a shrewd New Hampshire farmer with a keen interest in medical botany. According to his widely-circulated autobiography, he turned to the practices of root doctors following several episodes of failed regular medicine. His experience convinced him that herbs, not bleeding and purging, could clear the body of obstructions. He developed a theory that cold was the cause of all diseases and the remedy was heat, supplied by botanicals, such as cayenne pepper, and the emetic herb, *Lobelia* (well-known as Indian tobacco), along with steaming vapors. Thomson did not reject regular science; he confronted it with his own one-cause, one-size-fits-all theory.[24]

Thomson's motto was: "Every man his own physician!" In 1822 Thomson collected his recommendations into the *New Guide*, which drew ideas from Buchan's *Domestic Medicine* and Wesley's *Primitive Physick*. He sold the book for twenty dollars and included an exclusive right to use his system to treat others plus membership in the local Friendly Botanic Society, where practitioners could receive additional information. Those who used Thomson's system soon referred to themselves as doctors.

Thomson appealed to his customers' painful experiences with heroic therapy and their distrust of elitism in the *New Guide's* preface:

There are no doubt many exceptions among the practising physicians; but their manner of treating disease by bleeding and blistering, and administering mercury, arsenic, nitre, antimony, opium, &c. is directly opposed to nature, and cannot be justified by any principles founded on natural causes and effects. Another serious difficulty exists, which is that the people are kept ignorant of every thing of importance in medicine, by its being kept in a dead language, for which there can be no good reason given.[25]

Thomson's *New Guide* was a collection of remedies and a cult manifesto. The 1825 second edition contained 180 pages describing the author's life, his experiences with his system, his travails in defending his patent, and numerous endorsements from satisfied users. It offered only ninety-six pages of medical guidance, divided between instructions on preparing treatments and the management of specific conditions, including common injuries.

Thomson inspired and encouraged his customers. A family could care for itself by following his advice and maintaining a basic medical stock of common botanicals. According to Thomson, "This stock will be sufficient for a family for one year, and with such articles as they can easily procure themselves when wanted, will enable them to cure any disease, which a family of common size may be afflicted with during that time. The expense will be small, and much better than to employ a doctor and have his extravagant bill to pay." Thomson's family medicine chest consisted of well-known components. Regular physicians also used them, but not always for the purposes Thomson recommended.[26]

The appeal of Thomsonism was more than anti-mainstream cultism. Thomson and his followers saw themselves as nature's allies in the battle against illness: "for all the good that can be expected by giving medicine, is to assist nature to remove the disease."[27] Rural Americans appreciated the simplicity of Thomson's system and its rejection of heroic medicine and scholarly obfuscation; they also believed in his message that nature, Providence, and patients had a role.

Thomson sold thirteen editions of his book between 1822 and 1834 and claimed that he reached two million people. His vigorous promotion created a new medical sect with its own journals, such as the *Thomsonian Recorder* and, according to one historian, at least eighty-five other botanic medical journals by 1860.[28] Branching from Thomson's message of self-help, his followers and botanical competitors formed medical colleges, first in New York and then in more receptive states, such as Ohio. One of Thomson's admirers, Alva Curtis, started the first chartered Thomsonian medical college in Columbus in 1836, The Botano-Medical College of Ohio. Curtis parted ways with Thomson and moved his school to the larger city of Cincinnati in 1841, where it continued until 1880 as the Physio-Medical College. Cincinnati was the American home of botanic medicine and its successor, eclectic medicine.[29]

Thomson's attack on regulars roused heated counterattacks from America's regular medicine establishment, which focused on the inconsistencies of Thomson's science. In front of the Maryland legislature in 1835 one regular physician accused Thomsonians of "slander, foul abuse, and misrepresentations of regularly educated physicians" and possessing a system of "illogical and nonsensical reasoning and preposterous absurdities, mingled with sentiments of atheism and blasphemy." The speaker publicly called Thomsonians "boasting pretenders," in a word, quacks,[30] which implied that Thomsonians knew their therapies did not work. Whenever they could, regulars resisted Thomsonians' efforts to join medical societies, start medical colleges, and claim the title of Doctor. Regulars attacked Thomsonians and their eclectic successors as unscientific, whereas, to the public, these practitioners marketed less noxious therapies and patient self-empowerment.

As Samuel Thomson began promoting his alternative treatments, a regular German physician, Samuel Hahnemann, developed a different therapeutic approach, also cloaked in the language of science, which launched another medical sect. Frustrated by his medical practice, Hahnemann was working as a medical translator and chemist in Leipzig in 1789 when he experimented on himself with Peruvian bark, or cinchona (the source of quinine), widely used to treat intermittent fever (malaria).[31]

Hahnemann experienced coldness, palpitations and anxiety after ingesting cinchona. These symptoms were signs of quinine toxicity, but to Hahnemann they were symptoms of intermittent fever. He did more experiments on himself and his family and found several other drugs, that when given in ample amounts to normal persons, produced symptoms that, to him, approximated the diseases for which they were used.

Hahnemann concluded that he had discovered a law of nature that had been mentioned by the ancients, but not studied scientifically until his work. Maladies could be cured by the medication that most closely reproduced their symptoms in a healthy person. He summarized the law as "like cures like," or *similia similibus curantur*, and published his "New Principle for Ascertaining the Curative Powers of Drugs" in a respected German medical journal.

He pulled everything together in 1810 in his book, *Organon of Rational Therapeutics*. Here Hahnemann first referred to his theory as "the homœopathic law, [*sic*]" after the Greek word *homoion*, meaning "similar." Seeing himself in the middle of medicine's scientific mainstream, his book's title did homage to Francis Bacon's 1620 *Novum Organum Scientiarum*, which was, in turn, a reference to Aristotle.[32]

Hahnemann built his law of similars on data obtained from his investigations and two pivotal assumptions. The first assumption of the homeopathic law was: "only one disease can exist in the body at any one time, and therefore one disease must yield to the other." If the physician could find a medicine that would reproduce the disease's symptoms, it would, being the stronger force, drive out the disease. He cited, as an example, Edward Jenner's work, which showed that a mild disease, cow pox, prevented a much more serious one, smallpox.[33]

Hahnemann's second assumption was that the underlying sources of most diseases were unknowable and irrelevant to treatment. He told his readers that it was not necessary to discern the cause of a bullet's flight in order to stop it: "All that we need to know are the symptoms of the flight of this bullet, that is to say the force and the direction of its motion, in order to set against it a counter-force of equal strength in a direction exactly opposed, and so at once compel it to immobility." Because only symptoms mattered, he ran up a white flag of surrender in the search for disease causation: "When the physician maintains that research into such things is necessary, then he shows a misconception of the capacities of men and a misunderstanding of the requisites for the work of healing."[34]

Based on the two assumptions underlying his homeopathic law, Hahnemann's 1810

Organon presented 271 aphorisms to help physicians better treat their patients. One set of aphorisms set the wheels in motion for homeopathy's most long-standing confrontation with regular medicine. These aphorisms emphasized that the strength of a correctly chosen homeopathic treatment was improved by dilution: "even a drop of the highest dilution must possess, and does in fact show, a very considerable power."[35]

Homeopathy appealed to many regulars, unlike Thomsonism. One attraction was that Hahnemann's approach presented the appearance of genuine learning. For example, in his homeopathic formulary he told them far more about one of their important drugs, belladonna, than they could get elsewhere.

Regular physicians in Hahnemann's day might have had three pages of information on belladonna in their dispensatories.[36] In contrast, Hahnemann's formulary, his *Materia Medica Pura*, devoted fifty-two pages to belladonna. Because of its potency, Hahnemann classified belladonna as a "polychrest," a drug producing so many symptoms in healthy persons that it could treat a vast number of cases. He provided detailed instructions on its preparation, including thirty-fold dilution using the proper upward strokes of the arm. Next, he offered information on treating belladonna's untoward effects using opium, wine, and coffee, among others. He provided general recommendations, such as belladonna being appropriate for plethoric individuals and women and children, and persons with virtually any nervous disorder or inflammation. Finally Hahnemann provided a catalogue of 1,435 symptoms that belladonna induced in healthy people.[37]

Another attraction was that Hahnemann's method provided entrée to an upperclass clientele. Given information on preparation and general use, the homeopathic physician had to decide how the 1,435 symptoms attributed to belladonna matched up with his patient's symptoms. He wrote, "it is precisely the totality of the perceptible symptoms, and that alone which must afford the significant indication in disease for the selection of a remedy." After assiduously matching the patient's symptoms with the known effects of all homeopathic agents, Hahnemann told the physician to select the single best agent and use it in the lowest possible dose, typically a thirty-fold dilution.[38] Those who could afford to pay for their physician's attention loved the customized care and painless therapies of Hahnemann and his followers.

Hahnemann's presentation of homeopathy changed over the first third of the nineteenth century, although his law of similars remained intact. He began by seeing himself as an enlightened regular physician then responded to criticism by emphasizing the art of homeopathic medicine and capitalizing on his profession's mystical roots. By the fifth edition of the *Organon* in 1833, the last one published in his lifetime, he increasingly disparaged regular medicine, coining the word "allopathic" as a pejorative term for regulars or old school physicians.[39]

Homeopathy entered America in 1825 via Hans Burch Gram, who was born in Boston, but took his medical training in Denmark, where he was exposed to homeopathy. Gram returned to New York City in 1825 and practiced homeopathy exclusively. Over the next ten years eight more physicians joined him in New York and formed the New York Homoeopathic Society.

Shortly after Gram set up practice in New York, Henry Detwiller, a Swiss physician living in Pennsylvania, converted to homeopathy. He was joined by a German physician,

Dr. Constantine Hering, in 1833. These two men established a German-speaking homeopathic academy in Allentown, Pennsylvania in 1835, which closed in 1841. This was the first institution of its kind in the world. German immigrant physicians and German-speaking graduates of Detwiller and Hering's academy were the primary means by which homeopathy spread in America in the 1830s. Hering, considered the father of homeopathy in America, obtained a charter for the Homeopathic Medical College of Pennsylvania in 1848. This institution made Philadelphia, also the birthplace of America's first regular medical college, the home of homeopathic education for the world.

Even before Hering's arrival America's regular physicians disparaged homeopathy, using the same arguments and epithets they employed for Thomsonism. An 1831 editorial in *The Boston Medical and Surgical Journal* pronounced: "The leading idea of the doctrine, namely, that similia similibus curantur, or that diseases are cured by those remedies which produce the same symptoms, appears, in its obvious sense, to be utterly absurd." Regarding the dilutions used: "If M. Hahnemann seriously believes that such doses can control disease by any virtue which the article itself exerts, he presents a remarkable instance of mental hallucination."[40] Regular physicians later grudgingly admitted that Hahnemann forced them to re-examine their heroic therapies and to give more credit to nature,[41] but they persistently attacked the apostasy of any physician who even consulted with homeopaths for the remainder of the century, seldom appreciating that their battle was for the human side of medicine, not its science.

As regulars' privileged position deteriorated and competing medical sects entered the medical marketplace, a few American physicians tried to find a scientific path forward. One was a young Massachusetts doctor who had spent a year studying in Parisian hospitals and wanted to share his experiences. Edinburgh and London were popular sources of European medical education, but Elisha Bartlett encouraged American doctors and medical students to make the trip to France. In the 1820s, the huge Parisian hospital system established by Napoleon offered young doctors the chance to see more patients in a year than one might see in a lifetime. Bartlett began by writing a series of medical travelogues for his colleagues.[42]

Bartlett spent 1827 in Paris and in 1828 he published an article on the city's most important hospital, the Hôtel-Dieu, in America's most prestigious medical journal, the *American Journal of Medical Sciences.* The following year he told physicians about the second and third most important hospitals in Paris, La Charité and La Pitié. He noted that La Charité generally had a mortality rate that was almost half the other hospitals. He attributed this favorable result to its spacious wards and the "judicious arrangement of the patients," an observation that anticipated Florence Nightingale's work on hospital hygiene thirty years later.[43]

Bartlett did more than any American to encourage his medical colleagues to make the lengthy journey to France. Approximately one hundred American students and physicians visited Paris in the 1820s, but this number more than doubled in the 1830s. Bartlett portrayed several French physicians in his articles; however, he did not mention the man who would later become his and many American physicians' professional idol, the careful observer who most clearly showed how to utilize medical science's new opportunity. When Bartlett studied in Paris, Pierre-Charles-Alexandre Louis (1787–

1872) was collecting unglamorous autopsy and clinical data at La Charité and developing his "numerical method" of investigating medical diseases.[44]

American physicians were slowly learning the new French bedside techniques of percussion and auscultation via the stethoscope, along with an appreciation of pathology, but Louis devoted himself to quantitative clinical correlations, what would later become clinical epidemiology. He and his fellow French investigators could not have done their work without the French hospitals.[45]

The seeds of M. Louis' numerical method fell unevenly onto American soil and the story of their troubled growth became a major part of Reeves' professional life. French physicians led western medicine's transition from theories to a better approximation of Bacon's experimental methods, but many physicians resisted change. Some, like Bartlett, wanted to improve medicine's science, while other American regulars followed a different path.

⑃ 3 ⑃

Regular Medicine's Choice

Elisha Bartlett returned to Paris in May 1845 to pay his respects to Pierre-Charles-Alexandre Louis, the French physician whom he and others now regarded as the father of a new medicine. It was easy to see the breathtaking transportation advances that had occurred since his student days. His 1827 journey would have taken a month by sailing vessel. A steamship could make the Atlantic crossing in two weeks in 1845, in a direct line, with little regard for wind or tide. The mammoth iron steamship, Great Britain, arrived in New York harbor that year and thousands paid twenty-five cents to visit the vessel.[1]

While Reeves labored over his tailoring in a rural Virginia valley, regular medicine approached its scientific turning point. Louis developed a new method of answering medical questions: were all diseases the same; did bleeding cure patients or hurt them? Louis said the answers lay in the *méthode numérique,* sifting through the results of careful observation, not in theories.

Louis presented data from fifty cases of pneumonia in 1835. He cautiously suggested that bleeding might not always work: "the utility of bleeding has been very limited in the cases thus far analyzed. " The English translation of his paper circulated in America, joining many French papers that caught the attention of American physicians. Among others, and with the help of Louis' former pupil, Boston's Henry Bowditch, they were learning how to use Laennec's stethoscope to hear sounds inside the living body.[2]

Bowditch translated Louis' 857-page treatise on continued fevers into English in 1836. Louis used the term "typhoid affection" to describe the general nature of the diseases, but he found enough common features to delineate a unique form of continued fever, one that he called, "typhus." Louis was writing about typhoid fever, the archetypical-nineteenth century disease.[3]

Louis' conclusion that not all fevers were the same was controversial, as were his recommendations against heroic treatment. His observations, supported by mountains of data, that aggressive therapies did not make much difference, threatened many doctors' received wisdom and professional identities. A New England physician summed up his colleagues' response to Bowditch's 1836 translation of Louis' treatise: "Many a doubting glance was cast over its pages, and grave and respected elders were then heard to remark to each other and to the bystanders 'that it would be a disgrace to any New-England physician to treat fever as recorded in that work.'"[4]

Bartlett had taken Louis one step further. He advanced Louis' observations and challenged the way American physicians thought about fever in an epochal 1842 book, *The History Diagnosis and Treatment of Typhoid and of Typhus Fever*. Bartlett urged American physicians to replace the word fever in their lexicon and in their thinking with more precise concepts, ones that were based on the type of evidence that Louis analyzed. Tearing into generations of medical teaching, he wrote, "The word fever, when used, as it commonly is, to designate a disease, has no intelligible signification. It is wholly a creature of the fancy; the offspring of a false generalization and a spurious philosophy."[5]

The clinical thermometer was a cumbersome and rarely used instrument in 1842 and the term "fever" denoted prolonged bodily excitation and decline. It was a state of ill health, not a vital sign. Most physicians saw fever as a single condition with different forms, such as "continued," "yellow," or "remittent." If the fever had strong gastrointestinal components, it was also "bilious." Depending on the location, which affected the underlying but then entirely unknown modes of transmission, they also perceived regional variations, such as British, Continental, or American fevers. Without a clear understanding that one type of fever was different from another or that typhoid fever in Britain was also typhoid fever in Philadelphia, Physicians could not make sense of their experience. It was unlikely that they would find specific treatments or preventive measures. Quinine and cinchona worked in bilious remittent fever (typically malaria), thus it should be used to treat "fever." That it worked in some situations and not others was inexplicable.[6]

Bartlett reiterated Louis' correlations of symptoms and anatomy in his 1842 book. Autopsy results in patients with a clinical history of headache, abdominal pain, and an unusual rose-colored rash almost always showed the presence of redness, thickening, and softening of glands in the lower intestine known as Peyer's glands. These findings were not present in other patients. Bartlett's data-supported theory was that the characteristic Peyer's gland lesion was specific to a disease he called typhoid fever. The lesion was secondary to the true cause of the disease, which was unknown. Any further theories about fever causation were unproven hypotheses to Bartlett. He had to clear up confusion over the name of this disease, which Louis called typhus, others typhoid, meaning "like typhus," and still others called dothinenteritis, but that would come later.

Bartlett cited the practices of six well-known physicians, including Louis, and concluded that heroic therapy had no place in treating typhoid. He wrote, "I think, that all treatment, in any way decidedly active or perturbating, is to be avoided. The tendency of the disease, in all such cases, is towards a natural termination in health; and there is no evidence, that the dangerous complications, which are liable to occur, can be prevented by any active interference."[7] He then turned his attention to the frequently confused and, to him, totally different disease, typhus.

For typhus he cited the astute work of Louis' American pupil, William Gerhard. Gerhard observed a fever in 1836 that often accompanied ships into Philadelphia's busy port. This disease differed from typhoid fever, yellow fever, and remittent fever. It resembled a disease that had been called both typhoid and typhus among Napoleon's soldiers and British troops. Gerhard decided to apply Louis' numerical method to his studies of 214 cases in 1837. He chose to call the fever typhus, as the British had, and found that it was totally different from the typhus (typhoid) fever that Louis described.[8]

Using Gerhard's description, Bartlett wrote that typhus often began with vague symptoms, like typhoid, but soon showed pronounced neurologic disturbances, including severe headache, followed by confusion and often dizziness. The neurologic symptoms were much more a part of typhus than typhoid, although they occurred in both. The most striking difference between the two diseases was the distinct petechial (hemorrhagic) rash of typhus, which generally appeared between the fourth and seventh day and was totally different from the rose spots of typhoid. This characteristic rash could be overlooked in dark-skinned sailors. Another difference was the body temperature. Patients with typhus definitely felt warm, while those with typhoid felt less hot and could sometimes feel cooler than normal. At autopsy numerous organs showed signs of inflammation in typhus patients, but there were no specific findings and, most importantly, the inflamed Peyer's' glands that were present in typhoid were not present.

Bartlett pointed out other differences between typhoid and typhus, such as how they occurred in the community. Typhoid was virtually always present somewhere. It was a permanent malady, whereas typhus was not as common. Typhus tended to spread aboard ship, in military camps, and in jails. Bartlett called typhus a form of temporary epidemic. He did not know any more about the cause of typhus than he did of typhoid, but he was sure that it was worsened by crowding and poverty.

Bartlett was more favorably disposed to bleeding and tonics in typhus than typhoid, mainly because these treatments could ameliorate the severe headaches associated with typhus. But he admitted that with so much prior confusion about the diagnosis, it was hard to make sense of the various treatment recommendations. One of the purposes of his book was to remove this confusion so that future writers could comment on the treatment of typhus rather than another undefined illness.

Bartlett offered no theory of typhus, only an observation that all existing theories of the disease were, at best, speculative explanations or interpretations, not facts. To Bartlett more observation, not abstract reasoning, was the logical extension of Bacon's principles.

Bartlett's insights were based solely on the five physical senses physicians had used since Hippocrates. The difference was that he could report observations on hundreds of patients with similar symptoms by physicians who had time, energy, and skills to record and correlate their findings. Bartlett showed that careful observation provided an answer to a long-standing medical question, and the answer was: "No, all fevers are not the same."

Bartlett's friends at the *Boston Medical and Surgical Journal* admired the work, but speculated that Bartlett had kicked a hornet's nest: "he must not expect to sail on a summer's sea, with the reputation this book will give him, without encountering headwinds, and even hurricanes, before completing the voyage of authorship."[9] As it turned out, the book did well. Osler commented fifty years later, "From every standpoint, *Bartlett on Fevers* may be regarded as one of the most successful works ever issued from the medical press." The book enjoyed four editions, the last in 1857 after Bartlett's premature death.[10]

Bartlett's Kentucky students put the book's message into practice. There was an outbreak of typhoid in Elizabethton, Tennessee in May 1849. Dr. Abraham Jobe and one other physician were the only two in upper East Tennessee who had attended

Bartlett's lectures and, according to Jobe, were "qualified to treat that disease scientifically." Jobe noted how other physicians used heroic treatments with calomel, ipecac, and quinine, while he treated the disease mildly. Between May 1849 and December 25, 1849, when he developed the disease himself, Jobe saw 107 cases and only lost seven.[11]

After *Fevers* Bartlett turned his energies to the faulty science that was misleading medicine. He saw himself as a provocateur and knew he was kicking a hornet's nest. He published a 310-page *Essay on the Philosophy of Medical Science* in 1844, dedicated to the man he would visit in 1845. This was the first systematic presentation of Louis' philosophy. Its message was medicine must use the same approach that enabled progress in the physical sciences. Diagnosis and treatment must be guided by observation and facts, not theories.[12]

Bartlett attacked the medical practices of his day head on. He began his *Essay* with references to Bacon, including a Latin segment of one of Bacon's famous aphorisms, which would have been well-known to his readers, *Non excogitandum est quid natura faciat, sed inveniendum.* The full phrase, in English, was: "we are not to fancy, or imagine, but to discover what are the works and laws of nature."[13] Facts could only be discovered by experiment. They could not be inferred from hypotheses and theories. He continued, "Hippocrates himself held no general doctrine in regard to diseases, which can properly be called a theory; a circumstance which now constitutes one of the highest and most legitimate titles to the preeminent position, which he occupies."[14]

Before the mathematics of inferential statistics, Bartlett discussed the issue of sample size in drawing conclusions from statistical data. He also commented on the need for precision in medical diagnosis. When Dr. A says his treatment cures a disease, does he offer adequate proof that his patients actually have the disease? He urged his colleagues to test the value of even well-known therapies, such as bleeding, in a logical way. He called such tests "trials." He applied his advice to current practices and showed their deficiencies. Bartlett made it clear that he saw Louis as part of an historic continuum. Louis advocated an approach that had been respected since antiquity, but was being ignored by his colleagues:

> I have devoted no separate chapter to a formal exposition of what has been called the "numerical" method of observation. The reason of this omission must be obvious to every reader of my book,.... This method is no new thing. Its elements are as old as Hippocrates: and there is hardly an individual writer on practical medicine, of any authority or importance, from his period to our own— including those who have been most unsparing in their abuse of the method—who has not used it.[15]

Bartlett wrote that accurate diagnosis must precede treatment and, since most therapies of his day were derived from theory-based doctrines rather than observed facts, they were more likely to be harmful than useful. The good news was that improvements in diagnoses were happening and would eventually lead to better treatments. In the meantime, physicians should follow the golden axiom of Louis' mentor, Chomel: the first law of medical therapeutics was to do no harm.

Bartlett also counseled humility, admitting that some of nature's worst calamities might never yield their secrets: "I can see but small reason to believe, that the mysterious and overwhelming energies, constituting the causes of such epidemics, as the black death, the Asiatic cholera, the typhoid pneumonia and spotted fever of New England, will ever be counteracted, neutralized, or destroyed, by the skill or achievements of human science."[16]

The *American Journal of the Medical Sciences* lauded the book and accepted the challenges of impartiality and self-examination. Rather than blame his profession's troubles on its competitors, the reviewer admitted: "the imperfections of our art and the mistakes of its professors are more profitable subjects for consideration, inasmuch as we have more control over them, and if we but learn how to proceed, we can labour to remove them."[17]

In contrast, the editor of the *New York Journal of Medicine* resented Bartlett's criticisms of regular medicine and attacked the author's logic and conclusions: "Now, we think Dr. B. is entirely mistaken in imputing the uncertainties of medicine to the 'imperfection of our diagnosis, and the incompleteness of our knowledge of pathology.'" He derided Bartlett's respect for facts over theories as a blanket condemnation of human reason. He found nothing unique in Louis' work. In Bartlett's discussion of the failure of contemporary therapeutics, which also included scathing critiques of Thomsonism and homeopathy, he saw an endorsement of empiricism, which he equated to quackery.[18]

Historians have had mixed views. Some present Bartlett's 1844 *Essay* as an extreme, almost revolutionary response to existing medical doctrines even though Bartlett emphasized its place in medicine's historic continuum. Others have claimed that his emphasis on observation rejected Bacon's use of induction, despite Bartlett's masterful use of inductive reasoning in his *Fevers* and his clear statement in the *Essay* that facts were used to derive scientific laws.[19]

Whatever its historical relevance, Bartlett's 1844 *Essay* was a masterful exposition of the difficult choice facing physicians. He argued that they must follow the scientific road wherever it led, relying only on observable and impartial facts. Others countered that they could follow their own theories, their own reasoning, and the science that met their needs. This choice was more than a philosophical exercise; it had direct application to the medical marketplace and to physicians' societal position.

When Bartlett travelled to Europe in 1845 *The Southern Literary Messenger* published a harsh review of his *Essay* by a Baltimore physician. A Bartlett admirer wrote in the *Boston Medical and Surgical Journal*, "Fortunately for the reviewer, Dr. Bartlett is now in some remote part of Europe, and hence he [the critic] can thrash the shadow [Bartlett] with perfect impunity; but we opine that a day for a literary retaliation will come, when the charges made by Dr. A. will be fully refuted by one so well able to vindicate himself as Dr. Elisha Bartlett."[20]

Bartlett dined with Louis and his friends soon after his arrival in Paris. After leaving Paris, he and his wife spent the winter touring Italy and in the spring they visited London. On his return from Europe in 1846 Bartlett resumed his position as chair of the theory and practice of medicine at Transylvania University in Lexington, Kentucky, a position he had held since 1841. He was content with Lexington, making an adequate living from seeing patients and teaching. Soon he began work on a second edition of *Fevers*.[21]

As Bartlett revised his *Fevers*, a twenty-nine-year-old medical parvenu from upstate New York sought another solution for regular medicine's problems. Nathan Smith Davis was a self-educated product of rural America; in his case, a farm in western New York State. When Davis' father saw him reading a book while steering a plow, he sent Nathan to a nearby seminary. His father also supported Davis' decision to apprentice with a local doctor at age seventeen. Three years later, having attended three identical four-month courses of lectures, Davis graduated from the College of Physicians and Surgeons of Western New York and moved to Binghamton.[22]

An autodidact like Reeves, Davis taught himself Latin and botany. He organized the Lyceum Debating Society of Binghamton. He won prizes from the New York State Medical Society in 1840 and 1841 for essays on diseases of the spinal column and the physiology of the nervous system. The Broome County Medical Society elected him a delegate to the State Medical Society meeting in Albany in 1844. To Davis' surprise, the state delegates already knew the serious young physician from his writings.

The delegates debated the poor condition of medical education at the meeting and the Broome County representative made a motion to improve medical education. Davis felt that four months was not long enough to learn all the required subjects and, despite his own lack of secondary education, that preliminary requirements were too low. The delegates asked Davis to prepare a report for the next annual meeting.

Davis' 1845 report on medical education led to a lively debate, the crux of which was that New York medical colleges were afraid of losing students if they unilaterally raised their standards. This led Davis to move that the New York Society should convene a national meeting the following year to consider uniform changes to medical education. The state delegates considered this an impractically utopian idea, but eventually appointed Davis and two others to do what they could to convene such a meeting. Davis sent out copious correspondence to medical societies and medical colleges over the following year, with generally favorable results.[23]

The first national medical convention of the United States convened in New York City in May 1846 with representatives from sixteen states. America's most prestigious medical colleges, Harvard and the University of Pennsylvania, declined to send envoys. The scene was confusing. Davis and the other members of the organizing committee confessed that they were not sure whom to admit as delegates, but this problem was quickly and pragmatically resolved. Everyone invited was allowed to attend as a delegate.

Two delegates from the host institution, the University of the City of New York (now New York University), which had publicly stated that it did not want the state medical society interfering in its business, immediately moved to adjourn the meeting. After this motion was defeated seventy-four to two, the national medical convention got to work.

On the second day of the meeting the delegates agreed to four resolutions and appointed committees to implement them: 1) That the profession form a national medical association, 2) That a uniform and elevated standard of requirements for the MD degree be adopted by all the medical schools in the United States, 3) That young men should acquire a suitable preliminary education before being received as students of medicine, and 4) That the medical profession in the United States should be governed by a uniform code of medical ethics. A fifth resolution, that diploma-granting and licensure be separated, with licensure restricted to state boards, failed. Davis was appointed to a committee to organize the next meeting and Drs. John Bell and Isaac Hays of Philadelphia were tasked with developing a code of ethics. The delegates then voted to adjourn, with plans to reconvene as a national medical association in Philadelphia in May 1847.[24]

Davis recognized that the convention's goals represented the aspirations of a new generation of American physicians. He wrote soon afterwards, reflecting on himself: "it may be said with propriety that the Convention was composed of the younger, more active, and, perhaps, more ambitious members of the profession." Commenting that many medical schools may have distrusted his and the other organizers' motives because they sensed animosity towards their increasingly tolerant educational policies, Davis disingenuously observed that "such a feeling was without the shadow of a foundation in fact."[25]

Davis returned to his practice and set out to organize the first meeting of the new national medical association. This time he was helped by others who reprinted the convention's work in medical journals and promoted its efforts in speeches and valedictories. Editor Isaac Hays wrote in *The American Journal of the Medical Sciences*: "The results of this meeting are altogether gratifying.... A foundation has now been laid, and if a suitable superstructure be hereafter erected upon it, an enduring citadel will be constructed, which will serve for the protection of the honour and interests of the profession against assaults from any quarter."[26] The allegory of a city on the hill was very much a part of the young country's sense of exceptionalism and the image of a besieged citadel would become an enduring professional metaphor.

The 250 delegates who met in Philadelphia in 1847 represented twenty-eight medical colleges and forty-two medical societies and other institutions. Oliver Wendell Holmes, distinguished anatomist, poet, and pupil of Pierre-Charles-Alexandre Louis, represented Harvard University. The University of Pennsylvania sent George Bacon Wood, Nathaniel Chapman, and Samuel Jackson, men who taught and promoted the lessons of French medicine, even though they had not yet travelled to Paris.[27]

The medical colleges kept their options open, but there were no fireworks as had occurred a year earlier. Shortly after convening the chairman read a letter from Hampden-Sidney College in Richmond, a college that Reeves would soon attend. The college regretted being unable to send delegates, but "expressed the concurrence of the Faculty in the objects that brought the convention together."[28]

The delegates' first order of business was debating recommendations for medical education. If there was any doubt that America's practicing physicians held animosity toward the country's medical colleges, the report of the committee to address education standards erased it: "The possession of the diploma no longer tests the qualification of the man; and it cannot be doubted that the large number of Medical Colleges throughout the country, and the facility with which the degree is obtained, have exerted a most pernicious influence."[29]

Likewise, if there was any doubt that the real issue was unfettered market competition, this report erased that as well:

> To relieve the diseases of something more than twenty millions of people, we have an army of Doctors amounting by a recent computation to forty thousand, which allows one to about every five hundred inhabitants. And if we add to the 40,000 the long list of irregular practitioners who

swarm like locusts in every part of the country, the proportion of patients will be still further reduced. No wonder, then, that the profession of medicine has measurably ceased to occupy the elevated position which once it did; no wonder that the merest pittance in the way of remuneration is scantily doled out even to the most industrious in our ranks, and no wonder that the intention, at one time correct and honest, will occasionally succumb to the cravings of a hard necessity. The evil must be corrected.[30]

The convention agreed to ten resolutions for medical colleges, including extending the period of required lectures from four to six months, a minimum requirement of three months' training in dissection, and a minimum faculty of seven professors. The medical college delegates objected to the requirement that lectures be extended to six months, but the entire proposal was adopted by the group. Everyone knew that this was about planting a flag rather than upsetting apple carts. There was no way that the convention could bind medical colleges to its recommendations.

Another proposal to separate the functions of teaching and licensing caused more dissension. Some argued that there was a conflict of interest and a potential threat to the public in allowing professors who were paid by students to decide if the student should be licensed. This proposal remained so contentious that it was deferred almost to the next century.

The delegates turned their attention to a proposed code of medical ethics. Hays presented the work of the ethics committee, chaired by Bell, who wrote the code's introduction. The unassuming Hays drafted the code itself. Hays merged English physician Thomas Percival's 1803 *Medical Ethics,* a guide to professional conduct, with American physician Benjamin Rush's 1805 lecture "On the Duties of Patients to Their Physicians."[31]

Parts of the new *Code* represented long-standing principles that patients and physicians of any generation would recognize: physicians should be available to their patients when called, physicians should honor their patients' trust and confidence, and physicians should live moral lives. Much of the *Code,* however, dealt with how patients and society should treat physicians and how physicians should behave in public. In the former case, Bell, in his introduction to the *Code,* justified an inclusion of patient and societal (public) duties as part of a reciprocal social contract. Bell and Hays borrowed the language of contract from Rush. If physicians had duties to patients and society, then they had rights to something in return. This was the language of a mutually negotiated contract, but, as ethicist Albert Jonsen later observed, only one side wrote the document.[32]

The duties of patients included obligations to use regularly trained physicians, to not "weary his physician with a tedious detail of events or matters not appertaining to his disease," and to "send for their physician in the morning." The duties of society included the elimination of sectarian competitors, "to entertain a just appreciation of medical qualifications; to make a proper discrimination between true science and the assumptions of ignorance and empiricism.[33]

To improve their profession's standing in the marketplace, physicians must respect their seniors, refrain from arguing in front of patients, and oppose quackery and empiricism at every turn. They were also required to agree on fees and avoid advertising, self-promotion, secret patents, and proprietary nostrums.

The *Code of Medical Ethics* was the first national code of medical ethics for any country. One hundred fifty years later philosopher Robert Baker likened it to the American Declaration of Independence and opined: "The grand moral vision inscribed in the 1847 *Code of Ethics* established the newly founded American Medical Association as the preeminent moral and political voice of American medicine." Others have cast a more jaundiced eye on the document, describing it as merely decent etiquette or, more ominously, a monopolistic manifesto.[34]

The genealogy of the 1847 *Code* can be traced to Philadelphia's Kappa Lambda Society, a secret medical fraternity to which Bell and Hays both belonged. One of Kappa Lambda's goals was to improve physician fellowship. Like other fraternities and societies, Kappa Lambda used moral testimonies as part of its loyalty oath. Given the 1847 *Code's* fraternal heritage, it is not surprising that it became a loyalty oath for the American Medical Association. The physicians attending the Convention had few reservations. They sought to restore professional order and they adopted the *Code* with virtually no discussion.[35]

Having decided how medical schools, physicians, patients, and the public should behave, the delegates chose a name for their organization: "The American Medical Association." They elected Nathaniel Chapman of Philadelphia as the Association's first president and Hays as its first treasurer, along with six other officers. They charged themselves with preparing reports, agreed on bylaws for the new organization, and adjourned until 1848.

The first annual meeting of the newly formed American Medical Association (AMA) convened in May 1848 in Baltimore. The delegates heard about the wonders of anesthesia, widely publicized by an American the preceding year. President Chapman also reminded them of their lost golden age and the need to reclaim their position in society: "The profession to which we belong, once venerated on account of its antiquity, its various and profound science, its elegant literature, its polite accomplishments, its virtues, has become corrupt and degenerate, to the forfeiture of its social position, and with it, of the homage it formerly received spontaneously and universally."[36]

Chapman urged his profession to fight for its proper place: "We do not want, nor will condescend to accept of any extraneous assistance. Confiding in our own resources, we shall through them maintain the struggle till conducted to victory and triumph."[37] Chapman's combative rhetoric appealed to many for whom the slow progress of scientific medicine was not enough.

⑈ 4 ⑈

Becoming a Doctor

Reeves could hardly have been more removed from the centers of American medicine. He lived in a rural Virginia valley, unconnected by rail or ship to the world, where lives overlapped. Among others, his father had multiple real estate agreements with attorney and future United States Senator John Carlile and Carlile's law partner, future West Virginia Supreme Court Justice Samuel Woods. These men, whom Reeves saw almost daily, played pivotal roles in his life and in West Virginia history.[1]

Woods arrived in Philippi in 1848 with his wife, Isabella. The young lawyer had no trouble identifying with Reeves' difficult lot and the two became lifelong friends. Woods' parents had immigrated to Canada in 1818, where he was born in 1822. The family moved to Meadville, Pennsylvania, and, in a path similar to Reeves' boyhood, Woods apprenticed to his father's trade of plasterer. But, like Nathan Davis, Woods had more options than Reeves and a more sympathetic father. Meadville was home to Allegheny College and Woods worked as a plasterer during the summers and attended college during the academic year, completing his bachelor's degree in classics in 1842. After graduating, he studied law with a Pittsburgh attorney.

Reeves had already decided to become a doctor when Woods moved to Philippi. His career plans increased the friction between father and son. Ann described the challenges her brother faced: "His father thought him rather visionary regarding the adoption of a medical profession, and he received little encouragement and aid from him, and when I look back and think of his early struggles and small beginning, and his later accomplishments in his profession, I feel that even his youthful energy and ambition would not have been equal to his task had he realized its herculean nature."[2]

Reeves was industrious, determined, and frugal. At eighteen, he used some of the money he had earned as a tailor to invest in Barbour County real estate, buying a lot in Philippi for thirty dollars.[3] The following year, 1848, he asked Dr. Elam Talbott to teach him medicine and Talbott obliged. Talbott was more engaged in business and politics than medicine, but he was the only regular physician in Barbour County with a medical diploma.[4]

Reeves lived at home and served as Talbott's and his father's worker during his medical apprenticeship. The unmarried thirty-eight-year-old Talbott lived nearby with Daniel Capito, who owned the tavern next to Josiah's tailor shop. With this proximity Reeves' studies did not interfere with his tailoring. Reeves worked all day and often until late in the evening with his father, then studied medicine until he fell asleep and up again at four o'clock in the morning with his books. Reeves moved on after a year with Talbott. The two worked together in later years and Reeves referenced his first preceptor in a medical publication as "my friend, Dr. E.D. Talbott," suggesting the parting was amicable.[5]

Reeves left Philippi in 1849 and travelled across the mountains to his boyhood home of New Market where he continued his apprenticeship with Dr. Jacob Neff, a third-generation Swiss-American physician. Neff was a thirty-eight-year-old widower raising three young daughters. He had a busy practice and quickly put Reeves to work, providing a horse when Reeves needed to see a patient. Reeves spent a productive year and considered Neff a valued friend. According to Samuel Woods, it was a year in which "the metal [sic] of the young student was sorely tried." Reeves' difficulties were as much financial as professional. He had to work one or two days a week at his tailoring to pay Neff.[6]

Having completed his second year of apprenticeship in the spring of 1850, Reeves decided to try his luck in practice. He moved back across the Alleghenies and opened an office in Sutton, Virginia. Sutton was eighty miles from Philippi, where his family lived, and two hundred miles west of New Market, where he had trained with Neff, making it a peculiar choice. He may have seen a need. Sutton's Braxton County had only five other doctors serving 4,200 residents.[7]

Reeves roomed with two other Sutton physicians, twenty-eight-year-old Marcellus Byrne and twenty-one-year-old Thomas Camden, in a boarding house owned by Thomas' father, John Camden. Thomas Camden later graduated from Jefferson Medical College in Philadelphia and, with Reeves, became an early and vigorous member of the Medical Society of West Virginia. Like Reeves, he was also a Methodist who favored the South, but opposed the Civil War. His brother, Johnson Newlon Camden, a twenty-two-year-old attorney who also lived in the house in 1850, avoided Civil War partisanship, and became one of the wealthiest industrialists and most powerful Democratic politicians in West Virginia.[8]

In October 1850 Reeves used his savings to attend lectures at Hampden-Sidney Medical College in Richmond ("Sidney" was the common spelling at the time). Reeves' entry into formal medical training exemplified antebellum medical education. The Richmond medical college had virtually no admission requirements. It was typical of many struggling mid-nineteenth century medical colleges, admitting about seventy-five students, and graduating seventeen or eighteen per year. The school had six faculty members who taught anatomy and physiology, surgery, chemistry and pharmacy, *materia medica* and therapeutics, obstetrics and diseases of women and children, and theory and practice. Each professor charged twenty dollars per course per session, paid to the professor. Hampden-Sidney required its medical students to take anatomical dissection, with specimens usually being obtained by grave-robbing. Students had to complete two identical sessions of lectures, running from October 23 to mid–March to receive a diploma. If there was a thesis requirement, the faculty did not enforce it.[9]

None of the college's medical professors attended the inaugural meeting of the AMA in 1847, but they sent a letter assuring the AMA of their desire to make whatever alterations the profession and the schools deemed appropriate. However, the faculty looked after its own interests first. Two years later, having been asked by the AMA what changes it had made, the professors of Hampden-Sidney Medical College replied: "Our Faculty have never been represented in the American Medical Association and none of its recommendations have been formally adopted."[10]

Hampden-Sidney's laissez faire attitude toward entry standards, combined with the availability of operating rooms and dissection tables, was perfect for the energetic and self-educated Reeves. Having completed his initial course of studies in March 1851, he left Richmond and travelled back to Sutton.

However, he soon he headed east again, this time to Rockingham County, just a few miles south of New Market. Reeves came back from Sutton in June 1851 and married Lydia Martz at her family's home near Spartapolis (now Mauzy), Virginia. Lydia's mother had died in 1844 and Lydia's father, Jacob Martz, died shortly after Reeves left Richmond, in April 1851. Lydia was the youngest of thirteen children and, at her wedding on June 16, the only family member still living in the Martz homestead.

Lydia was raised as a Bible Christian and Reeves was raised as a Methodist, but the Rev. John Suman, pastor of the Harrison-burg Evangelical Lutheran Church, married them at the Martz family home. After the ceremony Jacob's heirs sold his property, as his will directed, and divided the proceeds equally among the seven living children. Jacob's property was assessed at $29,000 in the 1850 tax rolls, making Lydia's share of her father's estate a considerable dowry of at least four thousand dollars.[11]

Reeves and Lydia did not stay in Spartapolis, New Market, or Sutton. Instead they travelled northwest to Barbour County, where, in August 1851, now with Lydia's inheritance, they bought a house in Philippi from attorney John S. Carlile for $1,024. Shortly after buying the house, Reeves sold the small lot he had purchased in 1847 for fifty dollars, making a twenty dollar profit, which was, on a percentage basis, the best investment of his life.[12]

Reeves' new house was in the center of town, and, in his words: "a handsome residence fronting the east corner of the public square."[13] The couple lived two blocks from his father and mother and their remaining children. They were also close to community leader Samuel Woods and his family. Reeves first lived about four houses from the one Woods bought in 1848. But Woods moved to the square in 1856, one house away from Reeves. Both families were members of the

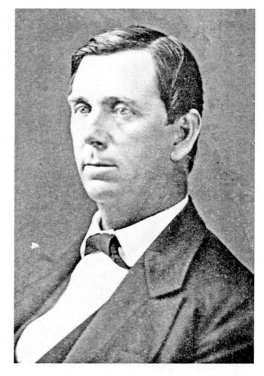

Philippi attorney, Samuel Woods (1822–1897), date unknown, Reeves' lifelong friend. Woods moved to Philippi, Virginia, in 1848, where he lived the rest of his life. Woods was widely respected for his intellect and sense of duty. He fought for the South during the Civil War and was appointed a justice on the West Virginia Supreme Court of Appeals in 1883 (West Virginia and Regional History Center, WVU Libraries).

same church and the Woods and Reeves children were similar ages.[14]

Philippi may have been little more than a western Virginia river crossing, but the tailor's son always presented himself well. A family photograph from the time shows him and Lydia as a trim and fashionable young couple, attired as for a *fête champêtre*. Reeves wore light slacks and a casual dark coat, with a white dress shirt and, perhaps an ascot. He sported a flat brimmed bowler hat and displayed the full beard that he carried his entire life. Lydia's dark hair, again in his words, "admired by all who made her acquaintance," was parted in the middle and pulled back under a bonnet featuring a chestnut leaf on it. Her dress was Victorian daywear reminiscent of a riding habit.[15]

Reeves settled into town while his former preceptor, Dr. Elam Talbott, pursued his political and business interests. The state decided to develop a turnpike through Philippi to Fairmont in 1850 and sought to build a three-hundred foot bridge so that the turnpike could cross the

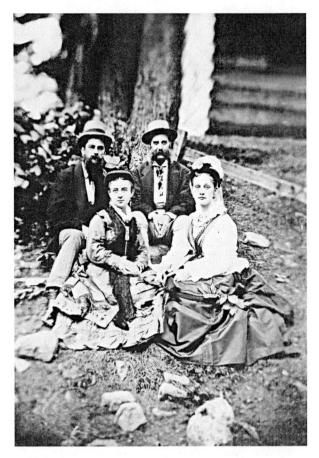

James and Lydia Reeves (*left*) and another unknown couple (*right*), date unknown. His biographers reported that Reeves always presented himself well. Lydia was noted for her long dark hair (courtesy Joan Webb).

Tygart Valley River. Talbott made several trips to Richmond to lobby on behalf of the bridge and a friend, furniture-maker and bridge builder, Lemuel Chenoweth. The state's choice of Talbott's comrade to build the Philippi covered bridge became local legend.[16]

Chenoweth had a rural education and was mostly self-taught, but he was a good engineer and a typically resourceful mountain man. When the day came to present bridge proposals to the state's Board of Public Works, he was the last one on the agenda. Having just arrived in Richmond on horseback, Chenoweth's appearance did not compare well to the more sophisticated Yankee engineers. He was preceded by a number of accomplished and poised individuals, with sophisticated drawings and models, "including iron structures, wire cables, cantilevers, stone arches, and wooden bridges of many kinds."[17]

But, as a furniture-maker, Chenoweth knew how to work with wood. He assembled a scale model of his proposed wooden covered bridge before the four-member panel, using no nails or screws. Then he placed his model bridge between two chairs and stood on it. After the competing architects declined his invitation to do the same with their models, the panel awarded Chenoweth the Philippi bridge and several other contracts.

When Reeves began his medical career in 1851, as work commenced on Philippi's covered bridge, he already enjoyed two advantages that eluded many American physicians. Many antebellum physicians sought new communities to begin their careers and, as soon as they arrived, they found a hostile welcome from their fellow physicians. Reeves had personal relationships with the citizens and doctors in his chosen community.

Another advantage was that Barbour County was less professionally competitive than many other American communities. An 1847 AMA survey, which included Thomsonians and homeopaths, found that Reeves' county had only one physician per 900 persons versus Virginia's average of one physician per 657 persons. Hyper-competitive Richmond City, the home of Hampden-Sidney Medical College, had one physician for every 368 people.[18]

The bridge provided a third advantage. The laborers building the bridge spent considerable time in the river and soon fell ill with typhoid fever. The disease struck the citizens of Philippi and, as sick workers returned home, it hit the countryside. After 1851 Philippi was never completely free of typhoid and Reeves soon had a large practice. The Philippi bridge was completed in 1852 and it barely survived the Civil War, floods, and a fire. Having been renovated and reinforced with steel and concrete, it is today a national landmark and the only covered bridge on a federal highway.

⑃ 5 ⑃

A Disease of Perennial Interest

There were at least 600 typhoid cases in Barbour County between 1851 and 1856 and Reeves treated 110 of them. The epidemic that helped establish his practice also put him on America's medical map. Typhoid was the archetypal nineteenth-century ailment, even more than tuberculosis, yellow fever, or cholera. Bartlett called it one of the nineteenth century's permanent maladies. Osler, speaking at the end of the century, said: "No other disease has possessed such a perennial interest." Typhoid fever drove major issues in medical science, sanitation, and practice and it induced Reeves to write his first book.[1]

Reeves got his typhoid knowledge from texts and journals, particularly Philadelphia professor George Bacon Wood's two-volume, 1,621-page *Treatise on the Practice of Medicine.*[2] Initially published in 1847, many American medical schools adopted Wood's *Treatise* as a standard text and, by 1852, it was in its third edition. The editor of Virginia's medical journal, *The Stethoscope*, noted its extensive use in 1852 and called it: "a splendid piece in the proud arch of American medical productions."[3]

The 1847 and 1849 editions, which most likely guided Reeves when he finished school and began practicing, devoted twenty-three pages to typhoid, which Wood called enteric fever. Wood based his approach on Bartlett's 1842 publication on fevers, but his *Treatise* showed how rapidly Bartlett's work was recognized in academic circles. Wood ignored the controversy Bartlett addressed, accepting his carefully reasoned answer as fact. For Wood, enteric fever and other generalized diseases, such as typhus and yellow fever, were clearly-defined entities, each with their own treatment. While he noted that therapies should be individualized, he provided well-defined boundaries and purposes. Wood's management of fevers was in step with the growing therapeutic trend, begun by Louis in France and led by Boston's physicians in America, that encouraged the expectant, non-heroic management of self-limited diseases.[4]

Reeves' practice showed Wood's writing and thinking. Reeves had no doubts in diagnosing typhoid fever. He saw several patients where other diseases were also present, such as pneumonia and erysipelas (acute skin inflammation), but he knew these were not part of typhoid fever, which was, to him, a distinct, and easily recognizable entity. He was quite comfortable distinguishing typhoid from other fevers. He wrote, "Typhoid fever, in this region of the country, has completely supplanted the bilious remittent form of bygone years."[5]

Like Wood, today's experts call the disease enteric fever, but the term typhoid fever is still widely used. Current authorities write, as did Bartlett and Wood, that it is a vague, slowly-developing febrile entity. The most common symptoms being headache (80 percent), loss of appetite (50 percent), and a coated tongue (50 percent). Two fairly specific physical signs, a rose-colored rash and a slow pulse (pulse-temperature dissociation), tend to occur in severe disease, where the clinical picture becomes more obvious. The inflamed Peyer's glands (patches) of the small intestine, which Louis described as the distinguishing feature of typhoid (enteric) fever in 1829, are lymphatic nodules. These tissue clusters are the body's first defense against the typhoid bacterium. If the battle is lost, they are typically the location of fatal intestinal hemorrhage or perforation. Most typhoid cases are mild, and today, even without treatment, 85 percent or more recover.[6]

Reeves' diagnosis of typhoid fever was probably bacteriologically accurate much of the time, although in the 1850s he knew nothing of bacteria. He likely underestimated its presence because, according to him, he seldom failed to observe the relatively specific rose spots. Rose spots only occur with more severe disease and are present in 40 percent or fewer patients who have bacteriologically-confirmed typhoid fever. They are quite rare in the other generalized febrile disease, such as malaria, yellow fever, and typhus that might have mimicked typhoid in his community.[7]

Patients with a persistent, lingering illness characterized by headache, gastrointestinal symptoms, and a rose-colored rash who died from intestinal hemorrhage or perforation in Barbour County in the 1850s almost certainly had typhoid fever. Once such a case appeared in the area it was a safe bet that other patients in the community with unremitting, slowly-developing fevers, headaches, and abdominal complaints also had typhoid fever unless they showed the well-known signs of typhus, yellow fever, or remittent fever (malaria).

Reeves was in step with the treatment approach recommended by Wood and Boston's medical leaders. He saw the disease as having mild, intermediate, and malignant forms, each of which required appropriate responses, but heroic therapies had no place. Demonstrating his scholarship, he wrote, "The old aphorism *aux grands maux les grands remèdes* [French: to great ills, great remedies] has proven itself to be wholly unsuited to the successful management of this disease; and we have learned to substitute for it, with much better encouragement, a reliance to the considerable degree upon the *vis medicatrix naturae*. [Latin: the healing power of nature]."

Reeves, like Wood, felt compelled to assist nature. He used bleeding in the early stages to ameliorate headaches. He applied cupping and mustard plasters for abdominal tenderness. He prescribed laxatives, such as calomel, to encourage loose bowel movements and Dover's powders (a source of opium) to treat diarrhea. He used stronger treatments if the disease became more severe, including opium for diarrhea, and quinine and alcohol as tonics. His treatment was tailored to the patient's circumstances, but it was circumscribed by what he recognized as good medical practice. It was neither completely unique for each patient nor idiosyncratic.

Reeves did not say whether his approach to typhoid differed from other physicians in Barbour County as it had for Bartlett's student, Abraham Jobe, in 1849, but evidence suggests that most physicians in Barbour County at the time were less heroically inclined, and probably more successful than Jobe's Tennessee colleagues. Reeves' mortality rate was nine of his first one hundred ten patients and he stated that the overall mortality for Barbour County's estimated six hundred cases was about sixty."[8]

The evolving concept that nature, not physicians, cured many diseases was accepted by the medical elite, such as Wood, and their students, such as Reeves, but many regular physicians resisted. The problem was more than dogged adherence to older treatment patterns. Thomsonians also preached the healing power of nature, but regulars saw them as unscientific quacks. Likewise, the minute doses recommended by homeopaths were seen as little more than the offerings of quacks who then handed their patients over to nature. For some regular physicians, the idea of letting nature take the credit threatened their claim to scientific stature.

The young Philippi practitioner wrote about his experience treating 110 typhoid cases and sent the paper to the *Buffalo* (NY) *Medical Journal* in 1856. Reeves offered his article so that: "country reports of any given disease, when truthfully made ... may be compared with city and hospital records, thereby affording the profession valuable data for determining its correct nature and treatment."[9] This was a worthy goal because Louis, Bartlett, and the *Journal's* previous editor, Austin Flint, dominated typhoid reports with their urban hospital experiences.[10]

Reeves followed the prevailing advice for good medical writing, handed down by Bartlett and the AMA.[11] He reported all of his cases, not just his success stories, and he included the relevant clinical information before he summarized his findings. What he did not do, although this was not common at the time, was justify his diagnoses. To him typhoid fever was so widely known that the diagnostic criteria were clear. He had some reason for thinking this. According to Blanton, typhoid fever was only first referenced by name in Virginia in 1851. But from then on, "no subject was so popular in the state."[12]

Reeves described his treatment methods and demonstrated his emerging appreciation of epidemiological concepts. He suspected that local conditions and patient susceptibility influenced the spread of typhoid, but he did not know how. It seemed to strike men and women about equally, with fifty-seven of his 110 patients being men. He confirmed that typhoid fever tended to occur in younger persons, with 77 percent of his patients being twenty-five years or younger. He noticed that the disease was never totally absent, but definitely more common in fall and winter months.

Reeves was convinced that typhoid fever was spread by personal contact. It was contagious, like smallpox. He wrote that everyone could see this: "The contagious feature of typhoid fever, together with another—the perfect immunity to subsequent attacks,—is well understood by the people at large throughout this country [meaning Barbour County]."[13] Despite his conviction, the contagiousness of typhoid was a controversial subject for most of the rest of the century because the disease sometimes appeared out of nowhere. The matter was not clearly settled until the twentieth-century demonstration of typhoid bacillus transmission by healthy carriers.

Reeves' report in the *Buffalo Medical Journal* caused a local stir and his Virginia colleagues urged him to expand his efforts. He sent a letter with his ideas to Philadelphia's George Bacon Wood, who also encouraged him. Wood advised Reeves to adopt the term enteric fever instead of typhoid. The word "typhoid" meant "like typhus." Since Louis' and Bartlett's researches proved that typhoid fever and typhus fever were two different diseases, typhoid fever needed a better name, perhaps one that reflected its unique intestinal pathology. Wood wrote to Reeves, "The name enteric fever, I think, is unobjectionable and will ultimately triumph."[14]

Wood's Philadelphia publisher, Lippincott, issued *A Practical Treatise on Enteric Fever* in 1859 and Reeves dedicated his first book to the Medical Society of Virginia, which he joined that year.[15] Much later Reeves' friend, Louis Wilson, and his niece, Anna Jarvis, wrote that Wood paid for its publication, but Wood's papers do not contain supporting letters nor did Reeves mention whether his *Treatise* had outside financial assistance.[16]

The slim two hundred-page work added twenty more cases to the 110 that he had already documented. Reeves also included the typhoid fever experiences of nineteen other Virginia physicians in his book. He reiterated that his purpose was to extend the existing literature on enteric fever with information from private practice, but he added that another purpose was to arouse his fellow practitioners to reflect on their experiences and contribute to their profession's knowledge. He exhorted his colleagues using a poetic simile, "like the sunlight on the wall":

> It is a lamentable fact that when the best of country physicians die, their experience, valuable sometimes, as it is hard earned, generally dies with them; they are of much service while living, but afterwards, for all the good they have done to advance the profession, it was as well they had not lived. They have been like the sunlight on the wall, which comes and goes and leaves no mark behind; or the shadow on the shore, which silently passes and disappears, leaving no footprint to indicate its course on the sand.[17]

The book did not contain much new information on Reeves' experience with typhoid, but it allowed him to reflect on the writings of others. He discouraged therapeutic creativity and urged physicians to follow the guidance of the experts: "an approximation to uniformity of practice is apparent, which was unknown prior to the works of Drs. Bartlett and Wood."[18]

Overall, his *Practical Treatise* read like a practitioner's cookbook, supplemented by opinions from other cooks, rather than a scientific investigation. Reeves intended it to be something a new Virginia doctor could use when he saw his first typhoid patients: how typhoid fever looks to your experienced colleagues and how they treat it. He provided practical advice supplemented with clinical suggestions. He deferred to other authorities where necessary and he noted that he had good outcomes, only eleven fatalities in one hundred thirty patients.

Several medical journals reviewed the book and appreciated its contributions. The *Boston Medical and Surgical Journal* thoroughly approved: "We have been much pleased by the perusal of this work, which is evidently written by a close observer and a man of judgment.... We know of no better or more graphic picture of this frequent disease.... Dr. Reeves' book is both interesting and valuable, and we heartily recommend it to the profession."[19]

Detroit's *Peninsular and Independent Medical Journal* responded favorably to Reeves' sensible approach and commended his industry: "This little volume ... is decidedly practical in its nature and will be appreciated by practical men.... The author, too, deserves much praise in setting a worthy example in keeping full and accurate notes of all his cases, and in reducing them to an available form."[20]

The most influential review came from Philadelphia's prestigious *American Journal of the Medical Sciences.* The reviewer lauded Reeves' goal of contributing new observations on a common disease. He praised the author's experience and advice: "the history it presents of the usual course, complications, terminations, and sequelae of the disease, the general sketch of its etiology, and we may add, also, of its most appropriate treatment, the work of Dr. Reeves may be consulted with much confidence and profit."[21]

But the *Journal* faulted Reeves' book for not being the scientific study that Reeves never intended: "His facts, from want of a proper collocation and comparison, do not always tell their own story, and are occasionally of no value, excepting so far as they are found to conform to the truths carefully developed and weighed by preceding observers.... The views of Dr. R. in regard to the actual nature of the fever he describes are purely hypothetical, and expressed in terms so vague and confused as to convey to the reader no very clear idea of even the author's meaning."[22]

A Practical Treatise on Enteric Fever left few footprints on the medical literature landscape. The AMA's Committee on Medical Literature acknowledged it in 1860[23] but it probably never became a medical school text or gained wide recognition as a scientific work. Given Reeves' connection with George Bacon Wood, who was a professor of medicine at the University of Pennsylvania, as well as Reeves' later connection with the school itself, it is telling that Wood's institution did not recommend his text nor did Wood mention it in his 1866 *Treatise on the Practice of Medicine.*[24]

Still, it was not totally ignored. The book was cited by footnote in an 1876 review of important American medical literature up to that time. When Reeves was nationally-known in 1888 Army surgeon Charles Smart referred to it repeatedly, along with the works of Louis and Bartlett, in his discussions of typhoid in the *Medical and Surgical History of the War of the Rebellion.* Much later, in 1933, after Reeves had been generally forgotten, medical historian and physician, Wyndham Blanton, assessed Reeves' *Practical Treatise* as giving "an excellent idea of the current view of typhoid fever." Nevertheless, even if it only occupied a niche position in American medicine, Reeves' *Practical Treatise* gained national recognition for the young Virginia physician and helped establish him as an expert on typhoid fever and public health.[25]

Reeves' approach to typhoid sat on one side of a professional divide. His medicine and his science were aligned with those of Wood, Bartlett, and Buffalo's Austin Flint. For these men, Bacon's methods existed to guide therapy and the results of inquiry must be accepted. The scientific message should be followed until a new message emerged. If medical science indicated that treatment should assist rather than combat nature, the physician must be humble enough to receive the message.

On the other side of the divide were the economic imperatives of medical practice. Science was what regular physicians sold and, for many, Bacon's language, not his philosophy, was what separated them from their competitors. Admitting fallibility, no matter how Baconian, did not serve those interests. It was the same schism that Bartlett surfaced in his 1844 *Essay.* A dispute over typhoid fever between two of the country's most brilliant physicians exposed the rift again in 1853.

Austin Flint initially rejected Bartlett's conclusion that typhoid and typhus fevers were separate diseases, but he did his own investigating beginning in 1851. Flint described his experience with 164 cases of typhoid and typhus in three annual volumes of the *Buffalo Medical Journal.* After completing his analyses, Flint retracted his dismissal of Bartlett and stated that there were enough differences to define typhoid and typhus as separate diseases. He presented complete descriptions and comprehensive recommendations for treatment. His typhoid fever studies occupied 376 pages, or 15 percent of the *Journal's* three year output.[26]

Based on his study, Flint was confident in his ability to distinguish the two diseases based on their different clinical presentations. Flint made his own autopsy correlations and these convinced him that he and other physicians could use clinical findings to make the correct diagnosis in living patients: "There can be no room for doubt that in every instance the *ante mortem* history, exclusive of the *post mortem* appearance, fully warranted the determination of type [author's italics]."[27]

Flint pulled everything together in a book in 1853, *Clinical Reports on Continued Fever,* to which he attached new information on the contagiousness of the disease. He asserted that typhoid was contagious, as was typhus. He acknowledged that the mode of contagion, which had to be some sort of miasm, was not known and was less predictable than some other contagious diseases, such as smallpox and measles.[28]

Flint's writings advocated the end of heroic medicine's fight with nature. He argued that physicians should use their limited capabilities to assist the healing process: "the plan of treatment most consistent with what knowledge we at present possess, is the *expectant,* as it is called [author's italics]." Even if patients might improve with no treatment, he did not advise the physician to walk away: "In saying that the treatment should be *expectant,* it is not intended to assert that the practitioner is to be merely a spectator of the phenomena of the disease, waiting for convalescence without any effort to render therapeutical aid [author's italics]."[29] Flint's treatment options were well-defined and limited. If the patient was in pain or experiencing diarrhea, the doctor should provide relief with opium. If the patient was weak, he could offer stimulants, such as alcohol. In all situations the physician must avoid any approach where the likely risks exceeded the benefits of doing less: "we should be hardly justified in resorting to those [treatments] which, if not successful, would be likely to impair the chances of passing through the disease with safety." In short, firstly do no harm.[30]

Flint referred to Louis, while channeling Bartlett. No existing therapy altered the course of the disease; science did not understand the cause; thus, there was no "point of departure from which to advance deductively toward a rational plan of cure"; and "In the majority of instances, the tendency of the disease was to end favorably."[31]

Some physicians were impressed with Flint's science. The editor of *The Southern Journal of the Medical and Physical Sciences* wrote, "As a model of close observation, and analytical exactness, these Reports are worthy of all imitation by those who would cultivate, with profit, the vast field of Medical Science."[32]

Others found his science threatening. AMA founder Nathan Davis reviewed Flint's *Clinical Reports* in the AMA's summary of medical literature in 1853 and brought the competing views of medical science into focus. Davis denigrated Flint's scholarship: "The *mode* of investigation adopted, especially in the chapter on the *Identity* of Typhus and Typhoid fever, we regard as faulty and well calculated to lead to erroneous conclusions [author's italics]." Davis scorned Flint's science along with the science of "Louis, Jenner, and many others."[33]

Davis spent two and one-half pages explaining how medical science should be done, in essence granting every physician the right to decide for themselves. He rejected Flint's, Wood's, Bartlett's, and Louis' premise that generalized diseases such as typhoid fever had well-defined and universal characteristics, characteristics that mandated a uniform approach to treatment.

Good medical science required consideration of *all* factors and medical treatment must allow for infinite variability based on each patient's specific circumstances. Davis asserted that each patient's doctor was free, even required, to use the findings of medical science as he thought best. The resulting therapeutic doctrine, which medical historian Warner labeled the doctrine of therapeutic specificity, differed from Flint's well-defined approach to typhoid and Wood's recommendations throughout his popular textbook. As Warner noted, many regular physicians found Davis' doctrine appealing. It provided them with a rationale to do whatever they wanted, while rejecting Thomsonism, homeopathy, and any other discipline that appeared to offer a predetermined and, hence, "unscientific" approach to treatment.[34]

⑾ 6 ⑾

Practice and Politics

Reeves and Lydia had four children: Nancy Frances, born in 1852, Ann Elizabeth, born in 1854, Joseph Cullen in 1856, and Charles Bell in 1858. Methodist Presiding Elders from Clarksburg, Moses Tichnell and Gordon Battelle, baptized the children. Tichnell and Battelle were members of the regular Methodist Episcopal Church and Battelle would become a leader in West Virginia's separation from Virginia. Reeves followed his family tradition of naming sons after famous men, although he chose physicians rather than politicians or clerics. He and Lydia baptized the boys after Charles Bell (1774–1842), a Scottish and later English anatomist, and William Cullen (1712–1790), also a Scot who profoundly influenced Benjamin Rush.[1]

Reeves treated whatever afflictions came his way. He rode out at two in the morning on February 1, 1856, to see a dangerously ill pregnant patient for the first time. The thirty-six-year-old mother of four, pregnant with her fifth child, was having convulsions. The hectic medical situation was a common scenario. Childbirth was a domestic event in many homes and, outside of the larger cities, families only called physicians for complicated pregnancies.[2]

His new patient had just recovered from her second seizure when Reeves arrived. She was twenty-six weeks into a difficult pregnancy. She had been troubled with morning sickness at first, but as these symptoms improved she developed severe headache, vertigo, facial discoloration, confusion, and lower extremity swelling. The evening before Reeves arrived she experienced the first of two convulsions, which prompted her family to send for the doctor. She was awake but confused when Reeves examined her. She asked him what happened. Her face was swollen and dark violet; her pupils were dilated and unresponsive to light; and her pulse was weak and rapid, at 120 beats per minute.

Reeves easily diagnosed the condition. Physicians had recognized and described the dangers of seizures during pregnancy for centuries. Churchill's 1850 textbook, *On the Theory and Practice of Midwifery,* cited the symptoms of puerperal (childbirth) convulsions that Reeves witnessed. Other authors commented that, once seen, there could be no mistake in recognizing the disorder. The disease occurred in about one in every 600 pregnancies and had an alarming 25 percent mortality rate.[3]

Churchill recommended treating puerperal convulsions with bleeding, purging with calomel and tartar emetic, opium, and cold water to the head. He strongly advised against interfering with the pregnancy. Ramsbotham, the other English author whom American physicians read, recommended a similar approach but noted that emptying the uterus, usually with forceps and loss of the baby, could be considered as an extreme measure to save the mother's life. The most esteemed American obstetrics textbook, written by William Dewees, was in its twelfth edition in 1853 and becoming dated. Dewees' description and management of puerperal convulsions differed little from Churchill and Ramsbotham. He too advised against interfering with the pregnancy.[4]

However, by mid-century younger American physicians were turning to the lectures and writings of Philadelphia's Charles Meigs, whose second edition of *Obstetrics—The Science and the Art,* was published in 1852. Reeves knew and admired Meigs' work. Years later he wrote, "I could wish especially the incomparable lectures of Chas. D. Meigs on the Diseases of Women had not so far been forgotten, for it is the most attractive book I have ever read in its department."[5]

Meigs vividly described the sudden onset of puerperal convulsions: "It is very well known that not a few instances do occur wherein the fatal blow is struck at the very onset, and that some women never speak, nor exhibit the smallest sign of reason or sensation from the moment of invasion, but sink at once into the stertorous apoplectic sleep that leads rapidly to the sleep of death."[6] Meigs used a term for the disorder that Churchill, Ramsbotham, and Dewees did not, "eclampsia." He likely borrowed the word from the French *accoucheur* Alfred Velpeau. The term eclampsia had first been mentioned in 1619, but in Reeves' day it was not commonly used in English or American medical texts.[7]

Meigs' basic treatment was the same as Churchill's with one noteworthy exception. In addition to bleeding and other depletive treatments for eclampsia, Meigs strongly favored termination of the pregnancy when possible. This was not a last-ditch effort, but a potential life-saver for mother and baby. He wrote, "We shall enjoy a far better prospect of rescuing the woman if she can be delivered, than we shall if the womb remains unemptied." He cautioned physicians not to attempt this unless there were signs of early labor, such as cervical dilation.[8]

Reeves followed the standard approach of bleeding and depletion, which helped. Her pulse decreased to ninety beats per minute and her mental condition recovered. He also ordered a laxative. Before leaving he advised her husband to pay attention to her bowels, to bleed her again if she showed signs of seizure, and to apply cold water liberally to her head and shoulders.

His treatment was likely beneficial. The bleeding and purgatives would have lowered his patient's elevated blood pressure, a cardinal feature of eclampsia, with bleeding being the more effective therapy. The treatment made physiologic sense, but physicians of the time were treating vascular congestion they could see in the patient's face and extremities, not hypertension. It was not until 1894 that Vinay showed a connection between increased blood pressure and the complications of eclampsia using a primitive sphygmomanometer.[9]

Her conditioned worsened two weeks later. She developed headaches, ringing in her ears, loss of vision, and vomiting. The family tried bleeding her again, but she suffered a series of convulsions. The desperate family summoned Reeves, who immediately drew twenty ounces of blood and applied cold compresses to her head and shoulders. His patient began experiencing a dramatic series of convulsions every twenty or thirty minutes throughout the evening. Her extremities grew cold and she appeared hopeless.

Reeves examined her pelvis and found the cervix slightly dilated. If he had followed prevailing wisdom he would have waited, but at seven in the evening, as Meigs advised, he ruptured her membranes and induced delivery.

The results were almost immediate. Within one-half hour she was in active labor and an hour later the baby emerged. Reeves had the pleasure of welcoming a healthy four pound and seven months' gestation baby boy. The placenta was delivered within ten minutes and the patient fell into a deep stupor. She awoke fourteen hours later with no memory of the events and, seeing her son, she asked whose child it was. Reeves treated her high pulse and headache with calomel and rhubarb powder as laxatives, along with morphine and cold strips to her head. He knew that he had saved the mother's and baby's lives.

Reeves used the British experts' language in his description of the episode. He never referenced Meigs' term eclampsia, but he was clearly aware of Meigs' newer approach to managing the disorder. His success was part of the American medicalization of obstetrics, which was being abetted by innovations in gynecologic surgery, anesthesia, and physician education. Unlike their English counterparts, American medical colleges increasingly required students to study obstetrics or, as it was more commonly called, midwifery. English physicians continued to recommend against early delivery for eclampsia, unless the baby was clearly dead, into the latter part of the nineteenth century.[10]

Reeves' management of another patient demonstrated his curiosity and his increasing connection to the larger world of American medicine. He treated a thirty-five-year-old man suffering from chest pains and shortness of breath in the spring of 1858. The fellow was a heavy drinker but had ceased alcohol use because of failing health. On listening to his chest, Reeves noticed "morbid sounds" in the lower lungs. The man began to cough up blood (hemoptysis) and, after several days of considerable hemoptysis, he coughed up a large bronchial cast, a fibrinous mold of his lower bronchial tree. The hemoptysis cleared after that and the man was well.[11]

The bronchial cast was a genuine medical curiosity. Instead of tossing it aside, showing it off to friends, or putting it in a jar, Reeves shipped it to the Pathological Society of Philadelphia. Philadelphia surgeon and society past-president Samuel Gross presented Reeves' report and demonstrated the specimen to his colleagues on September 14, 1859. This was probably the first bronchial cast that the Society members had ever seen. Gross noted that Britain's famous John Hunter had described a similar case and referred Reeves' specimen for microscopic examination. Much later, a house officer at Johns Hopkins Hospital reviewed the world's medical literature in 1902 and found only ninety-eight reported cases. Reeves was invited to join nationally-known physicians, including Austin Flint, as a corresponding member of the Pathological Society of Philadelphia.[12]

Reeves had to sometimes fight to get paid. He removed two diseased toes from seventy-three-year-old Thomas Skidmore's right foot in August 1856, but the disease progressed and in September Reeves amputated Skidmore's right leg below the knee. Reeves continued seeing Skidmore until his full recovery in January 1857. However, Skidmore refused to pay. Reeves, represented by Samuel Woods, finally sued Skidmore and his son in 1859 for $58.96¾ (*sic*).[13]

Reeves charged Skidmore $2.50 for each of fourteen calls, including medications, for a total of $35. Reeves rode six miles each way for these visits. He also billed $5 for amputating the toes and $15 for amputating the leg. He charged $.62½ for two items of medicine that he sent. The previous balance due from 1856 was $3.33¾, making the total, according to Reeves, $58.96¾. In 1856, $58.96 had the purchasing power of $1,650 in 2017.[14]

Reeves' charges were modest by existing standards. If he had adhered to an 1853 fee schedule from rural Nottoway County, Virginia, he could have charged Skidmore $8 per visit instead of $2.50, $10 for the toe amputations versus $5, and $40 for the leg amputation rather than $15. If Reeves lived in Richmond City and followed its fee schedule, he could have charged $12 per visit, $20–$50 for amputating the toes, and $40–$100 for amputating Skidmore's leg.[15]

Payment difficulties were a pervasive part of a nineteenth-century physician's life. Compounding his problems, the rural physician never asked for payment at time of service, only at the end of treatment or end of year. He did about average if he billed between $500 and $2,000 annually. He did better than average if he collected more than half of what he billed in cash or in kind.[16]

The AMA sought to address income problems in its 1847 *Code of Medical Ethics* by discouraging price competition, such as providing discounted or free services to the public. Elsewhere, physicians admonished each other to abandon the credit system and collect their fees at the time of service while local medical societies issued fee schedules to encourage consistent billing practices.[17]

Reeves and Woods thoroughly described the sequence of medical events and the itemized charges in their suit, but they also listed the many real estate transactions between Skidmore, his son-in-law, and several others, which led Skidmore and his son to claim destitution, while still controlling their land. It seems likely that Reeves was quickly paid, because the suit was dismissed a month after it was filed.

His father spoke for the family in Barbour County's political affairs while Reeves built his practice. Josiah was one of Barbour County's representatives to the Democratic Party state convention in 1853 and a year later he and Samuel Woods represented Barbour County at another Democratic convention.[18]

Reeves was also a Democrat, but he generally avoided partisan politics, even as he later participated in local government. The exception was prompted by the nativism of 1855 and the duplicity of his ex-neighbor, John Carlile. Virginia's voters directly chose their governor and other state officers that year for just the second time. Democratic Governor Joseph Johnson, a congenial politician from Clarksburg in neighboring Harrison County, and Virginia's first popularly-elected governor, could not succeed himself. His 1851 election had launched a relatively peaceful period in Virginia politics, which came to an explosive end in 1855.

Virginia's Whigs hoped that constitutional reforms enacted in 1851 might improve their standing, but political fortune was not on their side. The struggling Whigs were superseded in 1855 by a well-organized, clandestine faction that had originated in New York's immigrant cauldron, the secret Order of the Star Spangled Banner, popularly called the Know-Nothings.[19]

The Know-Nothings were the first political organization to exploit America's white Protestant anxieties on a national scale. The Order of the Star Spangled Banner began in 1850, pledged to fight for the election of Protestant and American-born political candidates. They were not the country's first or only nativist organization, but they were more private and more aggressive. The Order functioned like a secret fraternity, with lodges rather than party caucuses, which led to the group's public moniker, "Know-Nothing." The name reputedly reflected how a member of the Order was supposed to answer outside inquiries.[20]

The Order of the Star Spangled Banner merged with a larger nativist organization and began covertly supporting political candidates who opposed foreigners and foreign influence, particularly Catholicism. The Order had no stance on slavery. If anything, it co-opted the Whig party's pro-union agenda, with an endorsement of states' rights to make their own decision on slavery.

The group captured the public conversation by manipulating Anglo-Protestant fears of the growing numbers of Irish and German immigrants. The spark that lit the political tinder-box was the 1854 Kansas-Nebraska Act. This law effectively repealed the 1820 Missouri Compromise by permitting residents to voluntarily accept slavery in the Nebraska territory. Supposedly a concession from Democratic president Franklin Pierce to Southern slaveholders, the Act infuriated northern Democrats while stoking Southern apprehensions that waves of foreign immigrants would flood the new territories and oppose slavery.

The Know-Nothings' discipline and political focus produced results in Pennsylvania and New England. Know-Nothing candidates trounced incumbent Whigs in October 1854 and swept the Massachusetts ticket. The Know-Nothings felt that it was time to form a national political party and, for this, they needed visible Southern support. Know-Nothing leaders saw that Virginia's May 1855 election was the only major Southern contest before their newly minted American party held its national convention. Virginia's 1855 state election was a pivotal national event for them, "On which the great battle for the Constitution is to be fought."[21]

Virginia's Democratic Party recognized the Know-Nothing threat and chose energetic and combative Henry Wise as its gubernatorial candidate in November 1854. The state's Know-Nothings met secretly in March 1855 and nominated Whig Thomas Flournoy for governor and Democrat James Beale for lieutenant governor on the American Party ticket. This confounded Virginia politics and drove Virginia's Whig party from the field.

Before the Know-Nothings met the Barbour County Democratic Party convened in a packed room at the Philippi courthouse on February 5, 1855. The attendees chose Reeves as party secretary on his first venture into Virginia politics. Samuel Woods joined a committee of five to prepare the meeting's resolutions.

Reeves and his fellow Democrats spent more than two hours painting the Know-Nothings in demonic terms: "a secret cabal of despotic and proscriptive demagogues whose avowed object is to change the fundamental features of our political system." They castigated Know-Nothing unionism as nothing more than covert Yankee abolitionism: *"Resolved.* That we recognize Know-Nothing Whiggery as Abolitionism in disguise—the faithful representative of the fanaticism and dangerous vagaries of the North, and denounce it as such [italics in original]." To the Barbour County Democrats, abolitionism was far worse than foreign birth or Catholicism.[22]

The scathing language directed at abolitionism was standard sectionalist fare in western Virginia, typically used to stoke fears of external tyranny rather than reasoned concerns about personal property. Slavery barely existed in Barbour County in 1855. With a total population of almost nine thousand persons in 1860, Barbour County had forty-two slaveholders who owned ninety-five slaves.[23]

Philippi's Democrats met in the town's Methodist church in April, after the statewide races were underway. The gathering demanded that Reeves speak. The twenty-five-year-old doctor obliged the audience with an impassioned oration. He opened with the obligatory condemnations of the "great conspiracy against the liberties of the people concocted in the abolition sinks of the North." But he departed from standard sectionalist rhetoric and directed most of his firepower against conspiratorial nativism. He reminded the audience of the gallant sacrifices of foreigners, such as General Lafayette, in the service of the United States. He decried all secret political organizations as dangerous, and he implored the audience to meet the approaching struggle for civil and religious liberty.[24]

John Carlile made the ensuing electoral campaign personal. Carlile had sold Reeves his house and was Samuel Woods' original law partner. After representing Barbour County as a Democrat and son of the South at Virginia's 1851 Reform Convention, Carlile moved from Philippi to neighboring Clarksburg. Once he settled in Clarksburg, Carlile opened his law office and quickly joined the local Democratic Party.[25]

While Carlile touted his Democratic connections and Southern values, he secretly worked to secure Know-Nothing support for his candidacy for the U.S. House of Representatives. He stunned Virginia's Democrats in April 1855 by announcing his intention to run for Congress as a member of the American Party. The Parkersburg *News* recounted his previously staunch support for the Democrats, reprinting his earlier letters and describing them as: "false and treacherous beyond our furthest conceptions."[26]

When Carlile campaigned as a Know-Nothing in Philippi on May 10, 1855, Democrats denounced him as a traitor. *Cooper's Clarksburg Register* told the story, with no pretense of even-handedness: "The indignation of the people of Barbour County at the political treachery and duplicity of that gentleman was immense, and manifested itself in every form short of absolute insult." Carlile's duplicitous actions were offensive to Virginians' codes of loyalty and honor, but for Reeves, who knew the man well, his support of Know-Nothing principles was more akin to sin. He took the spotlight and pointedly called out Carlile. He avoided the *Register's* denunciations. Instead, he followed Methodist advice on reproving neighbors. Reeves cited Carlile's public professions and challenged him to repent, for he had clearly gone astray: "But alas, a change has come over the spirit of his dream."[27]

By May 24 weary Virginians were ready to vote in the most contested election since the presidential campaign of 1840. The Know-Nothings carried urban Richmond and Alexandria, areas with a long Whig history and strong press; however, they were soundly defeated in rural Virginia, particularly west of the Blue Ridge. Barbour County voted for Wise by more than two to one. Wise and his statewide ticket won by a 10,000-vote margin.[28]

Despite the American Party's defeat, smooth-talking John Carlile was a winner, the only successful Know-Nothing candidate in thirteen Congressional contests. The local numbers showed that Carlile ran well in places where he was least known, such as Charleston. He lost to his Democratic opponent 759 to 308 in his previous home of Barbour County, and in his present home of Harrison County he lost 1,038 to 899.[29] Soon enough, Reeves' mercurial and opportunistic former neighbor, Congressman Carlile, would lead West Virginia's separatist movement.

The Know-Nothing star faded after Virginia's 1855 gubernatorial election. The main reason historians offer, aside from its offensive secrecy, was that it came apart over slavery. Southern Know-Nothings interpreted their losses in Virginia as a referendum on slavery and insisted that Northern Know-Nothings disavow abolitionism. This fractured the organization, leaving the emerging Republican Party as the only political organization with a clear position on slavery.[30]

Virginia's 1855 election was a harbinger of 1860. The Know-Nothing doctrines of nativism and anti–Catholicism generated little enthusiasm in Virginia, but the group's third pivotal doctrine, unionism, did. Thus, Virginia's 1855 rejection of the American Party became an indirect referendum on preserving the Union, a referendum that the Unionists lost.

The 1855 election also demonstrated communication changes that were developing throughout the country. The successful Democratic candidate, Henry Wise, chose to follow his political predecessors and hit the campaign trail. His American Party opponent, Thomas Flournoy, wanted newspapers to win the contest for him.

A newspaper campaign was possible because of the industry's brisk growth. Virginia's population increased by 20 percent between 1840 and 1860, while the number of daily and weekly newspapers increased by more than 150 percent. This occurred throughout the country. Antebellum newspapers were local ventures, recording meetings, illnesses, civic events, and train schedules, and reflecting their owner's political or religious agenda. Seventy percent of Virginia's newspapers in 1850 had political affiliations, often announced in their names, such as the *Richmond Whig*.[31]

Political parties were the first to take advantage of the new mass medium, but other entrepreneurial Americans also understood their marketing reach, notably medical pitchmen. Even then regular physicians lamented newspaper peddling of fake medical miracles. An angry Massachusetts doctor wrote in 1853: "For a considerable time past, the public newspapers have contributed largely toward misleading and depraving the public mind. It is a lamentable fact that three quarters of all these papers derive their principal support from the proprietors of quack medicines."[32]

This was apparent in rural western Virginia and Reeves could not have missed it. A typical page from *Cooper's Clarksburg Register* in 1856 showed the usual notices of hotels, schools, and professional services, along with livestock and commodity prices, but more than 10 percent of the announcement space was devoted to medical nostrums and cures. These included endorsements for Holloway's pills: "a certain cure for termination of blood to the head," Dr. Scott's White Circassian Liniment for "Rheumatism," and Dr. Kinelin's treatment for male "diseases of a private nature." None of these "doctors" lived in Clarksburg.[33]

As mass communications were changing, so was transportation. Reeves was forced to respond to the new realities created by the B&O Railroad. The line's original Ohio River target was Wheeling, in Virginia, but once it reached Cumberland in 1842, company surveyors felt the most sensible means to the Ohio River was via western Pennsylvania, following the National Road, then on to the river at Pittsburgh. Progress stopped because the B&O could not get Pennsylvania's approval to cross the state; then the governor of Pennsylvania issued a proclamation in 1847 preventing the B&O from building to Pittsburgh. Had Pennsylvania done otherwise, Reeves' life might have taken a different path and the Civil War would have had a different beginning.[34]

The Virginia legislature allowed the B&O twelve more years to complete its line to the Ohio River, but, to protect a planned canal in the southern part of the state, it mandated that the terminus be Wheeling, in the state's remote northwestern panhandle. The legislature also required that the route pass within three miles of Three Forks Creek, empty pastureland on the Tygart Valley River, twenty miles north of Philippi. One legislature member who lived in the area understood the positive implications of a railroad line and added this requirement.

As the railroad approached Three Forks Creek in 1852, the locals offered land at a good price and the B&O set up shops and buildings for the crews. This area became the town of Grafton. From there the crews turned northwest to Fairmont, where the Tygart Valley River joined the Three Forks to become the commercially navigable Monongahela. The line reached Fairmont on June 22, 1852, and workers completed the seventy-seven mile push to Wheeling in six months. They drove the final spike at the edge of the Ohio River on Christmas Eve, 1852. One thousand Wheeling residents and dignitaries celebrated the event on January 12, 1853. The Atlantic seaboard was now as accessible to them as the Ohio River. Coal, timber, flour, and other western commodities began pouring east.[35]

The railroad's completion made winners and losers. Josiah Reeves hoped the tracks would come near his property, but they did not. Counties that were on the railroad line, such as Marion (Fairmont), Ohio (Wheeling), and Taylor (Grafton), prospered. Between 1850 and 1860 Marion County's population increased by 20 percent, Ohio's by 24 percent, and Taylor's by 39 percent. In contrast Barbour County, just south of Taylor County, but not along the rail line, lost 1 percent of its population.[36]

Philippi was surrounded by rails but not connected to them and Reeves knew he had to leave if he wanted to improve his fortunes. With no licensure laws in Virginia, a prestigious degree was the only proper way a doctor could convince a new town that he had something his competitors did not. Reeves had already completed one course of medical studies and required just a few more months to get a medical college diploma.

Reeves disparaged the abolition sinks of the North, but sectionalist arguments urging him to finish his schooling in the South did not convince him. He had corresponded with Pennsylvania's George Bacon Wood and Samuel Gross. He had published his medical articles in a New York journal and his typhoid book in Philadelphia. Philadelphia was the domestic alternative to Paris for many American medical students and if the seat of American medicine was Philadelphia, he would go there to complete his training.[37]

Reeves enrolled in the country's oldest and most prestigious medical college in October 1859. Compared to Richmond's Hampden-Sidney, where he had studied in 1851, the Medical Department of the University of Pennsylvania was huge, with five hundred students in his class instead of seventy-five. Many of the great names of American medicine were connected to the institution, including American Founding Father and advocate of heroic medicine, Benjamin Rush, Hunter's pupil and the father of American surgery Philip Syng Physick, the father of American Obstetrics William Dewees, the American physician who first defined the distinguishing features of typhus, William Gerhard, the first AMA president Nathaniel Chapman, and, in Reeves' day, the leading expert on materia medica, George Bacon Wood, and the country's foremost anatomist and medical microscopist, Joseph Leidy.[38]

Events in Reeves' state soon changed the nation's direction and induced many Southerners to leave Philadelphia. The conductor of the B&O's Night Express from Wheeling sent an urgent telegram to the railroad's transportation manager in Baltimore during the early morning of October 17, 1859: "Express train bound east under my charge was stopped this morning at Harpers Ferry by armed abolitionists. They have possession of the bridges and of the arms and armory of the United States."[39]

John Brown's nighttime assault on the federal arsenal at Harper's Ferry, Virginia terrified the South. Local militias quickly penned him in and soon U.S. Marines led by Army Colonel Robert E. Lee captured Brown. Virginia's bellicose governor, Henry Wise, ordered Brown transferred to nearby Charles Town, where he was quickly tried for treason and hanged on December 2, 1859.[40]

The fallout from Brown's raid did not to induce Reeves to sacrifice his medical education. When two hundred Southern medical students who were enrolled in Philadelphia medical colleges protested John Brown by leaving their schools in December 1859, Reeves was not among them. Nor were many others who had made the sacrifice to attend the University of Pennsylvania. Penn's matriculating class in 1859 was 7 percent Virginians (37/528) while Reeves' graduating class in 1860 was a little more than 12 percent Virginians (22/176). Penn's matriculating class in 1860, after Brown, but before the start of formal hostilities, was 9 percent Virginians (36/405), evidence that many Virginians still valued a Philadelphia medical education.[41]

Penn exposed Reeves to a city and to a group of men that played pivotal roles in his later professional life. He already knew Wood from his typhoid fever correspondence and Gross from his membership in Pathological Society of Philadelphia. The University considered Reeves a medical doctor when he enrolled because he had practiced medicine for eight years. He had also published a book and several medical papers. Reeves completed the required seven courses in March 1860 and, without authoring a thesis, received the Doctor of Medicine degree.[42] He returned home to plan a move that would provide a larger field for his professional skills and better remuneration for his services.

⑃ 7 ⑃

Duty, Honor,
Country, Statehood

Reeves set his sights forty miles north, on Fairmont, where he had connections. Samuel Woods' brother-in-law, James Neeson, was a well-known Fairmont attorney. Dr. Matthew Campbell, who was the chief surgeon to the B&O and lived in Grafton, had practiced in Fairmont from 1852 to 1853 and was Reeves' family physician.[1]

Fairmont provided communication with America's business and professional centers, if little else. It was on the busy B&O line between Baltimore and Wheeling and also had connections through Grafton to Parkersburg, Virginia, another Ohio River port. From Wheeling and Parkersburg, trains crossed the river via ferries to connections in Ohio and the West. Steamboats and flatboats could also navigate the Monongahela River from Fairmont north to Pittsburgh and then down the Ohio River.[2]

The town itself was the seat of Marion County and a farming community crossroads. Coal mining was not yet economically important and most of the residents inhabited the surrounding countryside. Only seven hundred persons lived in Fairmont. Nonetheless, the county was a growing home to thirteen thousand people instead of Barbour County's smaller and declining population of nine thousand.[3]

Except for the $30 Philippi lot he sold for $50, Reeves almost never made money on real estate. He sold the house he had bought for $1,024 in 1851 for $850 cash and a gold watch in June 1860. The family travelled to Fairmont in July, where Reeves purchased a home on the north side of Jackson Street for $1,000.[4]

But politics consumed everyone's lives. Vocal Southerners fanned fears of Northern tyranny after Lincoln won the 1860 Presidential election. South Carolina fulfilled its threat to secede from the United States on December 20. Virginia was at first reluctant to join South Carolina and Unionists in Reeves' area vowed to fight secession. Other westerners had different views. Some, such as Barbour County's Samuel Woods, leaned toward secession, but favored efforts to redress western grievances so that, if nothing else, Virginia's integrity could be preserved. Still others, such as Woods' former law partner and turncoat Democrat John Carlile, opposed secession but secretly sought Virginia's dismemberment.

Six other states had joined South Carolina by February, and in March 1861 the seven states formed the Confederate States of America. Rebel soldiers in Charleston, South Carolina fired on the U.S. Army garrison stationed at Ft. Sumter on April 12.

Although there were no casualties on either side, the fort's commander surrendered on the next day, to the delight of Charleston's onlooking crowds.

Newly inaugurated President Lincoln called for 75,000 volunteers on April 15 to quell the rebellion in South Carolina. Faced with Lincoln's request for troops, Virginia voted for secession on April 17, 1861. Lincoln offered Colonel Robert E. Lee command of the United States Army on April 18, which he rejected. Governor Letcher offered Lee command of the armies of Virginia on April 22 and Lee accepted.

Ohio Governor Dennison prepared to defend Ohio's interests, which, to him, began along the B&O rails in western Virginia's mountain passes. He offered a thirty-four-year-old railroad executive, George B. McClellan, command of the Ohio Volunteers on April 23 and on April 26 the Ohio legislature passed an act conferring war powers on Governor Dennison. McClellan assumed command of the U.S. Army's Department of the Ohio on May 3, 1861.[5]

John Carlile detoured to Washington City after Virginia's secession vote to share the news with President Lincoln. The only newspaper in Philippi, the pro–South *Barbour Jeffersonian,* again saw treachery: "The depravity of the human heart is most woefully displayed in the career of the traitor Carlile."[6] But Carlile was just getting started. After he returned to Clarksburg he wrote and distributed the "Clarksburg Resolutions," calling for a convention of western counties in Wheeling on May 13. Wheeling was the largest city in western Virginia and the center of Union support. Virginia men wishing to fight for the Union travelled there to join the United States First Virginia Infantry Regiment. They were housed at Camp Carlile, located on Wheeling Island in the Ohio River. The site was named in honor of John S. Carlile.[7]

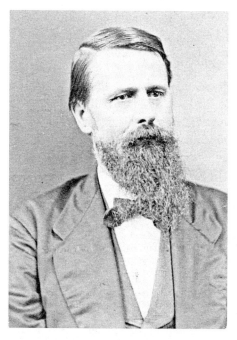

James Reeves in 1860. In the fall of 1859 Reeves enrolled in the University of Pennsylvania Medical College. Following John Brown's raid that October a number of Southern students left Philadelphia, but Reeves remained, obtaining his M.D. degree in March 1860. After returning to Philippi he moved forty miles north to Fairmont, on the B&O rail line from Baltimore to Wheeling (courtesy Joan Webb).

Western Virginia saw war two months before the rest of the nation felt its impact. Confederate troops gathered in Reeves' parents' town of Philippi in May, arousing the citizens with military bravado that their commander, George Porterfield, endorsed. Their strategic purpose was obvious to local Unionists. Carlile telegrammed Ohio Governor Dennison on May 20 that Philippi's assembling Confederate troops were heading to the railroad terminus at Grafton and then on to Wheeling to break up the loyalists.[8]

The first man killed in hostile action by organized forces in the Civil War was Union scout Thornsberry Brown, who was shot by a confederate militiaman near Grafton on May

22, 1861. On May 23, as Carlile had warned, Porterfield marched his cadre of 500–700 men to Grafton and began burning railroad bridges. Carlile surreptitiously took a train to the White House on May 24 to meet with Lincoln. He told the president, "Sir, we want to fight. We have one regiment ready, and if the Federal Government is going to assist us, we want it at once." Lincoln replied, "You shall have assistance."[9]

Railroad bridge-burning was all the provocation Ohio needed. McClellan ordered his regiments to cross the Ohio River into Parkersburg on May 27. This force joined soldiers who had crossed at Wheeling and loyal Virginians from Camp Carlile. When Porterfield learned that as many as 23,000 Federals were advancing on him, he left Grafton for the friendlier town of Philippi. Showing military energy that he subsequently lacked, McClellan ordered a rapid march on Philippi, sending two columns of three thousand soldiers each. Porterfield had no inkling of their presence.

The two sides met in Philippi on June 3, 1861. The preceding night delivered a torrential rainstorm, which delayed Union forces and convinced Confederate sentries that no one would be moving. The surprised Confederate soldiers panicked when artillery rounds crashed into town at four in the morning. Union commanders intended to encircle the enemy, but the delayed arrival of one column allowed Porterfield's men, along with local secessionists including Samuel Woods, to hurriedly escape. The entire affair lasted a few minutes, with no casualties and a total of ten men injured. The first land battle of the Civil War was a decisive Union victory, which became known in the Northern press as the "Philippi Races."[10]

One of the few wounded men was Confederate private James E. Hanger, an eighteen-year-old Virginia engineering student who had enlisted just two days before. Early in the morning of June 3, a six-pound Union cannonball tore into his left leg. Union doctor James Robison, of the Sixteenth Ohio Infantry, performed a battlefield amputation of the lower half of Hanger's left thigh in Philippi's Methodist church, without anesthesia. It was the first of thirty thousand Union Army amputations.[11] Hanger survived his operation and was medically treated as a prisoner of war in Ohio until August 1861. Then he was fitted with a wooden peg and allowed to return home. Unhappy with his Union stump, the enterprising Hanger developed a hinged prosthetic leg, which impressed other Confederate amputees. Later he founded the J.E. Hanger Company, which supplied prostheses to the Confederate Army.[12]

McClellan left Grafton on June 25 and spent the next several days at Reeves' sister's house in Webster. By July 4 McClellan occupied Buckhannon, forty miles south, astride a major route into eastern Virginia. As McClellan consolidated his position Lee replaced Porterfield with West Point graduate and career soldier Robert Garnett, whom he ordered to halt the Union advance into Virginia. McClellan was called to Washington after the disaster at Bull Run on July 21, but the North would not be denied its connections to the West.

There were several battles and skirmishes in western Virginia over the next months. Lee rode there on August 3 to chase out the Federals and secure the railroads for the South. However, he was defeated in his efforts to take a Union position on Cheat Mountain and failed to remove the Union Army from the southwestern Kanawha region, near Charleston. He was recalled on October 30. By year's end Union forces occupied most of western Virginia and Confederate forces directed their attention elsewhere.

Philippi and Fairmont fended for themselves. Maxwell described Philippi during the War: "When Union soldiers were not occupying the town, often not a human being was to be seen on the streets. The country people preferred to stay at home, and few citizens of the town occupied their houses."[13]

The Union occupation of western Virginia allowed West Virginia statehood to proceed, even if circumstances were hardly those of militarily-enforced stability. Soldiers faced persistent guerrilla warfare and civilians lived with friction and increasing shortages. The mountainous terrain of western Virginia offered ample opportunity for both sides to ambush their enemies and settle scores. As one observer saw the scene: "Every man's hand was raised against his neighbor until a spirit of armed resistance to all law largely prevailed."[14]

The subsequent sundering of Virginia involved men who were close to Reeves, including one of the ministers who had baptized his children. The leader was John Carlile, whose Wheeling convention on May 13, 1861, took no action. After charges and counter charges of treason, the group disbanded and agreed to call a second convention on June 4. Carlile delivered the meeting's valedictory. He told his audience that the erection of a new state was the only sure way to salvation.[15]

On June 4, 1861, following the Union victory at Philippi, thirty-two Northwestern and two Potomac River counties sent delegates to a Second Wheeling Convention, where Carlile confused everyone by arguing against separation. Carlile's logic was that the delegates should first reorganize Virginia and then dismember it. This action would be more likely to appeal to Washington because it was consistent with the U.S. Constitution's Article IV, Section 3: "no new State shall be formed or erected within the Jurisdiction of any other State ... without the Consent of the Legislatures of the States concerned as well as of the Congress."

The convention set the stage for one of the most extraordinary events in U.S. Constitutional history. It declared all Virginia government offices vacant and elected forty-six-year-old Fairmont lawyer, Francis H. Pierpont, Governor of Virginia. On June 25 Pierpont received a dispatch from Secretary of War Simon Cameron, effectively recognizing the Reorganized Government (also called the Restored Government) as the only government of Virginia. Following that the newly constituted legislature elected John Carlile and Waitman Willey as Virginia's U.S. Senators.[16]

The rest of the process was a convoluted and bitter exercise that could only have occurred during the Civil War. Along with the issue of slavery was the Constitutional question of legitimacy. If part of Virginia seceded from Virginia, this could be considered a justification of Virginia's secession from the Union, the cause of the conflict in the first place. U.S. Attorney General Edward Bates interpreted Virginia's proposed dismemberment as a revolution, one that should await the end of the war. Others, including Lincoln, saw an urgent need to bring western Virginia's men and resources into the Union war effort.

Thirty-nine counties voted on the question of secession from Virginia in October, and the outcome was a clear victory for dismemberment: 18,408 for, to 781 against, although the results did not represent Virginia or even the electorates. Six counties of the core thirty-nine did not vote at all and, of the counties that did vote, turnout was only 38 percent.

The next step was a Constitutional Convention, which began meeting in Wheeling in November. Some delegates wanted a large state of seventy-one counties, forty-five of which were loyal to the Confederacy and lay outside Union control. Others favored a smaller, Unionist state. Some opposed any efforts to limit slavery while others, led by Gordon Battelle, the Methodist Presiding Elder who had baptized three of Reeves' children, wanted emancipation language in the constitution. Eventually the Convention settled on a new name, West Virginia, state boundaries that included a realistic forty-four counties, and no emancipation language. The voters approved a new state constitution on April 4, 1862, and sent the contentious issues of statehood and slavery to the U.S. Congress.

The federal official charged with drafting the West Virginia statehood bill was West Virginia Senator Carlile, whose actions became confusing to the point of impenetrability. Carlile's Senate bill called for sixty-three counties in the new state, gradual emancipation, and a new constitutional convention to be ratified by the voters. Carlile specified the impossible constraint that gradual emancipation must be approved by a majority of all registered voters in the new, larger state.

The eventual solution was an amendment by West Virginia's other Senator, Waitman Willey, which proposed a smaller state and emancipation. The final form of the West Virginia statehood bill required that Willey's emancipation language be included in the state's constitution, which, in turn, had to be approved by the voters before it could be submitted for Presidential proclamation.

Lincoln asked his cabinet for its thoughts. The six men who had opinions were split on whether he should sign the bill. On the troublesome issue of whether the new state represented the will of the people of Virginia, which it clearly did not, Lincoln reasoned: "Can this Government stand if it indulges constitutional constructions by which men in open rebellion against it are to be accounted, man for man, the equals of those who maintain their loyalty to it?" Lincoln told Willey and the other Virginia representatives that he would sign the bill and issue the statehood proclamation once the voters ratified the constitutional changes.

The West Virginia Constitutional Convention inserted the required emancipation language as well as dates for the election of the state's new officials. The voters of western Virginia overwhelmingly approved the emancipation language on March 26, 1863. A month later President Lincoln issued a proclamation making West Virginia the nation's thirty-fifth state, effective June 20, 1863. Along the way Camp Carlile in Wheeling became Camp Willey.

Two of Reeves' closest friends took opposing sides in the conflict, consistent with their visions of duty, while Reeves took neither side. One was Samuel Woods, who was not an American by birth, much less a true Southerner. Still, Woods, who was also a devout Methodist, saw the contest as Southern resistance to tyranny. Honor and duty required that he join the Confederate Army, which he did in December 1861. Wood's wife, Isabella, accepted his choice while seeing larger issues. Isabella thought that slavery, which she disliked, was the real cause of the war. She argued that the South could not match the resources of the North and predicted that Virginia was certain to be the principal battleground of the upcoming conflict.[17]

Methodist Presiding Elder Gordon Battelle was morally bound to oppose slavery.

But, as an active member of the western Virginia political community, he was duty-bound to resist the intrusion of Yankee abolitionism. Like many Methodist itinerants, Battelle sought to reconcile opposing principles by preaching for Unionism while seeking to engage his Southern flock.[18]

At West Virginia's First Constitutional Convention Battelle opposed efforts to derail statehood. He understood the contentious ramifications, but he argued for emancipation. One observer noted, "I discovered on that occasion, as I had never before, the mysterious and over-powering influence 'the peculiar institution' had on men otherwise sane and reliable. Why, when Mr. Battelle submitted his resolutions, a kind of tremor— a holy horror, was visible throughout the house!"[19]

Battelle's efforts to add a gradual emancipation clause to the new constitution failed and he felt duty-bound to choose sides, even if his religious vows forbade killing. After the Constitutional Convention adjourned in February 1862, he enlisted as a chaplain in the Union Army. He died in Washington City later that year of camp fever, almost certainly typhoid. To Wheeling's *Daily Intelligencer,* Battelle was a loyal hero, who had devoted heart and soul to the interests of western Virginia. The Reverend Barnes singled out Battelle's faith and his sense of honor: "He was not only an able minister of Jesus Christ, but he was a man of true piety, true Christian piety, and a man of a high sense of honor."[20]

Reeves did not fight for either side, although he had medical skills that would have been valuable to both armies. Part of the reason may have been his wife's worsening depression. When he moved to Fairmont in 1860, Lydia was separated from her Philippi friends and further removed from her family in the Shenandoah Valley. Reeves wrote that he "at once entered upon an encouraging business; and this success went far towards counteracting Mother's regrets on leaving Philippi."[21] Lydia made new friends, but her health declined.[22]

Lydia's condition deteriorated in early 1862. Her main symptom was deep melancholy, with episodes of left leg and arm numbness and weakness. She told her husband that she constantly thought about her family fighting for the South. She asked Reeves why a good Christian would want to live in such times and confessed that she looked forward to her heavenly reward.[23]

On June 21, 1862, Lydia became acutely ill after having tea with a neighbor. She experienced a severe attack of "cholera morbus," a term now implying seasonal gastroenteritis.[24] She began vomiting and her left arm and leg numbness returned. Then her numbness progressed to severe left-sided pain. She became feverish and sleepy, in Reeves' clinical words, "semi-comatose." His friend and colleague, Dr. Matthew Campbell, came up from Grafton, but he could do little. Lydia intermittently awoke from her lethargy and at ten in the morning on June 26 she gave her husband a last embrace. She died six hours later, surrounded by friends and family. The funeral service two days after her death was led by the Rev. John Irwin, Presiding Elder of Fairmont's Methodist Episcopal Church.

Reeves prepared a diary-sized, sixteen-page book about his wife for their children. He had it bound in leather and titled the book, *Mrs. Lydia Reeves: A Letter to Her Children by Father.* Each child received a copy with their name embossed on the cover. The book described Lydia's family and recounted her last few months. It also listed those who were present during her final days.[25]

According to the book, Lydia died from congestion of the brain. By the 1860s this term, with its anatomical implications, was not a disease, but a description of a terminal event, like renal failure might be today. George Wood often used the phrase in his textbook to describe a state of stupor or lethargy, no matter what the presumed etiology. Wood made it clear that, unlike earlier physicians such as Benjamin Rush, he did not see vascular congestion as a causal explanation, but, instead, as an effect of a disease: "a vast deal of mischief has been done by looking to the blood-vessels exclusively as the seat or source of cerebral disorder."[26]

The group gathered for Lydia's passing, described in the book to her children, included Reeves' parents, Dr. Matthew Campbell, the Rev. John L. Irwin, Mrs. Ulysses N. Arnett, Mrs. Newton Pierpont, and Mrs. Ebenezer Mathers. The tableau of political loyalties present at this painful moment provides insight into Reeves' stance during the war.

Reeves' family was Unionist and most of those attending Lydia's death supported the United States. Methodist Episcopal minister Irwin served as the chaplain for the U.S. Army's Fourteenth West Virginia Infantry and Mrs. Mathers' husband, Methodist Protestant minister Ebenezer Mathers, was chaplain for the U.S. Army's Sixth West Virginia Infantry. Similarly, Dr. Matthew Campbell worked for the Union's lifeline, the B&O railroad in Grafton. Mrs. Pierpont's husband, Newton, was the brother of Virginia Governor Francis Pierpont and managed his brother's tannery while Francis ran the Reorganized Government of Virginia.[27]

In contrast Mrs. Ulysses Arnett's two sons, William and Jonathan, were soldiers in the Confederate Army. Many of Reeves' other close friends were also secessionists, including Lydia's family in the Shenandoah Valley, Philippi attorney Samuel Woods, and Woods' brother-in-law, Fairmont attorney James Neeson.[28]

Despite their opposition to secession, no member of the Reeves family fought in the Civil War.[29] Lydia's difficult circumstances may have obliged Reeves to remain a civilian practitioner in Fairmont, but his and his family's actions during the war were consistent with Methodist morality, not dictates of community loyalty and duty or personal honor. Methodist founder Wesley accepted the righteousness of armed self-defense but he did not use the term "war" and he opposed government actions that led to social disorder. He had experience with English civil war and would have abhorred the self-destructive impulses of the American Civil War.[30]

Reeves' sister, Ann Reeves Jarvis, provided the only public statements of the family's non-partisanship. After a Confederate militiaman killed Union soldier Thornsberry Brown near Grafton on May 22, 1861, Ann attended Brown's tension-filled funeral. All were silent around the body. Someone suggested that a prayer be said and so, surrounded by secessionists, Ann asked the Deity to be merciful to the soul of the departed Union soldier and patriot. Colonel James Smith later recalled, "She came forward with bowed head over that soldier and made the most beautiful prayer I have ever listened to."[31]

Ann organized Mothers Work Clubs to teach hygiene to local families on both sides and Reeves helped these efforts. When a Union officer asked her assistance with the wounded, she said she would provide it as long as it was clear that she and her Mothers Work Clubs did not have political allegiances. She told him, "General, we are composed of both the Blue and the Gray."[32]

Reeves quietly demonstrated his non-partisanship by risking reputation and personal safety to support Samuel Woods. After Woods left Philippi and joined the Confederacy, Woods' wife, Isabella, stayed to tend to their home and interests. When Philippi fell under Federal control, she was detested and harassed by local Unionists. Reeves sent money to Isabella and helped carry her correspondence with Woods through Union lines.[33]

Reeves favored the goals of Unionism, but supported peaceful reconciliation with the South. Publicly expressing this sentiment in Union-occupied Fairmont would have branded him a Copperhead, even worse than a rebel traitor. Open non-partisanship would have also put him in the same camp as his disreputable former neighbor, John Carlile. Reeves was quietly apolitical during the war.

Reeves remained a widower for a year after Lydia's death. He married twenty-seven-year-old Mary Frey, the daughter of Dr. William Frey, in her family home in Allegany County, Maryland, in July 1863. She was the sister of Dr. William Jr., also a Methodist and a physician, who was the same age as Reeves and lived in nearby Brandonville.[34] Mary helped raise Reeves' four children, but never bore children of her own.

The Civil War bypassed Fairmont most of the time, but Confederate generals John Imboden and William E. "Grumble" Jones launched coordinated campaigns in western Virginia in the spring of 1863. Their intentions were to disrupt the railroad, collect supplies for General Lee, and overthrow Pierpont's Reorganized Government. Jones' forces routed Union soldiers at Philippi and Beverly on April 24, 1863, driving them back to Grafton. Jones then marched to Morgantown and Fairmont. Along the route, his Confederates received support from local secessionists and bushwhacking from Union loyalists. On April 29, Grumble Jones led his army of 6,000 men against 300 Union defenders in Fairmont.[35]

Fairmont's Union soldiers surrendered after a short defense and Confederate

Reeves and Lydia's children, about the time of Lydia's death in 1862. Left to right, Joseph (b. 1856), Nancy (1852), Charles (1858), and Ann (1854). After Lydia died Reeves wrote a short volume for each child telling their family history: "Mrs. Lydia Reeves: A Letter to Her Children by Father," which he had professionally printed and bound in leather (courtesy Joan Webb).

troops quickly destroyed the B&O's 615-foot iron bridge over the Monongahela. Jones' forces looted the deserted town, showing no distinction between Union or secessionist property. The Confederate army withdrew within days, leaving ill-will on both sides and cementing Union sympathies in the northern counties of the soon-to-be state of West Virginia. Federal engineers replaced Fairmont's bridge with wooden trestles and, in short order, Union trains began running between Wheeling and Washington.[36]

Reeves avoided serious consequences from wartime hostilities, but his 1850 Sutton house-mate, Dr. Thomas Camden, was less fortunate. Camden's fate typified the turns of civilian life in western Virginia and the source of many civilians' postwar bitterness. Camden lived in Weston, forty miles south of Philippi. He was Reeves' age and also a Methodist and Southern sympathizer who found the war senseless. Camden did not enlist and cared for citizens from both sides. However, on May 19, 1863, after the Jones-Imboden raids, Union soldiers arrested him for treason, based on testimony from his Unionist neighbors.[37]

The Union Army dispatched Camden, his wife, and three young children to Camp Chase, near Columbus, Ohio. Weston's less partisan citizens wrote to West Virginia's incoming governor Boreman seeking his return and, on June 17, 1863, three days before West Virginia became a state, Boreman ordered that Camden be allowed to leave Camp Chase after swearing a loyalty oath to the Union and, with his wealthy brother Johnson Newlon's help, posting a thousand dollar bond. In an ironic twist, Federal troops garrisoned in Weston soon offered him the position of post surgeon. Camden survived the war and was an early member of the West Virginia Medical Society. He died in 1910, at age eighty-one.

⑃ 8 ⑃

Army Medicine
and Public Health

While Reeves was dealing with Lydia's death, part of America's public health future passed through western Virginia. Several of the nation's leading sanitarians, later Reeves' professional allies, advocated for an obscure Union Army physician who was stuck in Grafton in 1862.

Before the Civil War mid-century American sanitarians issued thoughtful reports and fought lonely battles because legislators paid them little mind. The laws and the legislators who created them did not require or even want medical expertise.[1] After Fort Sumter, Northern women's groups organized benevolent organizations to support the soldiers. The New York City women's group inspired Unitarian minister Henry Bellows and public health advocate, Elisha Harris, to work with the women to develop a formal medical relief effort for the coming war. U.S. Secretary of War Simon Cameron, over the misgivings of the Union Army's Surgeon General and President Lincoln, approved the New Yorkers' newly formed U.S. Sanitary Commission (USSC) as a nonmilitary medical support organization in June 1861. Sanitation became patriotic.[2]

The USSC volunteers were motivated by reform experiences in English manufacturing towns and Florence Nightingale's successes with sanitation and hygiene in the Crimean War (1853–1856). Physician members such as Harris also knew the analytic messages of Pierre Louis, his American followers such as Elisha Bartlett and Oliver Wendell Holmes, and his English pupils, such as sanitarian William Farr. Even if they did not understand the bacteriological causes of disease, USSC members were well aware of the casualties that accompanied the overcrowding and filth of the English and French armies in Crimea.[3]

The USSC's civilian leaders began documenting the state of military facilities in the District of Columbia. Harris and the Commission's newly appointed General Secretary, Frederick Law Olmstead, who had taken off from designing New York's Central Park, performed the initial inspections in July 1861. Olmstead noted that troop discipline was terrible, Army camp drains were inadequate, personal hygiene was nonexistent, and, since vegetables were forbidden, that scurvy and dysentery were soon to be commonplace. Olmstead's opinions and predictions were accurate and indicative of almost all military facilities, North and South, in the first months of the war. The USSC sounded an alarm, but military and civilian officials ignored it.[4]

The calamitous Union defeat at Bull Run on July 21, 1861, made the Army's lack of preparedness visible to all. Olmstead described the aftermath in Washington City, as injured soldiers were left to die on the battlefield and others straggled back: "a most woe-begone rabble, which had perhaps clothed itself with the garments of dead soldiers left on a hard-fought battle-field. No two were dressed completely alike; some were without caps, others without coats, others without shoes. All were alike excessively dirty, unshaven, unkempt, and dank with dew."[5]

Lincoln's response to Bull Run was to appoint the Young Napoleon, George McClellan, to command the capital's defenses. McClellan was receptive to the USSC's medical messages, one of which was a call for more hospital beds, to be located in permanent buildings and designed on the open pavilion plan recommended by Nightingale. Another USSC message was the need to establish and enforce scientifically-based medical professional standards. A third USSC message, one on which the first two depended, was that the Union Army required an immediate change in size, organization, and leadership. For the Army to succeed, it needed to centralize and improve its medical and sanitary practices.[6]

Congress had to reorganize the small Medical Department before the Army could choose a new medical leader. The existing arrangement was designed for frontier campaigns against American Indians, not the challenges of a large-scale land and naval war. The USSC's medical reform efforts advanced through Congress as the Wilson Bill, which passed in April 1862. Senator Wilson's "Act to Reorganize and Increase the Efficiency of the Medical Department of the Army" authorized twenty new military surgeons and an increase in rank of the Surgeon-General from colonel to brigadier general. In acknowledging the crisis Congress directed the Army to appoint its Surgeon-General on job qualifications, not seniority. The Act gave the Surgeon-General more authority over the regular army's medical staff and medical supplies, while it created a group of inspectors to enforce the "sanitary condition and wants of troops and of hospitals, and to the skill, efficiency, and good conduct of the officers and attendants connected with the medical department." The USSC got most of what it wanted.[7]

After the USSC's legislation passed, the Army needed a modern Surgeon-General. This was the connection to western Virginia. Lieutenant William Alexander Hammond was only thirty-three years old, but he had ten years of prior Army service, during which he had travelled to Europe and studied the construction of military and civilian hospitals. While on active duty the doctor had also conducted a series of experiments on himself, evaluating the physiologic and biochemical effects of dietary albumen, starch, and gum Arabic, and receiving the AMA's 1857 scientific essay prize for this work.[8]

Hammond had resigned his commission in 1860 and, with the outbreak of war, re-enlisted, putting his name at the bottom of the Army's seniority list. Worse, after rejoining the Army in 1861 Hammond made no bones about the poor levels of preparedness he saw. For this he caught the attention of sixty-four-year-old Surgeon-General Clement Finley, who had him re-assigned from the mid–Atlantic region to General Rosecrans' remote Department of Western Virginia. The civilians on the USSC had a different opinion. They wanted Hammond to replace the aging and conservative Finley.

Rosecrans ordered Hammond and his thirty-seven-year-old colleague, Jonathan Letterman, to survey the medical facilities at Grafton, Virginia and Cumberland, Maryland in early 1862. Their report was forwarded to the USSC. It exemplified the medical issues facing the Union Army and showed Hammond to be an energetic, modern physician.[9]

Hammond and Letterman visited Grafton and Cumberland around March 10, 1862. Grafton was the encampment for the nine hundred fifty soldiers of the Ohio Fifty-Fifth Volunteers. The sanitary conditions of the camp were marked by overcrowding, six to eight inches of mud, and tents placed over boards situated directly on sodden ground. A latrine trench was located between the tents and the Three Forks River; however, the soldiers often used any piece of open ground to relieve themselves. The inspectors noted that the camp's wretched conditions were not likely to improve so long as the regiment's officers were billeted in light and airy houses half a mile away.

Hammond and Letterman described the health of the Ohio soldiers and the poor state of the camp's medical facilities. They documented the presence of measles and noted that between measles and several other illnesses, one-seventh of the regiment was medically unfit for duty. The camp hospital was not a real hospital, but a series of private homes supplemented by five tents. Following Nightingale's advice, Hammond and Letterman recommended that there be at least twelve hundred cubic feet of air per patient. In one overcrowded house the amount of air was one hundred sixty-three cubic feet per patient. After the regiment arrived in Grafton eight soldiers died of measles who, they argued, with clean bedding and adequate ventilation, would have survived. The inspectors recommended short-term corrective steps, but their preferred action was to move the entire regiment to another site with less filth and better medical capabilities.

Their report was equally harsh on the fifteen permanent hospital facilities in Cumberland. In one case the reporter, likely Hammond, who had no trouble expressing severe judgments, wrote "I do not hesitate to say, that such a condition of affairs *does not exist in any other hospital in the civilized world;* and that this hospital is altogether worse than any which were such *opprobria* to the allies in the Crimean War (author's italics)."[10]

As Hammond was inspecting Grafton in March, the leaders of the USSC offered his name to newly appointed Secretary of War Edwin Stanton. Stanton resented the civilians' interference and blocked any mention of promoting Hammond. Following Stanton's rebuff, the USSC went to McClellan, Commander of the Union Army of the Potomac, who trusted Rosecrans and knew Hammond's work. McClellan was also a young outsider who had no trouble identifying with Hammond's situation and supported him. The tie-breaker went to Stanton's superior, President Lincoln, who backed McClellan. Immediately after passage of the Wilson Bill in April 1862, Surgeon-General Finley retired and McClellan appointed first lieutenant Hammond to brigadier general, for which Hammond earned the undying enmity of the Secretary of War.

Northern regular physicians were elated that one of their own was called to the country's service. *The Cincinnati Lancet and Observer* stated, "no selection could have been made that would have so fully commanded the confidence and esteem of the profession of the country."[11] The *Boston Medical and Surgical Journal* was "glad to learn that Dr. William A. Hammond has been appointed by the President to fill the important post of Surgeon-General."[12] *The American Medical Times* of New York City effused, "No man could be selected, who so happily combines in his professional relations, the confidence and esteem of both the Medical Staff of the army, and the profession of the country, as Dr. Hammond."[13]

Hammond summoned his fellow hospital examiner, Jonathan Letterman, to his side then bypassed the seniority lists and promoted Letterman to Medical Director of McClellan's Army, the post vacated by Charles Tripler. McClellan was impressed with his new medical officer's energy and administrative competence. He wrote about Letterman, "I never met with his superior in power of organization and executive ability."[14]

The capable Tripler summarized the difficulties Hammond and Letterman faced. The Union's large volunteer army was under the command of state governors and in many cases the physicians assigned to this force, who had been enrolled as rapidly as they could be found, were incompetent. These new military physicians knew nothing of the Army or military medicine and their commanding officers were not much better off: "The [volunteer] regimental medical officers were, for the most part, physicians taken suddenly from civil life, with little knowledge of their duties, which had to be taught to them from the very alphabet. The line officers were equally ignorant with themselves in this respect, and hence confusion, conflict of authority, and discontent, very seriously impaired efficiency in the medical department."[15]

Tripler's harsh assessment was an understatement to many civilians. As the war gathered momentum and newspapers recounted medical horror stories, angry voters besieged their Congressmen. During debates leading to passage of the Wilson Bill, Congressman Harrison Blake of Ohio quoted an editorial in the *Cincinnati Times*, decrying the state of Army physicians and their capabilities. From his own experience Blake added, "I was in the Army for a little while and there I found that a good many incompetent men have obtained positions as surgeons.... We have surgeons in the Army who have no right to be there."[16]

New York physician and Republican Representative Socrates Norton Sherman, himself a member of the Thirty-Fourth New York Volunteers, consistently opposed these attacks on his profession. Sherman was a capable surgeon, but as Congressman Sherman he did not see discussions of the Civil War's medical catastrophes as opportunities to improve Army medicine.

From the floor of Congress Sherman derided the need for hospital inspectors. These new officers would have little to do because "there are no officers of your Army who are more faithful and competent than the medical officers." He eventually and grudgingly agreed with Congressman Blake that there "are many men in the medical staff of the Army who are incompetent," but dismissed this as irrelevant because doctors could not be held to a higher standard than anyone else: "So there are many incompetent colonels and captains.... I challenge, as a class, a comparison between the surgeons of the Army and any other corps for usefulness, ability, and fidelity."[17]

Sherman's arguments did not carry the day, and the Wilson Bill included authorization for hospital inspectors. Recent medical historians have explored the pathbreaking organizational changes that the USSC and Hammond initiated and his successors followed, which included a massive hospital construction and staffing program, an organized ambulance corps, rigorous morbidity and mortality records, a pathological museum, a national medical library, the use of disinfectants for gangrene, and the standardized production of drugs.[18] However, one disastrous episode also brought regular medicine's persisting scientific schism out of meetings and journals and into public view.

As a scientifically-oriented physician, the energetic Surgeon-General found time in 1863 to publish a 504-page *Treatise on Hygiene with Special Reference to the Military Service,* which one reviewer considered the most important treatise on hygiene in the English language. Hammond declared his therapeutic leanings in the book's preface. To him, hygiene had been too much neglected and drugs too much administered.[19]

Hammond was disturbed by what he felt was Army physicians' abuse of two staples of heroic medicine's aging armamentarium: calomel (mercurous chloride) and tartar emetic (antimony potassium tartrate). Calomel and tartar emetic were used to treat dysentery, probably with positive benefit. However, as with typhoid, better-educated physicians now accepted that the ever-present dysentery was a self-limited process, which tended toward recovery and needed only symptomatic support. Union Army physicians had access to calomel and a less toxic form of mercury, blue mass (also called blue pill), and many reported that calomel was not particularly helpful for dysentery. In the face of ample evidence that the drugs were far less useful than once thought, Hammond received field reports that some military surgeons pushed calomel and tartar emetic to heroic doses.[20]

He issued Medical Department Circular Number 6 on May 4, 1863, ordering the removal of calomel and tartar emetic from the Army supply table, leaving blue mass available. Hammond stated, "No doubt can exist that more harm has resulted from the misuse of both these agents, in the treatment of disease, than benefit from their proper administration."[21]

Hammond's only realistic option for influencing his doctors' practices was managing their supplies. During the Civil War approximately 12,300 of the Union's 31,000 regular physicians served in the Union Army and almost all of these men (and three women) were volunteers, sometimes for brief tours.[22] Hammond sought to bring this unwieldy group under his control and establish medical proficiency examinations, but that task was impossible in the war's chaotic conditions. He battled to get matériel, staff, facilities and operational control. But, as a new-generation physician and therapeutic conservative, Hammond also wanted to protect Union soldiers from what he saw as outdated medical practices.

The response to Hammond's internal directive was a civilian medical firestorm that was quickly reported in the lay press. The New York *Times* wrote on June 7, 1863, "The recent order of Surgeon-General Hammond, prohibiting the use of calomel and tartar emetic in the army, has produced a good deal of lively discussion in medical circles, and is meeting with much criticism and opposition." The *Times* brought the matter home: "Now that we are all liable to become conscripts, the question of our medical treatment in the field and hospital is one which comes very close to us."[23]

The more common historical view of Hammond's order and its professional reaction is that it exemplified nineteenth-century struggles to introduce rational and conservative therapies. Arguments against Hammond represented the dying logic of prescientific heroic medicine.[24] But, there is an alternative interpretation that goes to medicine's rift over the ownership and purpose of medical science, the issue that Bartlett exposed in 1844.

Physicians who approved of Hammond's actions presented their case with logic-based rationale.[25] New York's Stephen Smith, editor of the *American Medical Times*, wrote, "Students in the school of modern pathology and physiology look on with indifference, feeling that they have little or nothing at stake in the issue." According to the *Times*, the Surgeon-General had acted within his legitimate capacity. Moreover, calomel was certainly being abused and its removal did not affect the judicious use of mercury within the Army because several other "more eligible and useful" mercury preparations were still on the supply table. The *Medical Times* concluded, "We are compelled to regard the order of the Surgeon-General as a judicious, and even a necessary measure."[26]

Those who resisted Hammond were not outraged about calomel. They saw a larger threat to the patrimony of regular physicians: their right to use medical science as they saw fit. Hammond's action argued otherwise and justified thirty years of claims by medicine's sectarian competitors that regular physicians overused harsh treatments. In the hyper-partisan climate of the Civil War, this was professional treason. Thirteen medical journals quickly and vehemently attacked the Surgeon-General.[27]

The Cincinnati Lancet and Observer led the charge. The *Lancet* announced Hammond's appointment a year earlier with unqualified approval. Now it began its castigation with: "We felt at the time that great injustice was done to the medical staff of the regular army in his appointment." The journal accused the Army's chief physician of insulting every man in the profession with his Circular Number 6. It denounced the evidence on which he based his removal of calomel and tartar emetic and then said, even if such evidence existed, Hammond had no business restricting access to a drug that could be abused because any drug was subject to abuse. Another offense, in the eyes of the Ohio editor, was that Hammond relied on reports prepared by men from Massachusetts. There was no room for further discussion: "The Surgeon-General has inflicted a grievous wrong upon his profession.... He must either recall Circular No. 6, or he must resign, the smallest atonement he can make to an insulted and outraged profession."[28]

Events at the AMA's annual meeting demonstrated that the issue was more than a therapeutic controversy. The Association had not met in 1861 or 1862 because of the war. The meeting that began on June 2, 1863, in Chicago was a tense affair, with only two physicians from the Confederacy present. AMA President Jewell spent most of his prepared address advocating for a greater appreciation of hygiene and preventive medicine. He used Hammond as a good example, mentioning his book on hygiene and citing as an illustration of the topic's importance the Surgeon-General's commendable order requiring that all applicants for the Army medical staff attend at least one course of lectures on hygiene. Shortly after Jewell's speech, an Ohio delegate raised the matter of the Surgeon-General's order prohibiting the supply of calomel and antimony in the Army. The chair appointed a committee to examine the matter.[29]

Before the committee presented its findings, the delegates heard from the AMA's education committee, which lauded recent advances in medical science, lamented the medical profession's lack of public esteem, and pointed to the high failure rates of applicants to the Army Medical Department as evidence of the poor quality of medical education. The delegates were reminded that the country was flooded with inadequately trained physicians.

On the third day the committee declared that Hammond's order was a blanket accusation against physicians in general. If some doctors were guilty as charged, then two valuable drugs should not be withheld from all, instead the malefactors should be removed. The committee made it clear that the matter was not just an Army issue. Hammond's action was "a most grievous offense against the dignity, usefulness, and humanity of our profession." It insisted on the order's revision.[30]

Spurred by AMA actions and *The Cincinnati Lancet and Observer*, other physicians and their journals called for Hammond to resign. Despite Hammond's battlefield results, where Army doctors, hospitals, and ambulances, aided by USSC volunteers, were overcoming monumental challenges, Secretary of War Stanton also wanted to remove his abrasive Surgeon-General. Hammond's supporter, General McClellan, no longer commanded the Union Army and, despite the USSC's positive role at Gettysburg and elsewhere, Stanton had little use for Hammond's civilian advocates. Stanton ordered Hammond on a series of long inspection tours during the fall of 1863 and when Hammond was finally allowed to return to Washington, Stanton's surrogates began court-martial proceedings in January 1864.

Later evidence showed that Hammond's court-martial charges were minor and mostly fabricated,[31] but they led to successful verdicts of disorder, neglect, and conduct unbecoming an officer. Hammond was dishonorably discharged in August 1864. His friends were stunned and *The Boston Medical and Surgical Journal* glumly took the matter as "a reproach on the whole profession."[32] In contrast, *The Cincinnati Lancet and Observer* crowed that the court-martial's findings were an unimpeachable damnation of Hammond alone, while reminding its readers of the Surgeon-General's offense: "that he had dishonestly violated his faith to his profession."[33]

Hammond was disconsolate after his dismissal, but he rebounded. He established a successful and lucrative neurological practice in New York City, serving as one of the American founders of the specialty. His strong opinions led to medical-legal clashes over the definition of insanity, but historians generally acknowledge that, during the Civil War, Hammond's short tenure produced measurable success and permanent improvements in Army medicine. Congress reversed his court-martial and returned his rank to him in 1879.

Letterman requested reassignment after Hammond's removal and then resigned. However, the USSC, the new Surgeon-General, and the other men Hammond had chosen continued their work. Importantly for the public and the next generation of American physicians, Surgeon-General Barnes, Hammond's replacement, saw to it that Army research continued and Hammond's visions of an Army Medical Museum, later the Armed Forces Institute of Pathology, the Army Medical Library, later the National Library of Medicine, and a substantial six volume report on the medical side of the war, were fulfilled.

Hammond's advocate in New York, Stephen Smith, helped wartime New York City become the birthplace of America's public health profession. Smith used his weekly journal, *The American Medical Times,* as a bully pulpit, partly for Hammond, but mostly for urban sanitation reform. He wrote in 1860, "New York and our larger American cities successfully vie with the great cities of Europe in all that relates to commercial enterprise, manufactures, popular intelligence, and the practical applications of science and art, but where and what are our sanitary defences?"[34] Smith was ready to place blame on New York City's Democratic machine, writing in January 1863, "Many of the Health Wardens, the most important officers in the [New York] city government if they rightly discharge their duties, are registered among the most disreputable class in the community."[35]

Smith used *The American Medical Times* to lobby for a state solution to what he saw as New York City's mishandled sanitation while he also participated in the war, writing a manual for military surgeons and serving a stint in a military hospital. To Smith the wartime message was clear, the only solution to New York's squalor and appallingly high death rates was a strong public health enterprise, removed from politics, and firmly based in the emerging discipline of sanitary science.[36]

A group of prominent New York citizens, including Hamilton Fish and John Jacob Astor, Jr., formed the Citizens' Association "for purposes of public usefulness" in December 1863. The group asked Smith, Elisha Harris, Austin Flint, and other prominent New York physicians for information on the city's public health. The physicians sent back an immediate response that the situation was terrible, emphasizing New York City's high mortality rates compared to other major cities. These data were compelling, but they were not enough to overcome public apathy and convince the Republican legislature to impose itself on New York City's Democratic politicians.

The Citizens' Association decided to overwhelm the opposition with facts. It organized a Council of Hygiene and Public Health in April 1864 to gather more information on the health and sanitary needs of New York's 750,000 inhabitants. Smith directed a massive survey by thirty-one volunteer physicians that was completed by year-end. He delivered a seventeen-volume report, with a 360-page summary and a 143-page introduction written by Elisha Harris in April 1865. This document, which was prepared in the middle of a catastrophic civil war, became a landmark in American public health and epidemiology.[37]

Smith's report added detail to the previously episodic efforts to reduce New York City's sordid conditions. It cited data from every section of the city on sickness rates, crowding, and general filth. It repeatedly showed that New York's mortality data were alarmingly bad, not only between sections in the city, but compared to numerous other cities. And it made no bones about where the blame lay, faulting the city's lack of political action and its lack of a scientific approach: "it is found that the subject of sickness rates has received no attention from the Health Department of the City Government, and that the records of Medical Charities of the City remain unstudied by any official authority."[38]

To Smith and most others, the reasons for correcting the city's sanitation and health problems were partly economic, it was less expensive to prevent disease than to cure it, but also moral. Poor health led to a city's social and moral decay: "such excessive unhealthiness and mortality is a most prolific source of physical and social want, demoralization and pauperism." Summing it up, Harris quoted Ben Franklin, "Franklin's aphorism that Public Health is Public Wealth, finds ample confirmation in the experience of all populous communities."[39]

The report had not been printed when Smith presented its findings to the New York legislature on February 13, 1865. Smith cited the results of his coworkers and lambasted the city's health inspector. He recounted a painfully amusing episode where a civilian health warden foolishly told a smallpox patient's care-giver to stay away and: "Burn camphor on the stove, and hang bags of camphor about the necks of the children." The proper answer was vaccination and isolation. Smith asked the members of the Senate and Assembly: "To what depth of humiliation must that community have descended, which tolerates as its sanitary officers men who are not only utterly disqualified by education, business, and moral character, but who have not even the poor qualification of courage to perform their duties?"[40]

Smith helped draft the law he wanted, but favorable editorials by the New York *Times* and *Tribune* and the printed copy of the Council's report were not enough to sway the legislature. Then, on April 14 Lincoln was assassinated and the bill was lost for the year. What finally decided the matter was a cholera outbreak in early 1866. The threat of a public health disaster made Democratic opposition look self-serving and the Republican legislature passed the Metropolitan Health Act in February 1866. The act was not just a landmark event in public health; the effort to pass it added momentum to a reform movement that deposed Tammany Hall's Boss Tweed in 1872.

The 1866 New York law helped reshape America's public health infrastructure as the 1862 Wilson Bill upended American military medicine. It professionalized the city's health department, creating a pathway for improved data collection and the emerging lessons of medical and sanitary science. The new Board of Health consisted of five health commissioners, four of whom had to be physicians, and four police commissioners. One of the commissioners was the Sanitary Superintendent, who had to be an experienced physician. The Board had authority to hire up to fifteen sanitary inspectors, at least ten of whom also had to be skilled physicians with professional experience in their district.[41] Although it was forced to do so by the state legislature, New York City was the first government entity to recognize that public health required more than law enforcement and street cleaning. Business interests quickly challenged the Board of Health but, following the 1866–1867 cholera outbreak, the Board enjoyed broad popular support. Stephen Smith was appointed a city health commissioner in 1868, a post he held for seven years.

Jane Boswell Moore, a civilian volunteer for the United States Christian Commission, visited Grafton's new pavilion-style hospital in March 1863. She pronounced it excellent: "we must accord the first rank to this hospital of the many we have seen." Surgeon (Major) Socrates Norton Sherman of the Thirty-Fourth New York Volunteers commanded the hospital in 1864, the same (former) Congressman Sherman who had opposed hospital inspectors in 1862.[42]

The Grafton Army hospital, as many other Army hospitals, was closely connected to the local community. Grafton's citizens provided the hospital with supplies and volunteers and the hospital reciprocated. Sherman attended a train accident on October 24, 1864, where, according to one injured participant, "He appeared like a ministering angel going about, doing good to his fellow man ... the skill and care of Dr. Sherman will long be remembered by the wounded."[43]

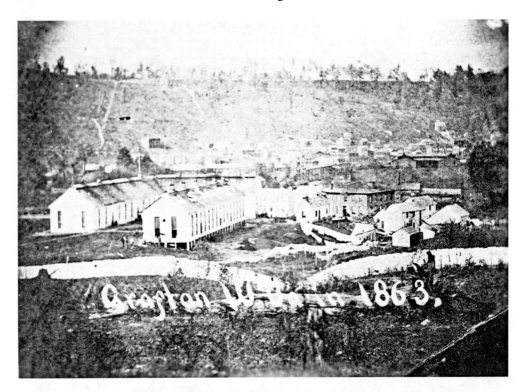

The Grafton Army Hospital in 1863, with Grafton faintly visible in the background. The recently constructed facility had 342 beds, and like many other Union Army hospitals, was based on the pavilion design. In July 1864 the hospital's commander was Major Socrates N. Sherman, of the Thirty-Fourth New York Volunteers. Union Army physician Sherman and Confederate sympathizer Reeves collaborated on a successful ovariotomy (salpingo-oophorectomy) that year (West Virginia and Regional History Center, WVU Libraries).

Reeves' involvement with Sherman began on July 12, 1864. His friend and colleague, Matthew Campbell had moved from Grafton to Parkersburg but still cared for a twenty-nine-year-old woman in Fairmont. He asked Reeves to help him see her. Campbell's patient had been troubled by an enlarging abdominal mass for more than a year.[44]

Reeves diagnosed an intra-abdominal cyst and recommended that Campbell drain the mass. Campbell did this, removing eight quarts of fluid. Afterwards Reeves could feel a soft movable tumor, about six inches in diameter. He and Campbell considered injecting iodine into the mass to prevent recurrence of the fluid, but felt that this was only slightly less risky than surgical removal, so they decided against this step. Following the procedure, Campbell asked Reeves, as a local physician, to monitor the patient's recovery.

The unfortunate woman did well for several days, with no evidence of fever and some return of her appetite. However, within two weeks the fluid reaccumulated and she felt progressively worse. Campbell and Reeves suggested that she should consider surgery. They had no reluctance in asking the accomplished Union Army physician, S. N. Sherman, stationed in Grafton, to see her and Sherman responded. He quickly concurred that surgery was needed. On October 1, 1864, the doctors explained the operation "and its terrible character" to Campbell's patient. She consented to the surgery, which occurred on October 6.[45]

Campbell and Sherman arrived on the train from Grafton, accompanied by Reeves' brother-in-law, Dr. William Frey of Brandonville. Like most surgeries of the time, the operation was performed in a convenient building, in this case, the patient's house. Reeves prepared a mixture of ether and chloroform and served as the anesthesiologist. He began administering the anesthetic at 2:45 p.m., switching to pure chloroform "on account of its slow effect." Shortly thereafter, the sedated patient was transferred from her bed to a table.[46]

Sherman and the other physicians called the procedure they performed an "ovariotomy," which referred to any procedure involving ovarian removal. The operation they performed in 1864 would now be considered a salpingo-oophorectomy, the removal of an ovary and its attached Fallopian tube. Prior to the development of surgical anesthesia in 1847, physicians seldom performed this high-risk abdominal surgery and generally attacked those who did. One notable exception was a backwoods Kentucky physician, Ephraim McDowell, who stunned the European medical world by performing a successful ovariotomy (salpingo-oophorectomy) in 1809.[47] With anesthesia but without antisepsis, the procedure was risky and controversial in the 1860s. In a three-year series comprising all ovariotomies in London, only nine of twenty-two patients survived the operation. The European and American medical literature recorded only 787 cases of ovariotomy by 1864.[48]

Campbell began the operation with a midline abdominal incision and quickly found a large left ovarian cyst. He removed ten quarts of fluid from the cyst and the sedated patient began vomiting. The surgeons waited for her vomiting to stop and then continued. Sherman did the remainder of the work, using his bare hands to free several adhesions and eventually bring the ovarian mass to the surface. As they proceeded Campbell and Sherman followed steps that British surgeon Spencer Wells outlined in 1861.[49]

There was no antisepsis or disinfection. The operators dressed the patient's wound with flannel and returned her to bed at five p.m., one and one half hours after beginning surgery, fully alert, with no effects of anesthesia. Her pulse was rapid and her breathing slightly labored, but she appeared stable. The physicians used opium for pain and offered her ice and toast water.[50]

Reeves and the surgeons stayed with their patient for the next day. She had some pain in her right thigh, her pulse was rapid, and she was restless. They treated her with opium and gave her liquids by mouth. They used a bladder catheter to help her void. Reeves remained to care for her after the second day.

Reeves visited her daily for the next eleven days as she gradually improved. He treated her pain with opium, the resulting constipation with spirits of ammonia, and ordered her family to regularly catheterize her to avoid bladder distension. He removed the dressings, pins, and the ovarian pedicle clamp four days after surgery. He only allowed her fluids for the first five days post-surgery then he slowly increased her diet to solid food.

She felt much better within two weeks. Reeves wrote, "She was able to quit her room, and take food more liberally. Opium was now entirely discontinued; and from this date her recovery was rapid and without drawbacks." On October 31, 1864, three and one-half weeks following major abdominal surgery with chloroform anesthesia and no use of antiseptic technique, she was discharged from further care. Seven months later she was back to normal health, with her first postoperative menstrual period occurring in May 1865. Her cyst recurred several years later and she travelled to Philadelphia for treatment, where she died.[51]

Reeves' successful case was the first ovariotomy in West Virginia. Two years following the surgery he described the events in *The American Journal of the Medical Sciences.* The patient was in good health at the time and Reeves stated that his delay in publishing the case was to confirm her complete recovery.

From an historical perspective, Reeves' and Sherman's ovariotomy demonstrated more than a small milestone in the development of American surgery. It illustrated overlooked aspects of Civil War medicine. As Ohio Congressman Blake complained in 1862, the war's early days were marked by catastrophic levels of ill-preparedness. Yet, Civil War medicine was much more than disasters on the battlefield and piles of amputated limbs.

James E. Hanger, the newly enlisted Confederate soldier whose left leg was amputated at the thigh by Union surgeon James Robison in Philippi's Methodist Church on June 3, 1861, would likely not have been as fortunate if he had been injured in a similar European conflict. French, German, and British doctors recorded an 80 percent fatality rate for lower extremity amputations during the earlier Crimean War. French physicians reported an 82 percent lower extremity amputation mortality rate in the later Franco-German War (1870–71). The Union Army performed 6,238 thigh amputations and 3,736 lower leg amputations during the American Civil War, with a 33 percent mortality rate, far surpassing contemporary European wartime accomplishments.[52]

Civil War surgeons, such as Sherman, gained precious experience and made considerable contributions to medical knowledge. Sherman reported more than twenty cases that were later described in *The Medical and Surgical History of the War of the Rebellion.* These cases ranged from soft-tissue injuries, to amputations, to neurosurgery, to vascular repair.[53] Sherman's management of Reeves' patient benefited from his wartime work, as all did all fields of American surgery from lessons learned in the war.

Germany's physician-scientist Rudolph Virchow was amazed by the Union Army's Medical achievements. He compared the American Civil War experience with the supposedly more medically sophisticated French experience in Crimea and concluded:

> That the French learned little or nothing in the Crimea, and the North Americans so much in their civil war, that from that date onwards begins a new era of military medicine—this depends not on the magnitude of the necessity which the Americans had to undergo, which in truth was not greater than the French underwent in the Crimea. It was far more the critical, genuinely scientific spirit, the open mind, the sound and practical intelligence, which in America penetrated step by step every department of army administration, and which under the wonderful cooperation of a whole nation reached the highest development that, relative to humane achievements, had hitherto been attained in a great war.[54]

Soldiers fought the Civil War throughout the country and their medical experiences served to break down sectional barriers. New York physician Sherman's caring for West Virginia train accident victims and treating rural physician Reeves' civilian patient was not unique. The war brought disparate physicians and communities together in ways that would have never happened.

DeWitt Peters, born in New York, but a Union physician from the western frontier who had published a personal biography of Kit Carson, was assigned to Fort Pickens, off the coast of the swampy Florida panhandle in 1862. The physicians in nearby Pensacola left to join the Confederate Army so Peters' commander charged him to care for the town's inhabitants, which he willingly did. He wrote, "In giving my services to these poor people, mostly women and children, I found them ever grateful and it was a source of satisfaction to me to aid in alleviating their sufferings."[55]

George Cooper, a Union Army surgeon originally assigned to Michigan, found himself in the rice fields of Georgia in 1862, where Southerners swore Northerners could not survive. Yet, with fresh vegetables, sanitation, and quinine, Cooper's soldiers did well, dispelling a pervasive myth about Southern diseases and Southern constitutions.[56]

The war also changed the way Americans looked at hospitals, paving the way for post-war hospital expansion. Hospitals before 1860 were restricted to major cities and were most often used for quarantine (pest houses) and care of the poor (almshouses). North and South, the Civil War's needs brought concerned and caring civilians by the thousands inside military hospitals and changed the conception of hospitals from unseen repositories to visible, community-based proving grounds for the new disciplines of hygiene, nursing, and medical efficiency.

The 342-bed Grafton Army Hospital, located in a rural West Virginia railroad town of only 891 persons, exemplified the scope and rapidity of the Union Medical Department's wartime accomplishments. In 1861 the Union Army had no fixed general hospitals where patients, physicians, and supplies could be serviced by train or steamboat. Within four years it had created 192 such hospitals with 118,000 beds. These hospitals were built from Wisconsin to Louisiana and from Maine to Florida. Three of them were in Grafton, Parkersburg, and Wheeling, West Virginia, a Union state that did not even exist when the war began.[57]

Hospitals closed after the war ended, volunteer soldiers returned home, and governments decommissioned their military machines. Reeves and West Virginia had to get down to business. Reeves was a resident of the oldest, most respected, and most traditional state in the country as the war began. When it concluded, he lived in a small mountainous state with untapped resources and, on its surface, a clean slate.

9

Medical Organizing

West Virginia's clean slate was an illusion. The state was fractured on the same lines as the rest of the country. The railroad divided West Virginia between Republican industrialists in the northern and Ohio River counties and former secessionists, mostly rural Democrats, everywhere else. The B&O brought mobility and promise to the state's northwestern area, particularly the state's capital Wheeling, while two-thirds of West Virginia's inhabitants were isolated farmers, distrustful of outsiders. West Virginia was run by the minority Republican Party.

West Virginia furnished as many soldiers and took as many Civil War casualties for its 400,000 people as other combatant states, but it did so for both sides. Thirty-two thousand West Virginians, including 200 blacks, served in the Union Army, with a 12 percent casualty rate. Likewise, although there are few surviving records, an estimated 10,000 men joined the Confederate Army, presumably with a similar or higher casualty rate.[1]

Reeves' friend, Samuel Woods was one of the returning Confederate soldiers. Woods travelled to Philippi from his military service in the spring of 1865 with fifteen-year-old son Frank. As they neared Philippi seven former Union soldiers on horseback stopped them. The leader challenged the buggy's driver: "Mr. Woods, by what authority do you presume to come back into this country, after having taken up arms and given aid and comfort to those who had taken up arms against the Government of the United States, and as a soldier, and Captain yourself?"

Woods sat with a revolver in each pocket: "Gentlemen, I come back into this country by authority of law to resume lawful possession of my home at Philippi and of my lands and properties in Barbour County, as I have a lawful right to do. It is true I have been a soldier in the Confederate Army for four years, but I am now paroled, and have the parole given me by authority of General Grant in my pocket, and that parole guarantees me my security and my property as a citizen of the United States while I am obedient to its law."[2]

Sitting, as he later did on West Virginia's Court of Appeals, Woods could still be a commanding presence. The former Union soldiers parted and Woods proceeded. He found his house occupied by a neighbor, but soon regained the property and brought his family back. However, West Virginia's post-war loyalty laws prevented him from voting or practicing law. Woods started by cleaning up Philippi's Methodist church, which had been variously used as a barracks and hospital, and providing legal support to a Taylor County attorney who had not joined the Confederacy. He impressed upon former Confederate sympathizers that they should work within the law for their rights, but some of his fellow citizens were slow to forgive. One of them wrote anonymously to the Wheeling *Intelligencer* in 1868 that Woods was "despised and execrated by all good citizens, as a traitor, whose character is the counterpart of those of Judas Iscariot and Benedict Arnold."[3]

Most West Virginians did not feel the animus of Woods' unknown neighbor and in 1869 the state passed a bill exempting Woods from the lawyers' test oath, as it did for many others. Woods resumed his legal practice and quickly re-entered state politics. When the resurgent Democrats forced a new constitutional convention in 1872 Woods attended, along with another man Reeves knew, Johnson Camden.

Attorney Johnson Newlon Camden, Reeves' 1850 Sutton housemate, was a rising businessman who sat on the Civil War's sidelines while he ran The First National Bank of Parkersburg. Union forces considered him safe enough in 1863 to allow passage to visit his younger brother and suspected Confederate sympathizer, Dr. Thomas Camden, who was interned at Camp Chase, Ohio.

Johnson Camden made a political move when the war ended that foretold the state's Democratic resurgence. To Camden West Virginia's future lay in oil drilling and railroads; a future which could best be realized by electing a successful banker and oil man like himself governor. Despite considerable voter disenfranchisement, Democratic-Conservative Camden lost an unexpectedly close gubernatorial race in 1868 to Union Republican William Stevenson. In his inaugural address Stevenson spoke of the need for industrialization and a lessening of wartime tensions.

Camden and his fellow industrialists took the reins of West Virginia's political parties. As John Alexander Williams told the story in *West Virginia and the Captains of Industry*, Democrats Camden and Henry Davis and Republicans Stephen Elkins and Nathan Scott controlled state politics and represented West Virginia in both houses of Congress for the latter third of the nineteenth century, even as they built fortunes by shipping West Virginia's resources out of state. In Camden's case, he sold his oil properties to John D. Rockefeller in 1875 and became Standard Oil's man in West Virginia. By the time Reeves left West Virginia in 1887 the state's extraction-based businesses and outside ownership had reduced it to a colonial economy.[4]

West Virginia's Second Constitutional Convention began in January 1872. The delegates convened in the new capital of Charleston because the ascendant Democrats had no use for Republican-dominated Wheeling. Major issues were black enfranchisement, the organization of government bodies including the courts, and land reform. In August the delegates reluctantly accepted black suffrage and produced an updated version of the 1851 Virginia constitution. This document still serves as West Virginia's constitution.[5]

The 1872 convention exposed a split in West Virginia's Democratic politics between what historian Williams and others have termed Regulars, ambitious industrialists like Camden, and Redeemers, mostly former Confederates like Woods. The Redeemers fought to preserve previous relationships and agrarian values as they opposed the monopolistic efforts of the Regulars. Williams observed that Regulars did well in business and politics and Redeemers, often successful land speculators, did better in seeking judgeships. The only written record of the convention was Samuel Woods' letters to his wife, which, among other details, made it clear that Woods distrusted Camden and his friends. When Reeves expressed political views, he leaned toward Woods and away from the industrial monopolists.[6]

The Second Constitutional Convention marked the end of West Virginia's reconstruction. Former Confederates returned to the fold and the state avoided most of the anti-unionist unrest and racial politics that tormented the defeated South. The Democratic governing coalition that emerged and dominated West Virginia for the rest of the century was known as a Bourbon Democracy. The name, which also applied to other states, was originally a Northern pejorative referencing France's reactionary Bourbon monarchy and its restoration that followed the fall of Napoleon, coupled with a pun on the preferred alcoholic beverage of Southern Democrats. West Virginia's Democrats willingly accepted the appellation. Their ruling culture favored institutionalized racial discrimination and Jacksonian rugged individualism, which, in turn, fostered environmental and human exploitation. Thus, as Curry later wrote, "West Virginia, like the rest of the nation, entered the 'Gilded Age' woefully unprepared to meet the social, political, and economic problems caused by the transportation and industrial revolutions."[7]

While West Virginia's reconstruction unfolded, Reeves moved to increase his professional visibility. He successfully applied for permanent AMA membership in May 1866. The organization included less than 10 percent of the country's regular physicians, and permanent membership, which required a vote, brought contacts and professional prestige.[8]

He also gave public lectures. Reeves helped his sister Ann during the war by talking on hygiene to her Mothers Work Clubs. He made the trip from Fairmont to Clarksburg in August 1866 to read a paper on physical culture to the annual meeting of the West Virginia State Teachers Association. Lay audiences appreciated such talks, which provided vehicles for regular physicians to garner public recognition without engaging in unethical self-promotion. The newspaper announcement of Reeves' presentation simply described him as "Dr. Jas. E. Reeves," with no embellishment of his qualifications.[9]

Regular physicians were ethically mandated to refrain from newspaper promotion, the arena of eclectics, botanics, homeopaths, Galvanists, hydrotherapists, and nostrum pushers. Still, regulars used the papers as much as they could, getting their names in front of potential patients for their civic and social activities and attending noteworthy accidents; all of which was ethically permissible. Occasionally newspaper accounts drifted from reporting to subtle physician promotion, which created professional resentments. This happened in Wheeling on January 11, 1866, when Dr. J.C. Hupp treated a B&O brakeman with an injured leg and a young man whose arm had been caught in a circular saw. The reporter wrote that Hupp was called to treat the injuries and then added, "under his skillful management both are doing well." Likewise, On July 17, 1866, Wheeling's Dr. W.J. Bates provided "skillful treatment" to a person with heat stroke.[10]

These modest embellishments implied that one doctor might be more competent than his peers. To many regulars, any attempt to call attention to oneself smacked of elitism or worse, quackery. The AMA's 1847 *Code,* which each state and local medical society had to accept verbatim if they sought AMA participation, clearly proscribed physician advertising and self-promotion.[11]

Physician self-promotion, including the claiming of special skills, was one of the topics that divided regular physicians. The problem was in clear view at the AMA's 1866 Baltimore meeting in the matter of AMA member Julius Homberger. Homberger helped form the American Ophthalmological Society in 1864, America's first specialty organization. Shortly thereafter he published a newspaper advertisement saying he was "prepared to perform all surgical operations necessary to restore sight or correct deformity. In no case will he make a charge unless perfectly successful." This promotion implied that Homberger possessed greater eye treatment skills than other physicians, while potentially discounting his fees. It crossed the profession's ethical boundaries in two places. The AMA had to consider whether physicians could confine their practices to certain areas and, if they could, how they should promote themselves.[12]

AMA President and Harvard Professor David Storer devoted his 1866 Presidential Address to specialization. Storer acknowledged that some physicians were more adept at handling certain problems, while their colleagues resented any implication that they might be less capable. He observed that it was human nature for patients to assume that one who specialized in a certain disease or procedure must be better than one who did not. Yet, if the patient chose a separate doctor for each disease, this would hardly improve his overall care. Finally he noted that it was also human nature for younger, newly-educated physicians to be impatient in the face of what they regarded as their older competitors' outdated practices. He told his audience to ask itself what would best serve the interests of the profession and humanity.[13]

In the end Storer endorsed the activities of the American Ophthalmological Society. To Storer the issue was not specialization, but how specialists treated their fellow physicians: "the only question which can arise relates to the manner in which the specialist shall proceed; whether any or no attention shall be paid to the feelings and wishes of the profession; whether an individual shall pursue that course which is generally considered gentlemanly and honorable, or assume an ideal superiority over his brethren, and thus temporarily obtain a meretricious reputation and an undeserved reward." He accepted specialization and referred AMA members to their *Code of Medical Ethics* for guidance on how to manage it.[14]

The AMA's Committee on Medical Ethics and Medical Specialization was split on how to handle advertising so it issued majority and minority reports, both of which the delegates accepted. The majority report from Connecticut's Worthington Hooker masterfully summarized the fundamental issues: "The oftener one performs any operation, even though it be a simple one, the better he can do it." Hooker predicted that specialization, which barely existed at the time, would lead to fragmented care and increased costs: "The tendency is to confine the attention very much to certain organs, and to forget that it is a congeries of organs, a system, a person, that is to be examined and treated…. The specialist is also tempted, by the position in which he stands before the community, to charge, in some cases, unduly large fees for his services, and the tendency of human nature is to yield to such temptations." Hooker's solution was that specialists, with few exceptions such as dentists, should remain generalists with a part-time specialty practice.[15]

The reports agreed with Storer that specialization, for better and worse, was part of regular medicine. They disagreed on how to handle advertising and self-promotion. Hooker was against any form of advertising, including subtle self-promotion in newspaper stories: "Getting advertised by puffs in newspapers is worse than a formal advertisement, because it is covert." Hooker believed that the real problem was a lack of objective evidence for special competence and anticipated America's first specialty board of ophthalmology by fifty years: "There would be no objection to advertising, if tests of skill were applied by the community as easily in medicine as in other kinds of business."[16]

Henry Bowditch, the iconoclastic Boston physician who translated Louis' work on typhoid fever in 1836, disagreed. He found the debate filled with wasted energy. His advice was not to agonize over nuances of physician advertising. He argued that unless an advertisement was clearly "of the mountebank character," that the AMA should forget the matter. Resembling Bartlett's observation from twenty years earlier that the profession's future lay in improving medicine's science, he wrote that the AMA would be best served "in the hearing of able papers and in discussions on all subjects connected with medicine than in any movements for the mere discipline of erring members."[17]

Arguments over physician self-promotion persisted until the late-twentieth century and often dominated Reeves' professional work. The AMA reports from 1866 offered several suggestions, but only one resolution for the delegates' vote, that the consideration of the subject of medical specialties be indefinitely postponed, which the delegates accepted. In a show of determination and organizational caprice, the AMA angrily expelled Dr. Homberger in 1868 because of his ongoing advertising, over the objections of Bowditch who noted that Homberger had already resigned.[18]

Although Reeves was a new AMA permanent member, he did not participate in the 1866 Baltimore meeting; none of the seven West Virginia permanent members attended the sessions. AMA rules precluded these members from voting unless they participated as delegates from medical societies, medical colleges, hospitals, or other recognized medical institutions. There were no organized medical societies or medical schools, just one small hospital, and no other recognized medical institutions in West Virginia. Thus, Reeves and his fellow West Virginia regular physicians were prevented from participating in AMA decisions, even if they were members. Reeves wanted to change this and bring the benefits of a medical organization to his new state.[19]

Reeves and several Wheeling physicians attended a preliminary meeting at Wheeling's McClure House on February 27, 1867, for the purpose of organizing a state medical society. The group chose Wheeling's William Bates temporary president and Reeves temporary secretary. They asked Reeves and Wheeling's John Hupp to send a call to the state's physicians to attend an organizational meeting in Reeves' town of Fairmont.[20]

Reeves drafted the call, which went out the next day. Sixteen physicians signed it, nine of whom were from the Wheeling area and all but one from northwestern B&O towns such as Fairmont, Grafton, and Morgantown. The call proposed to elevate "the standard of Practical Medicine and Surgery in West Virginia, and to render quackery odious, as it deserves." The founders hoped to establish their new society in time to send delegates to the AMA's May meeting in Cincinnati.[21]

The closely-knit group was controlled by Wheeling Republicans, which did not sit well in other parts of the state. To further complicate the organization's birth, Hupp's father-in-law, Dr. Archibald Todd, was also included. Todd was well-loved in Wheeling, but for more than forty years he had marketed A. S. Todd's Antibilious or Liver Pills. The newspaper advertisements for Todd's pills were often accompanied by letters to the editor endorsing his product's virtues. Todd's professional life conflicted with the AMA's ethical proscriptions on advertising and dispensing patent medicines. If Todd were a member of the state medical society, it would be in open violation of the AMA's *Code* and subject the new society to AMA expulsion.[22]

Twenty-two regular physicians, counting Reeves, responded to the call and convened on April 10, 1867, in Fairmont to organize the Medical Society of West Virginia. These physicians lived in the northern tier of the state, either on or near B&O lines. They represented just 6 percent of the state's approximately 390 regular physicians and ten of its fifty-two counties. Notably, Archibald Todd from Wheeling was not present, although his son-in-law Hupp was.[23]

As Chairman of the Arrangements Committee, Reeves spoke first and offered his vision for the new organization. It would a temple to nature where "none but the worthy will be allowed to enter its lofty portals." His temple would work with the public so that citizens would one day demand the society's approval before allowing a new candidate to enter medical practice. He described the enemy as charlatanism, naming homeopaths, eclectics, and botanics, but saving his strongest damnation for strutting regulars who boasted "knowledge and skill superior to that possessed by *gentlemen* who toil unceasingly in the vineyards of science"[24] (author's italics).

Reeves recounted the scientific accomplishments he and his colleagues had seen in their medical lifetimes: the invention of the stethoscope, laryngoscope, and ophthalmoscope; the development of microscopy and cellular pathology; the passing into oblivion of indiscriminant bloodletting and mercuralization. He lauded the achievements of the AMA and of American medicine and he reminded his audience of the triumphs of Civil War surgeons.

Reeves assured his listeners that their state medical society would bring West Virginia's physicians into the medical mainstream. In his address he said, "Conventions and associations of medical men are now the order of the day; and when the Medical Society of West Virginia shall have been organized, every State, I believe, will have its Medical Society." He urged the other twenty-one attendees "to go manfully forward in the discharge of the duties which we owe to humanity, to ourselves, and to West Virginia."[25]

Finishing his address, Reeves read a flattering letter from the ticket agent of the B&O Railroad, on behalf of the company president: "who, in keeping with his reputation for the largest liberality, and respect for the legitimate profession of Medicine and Surgery, was pleased to encourage the objects of the Convention," by offering the delegates free return passage from Fairmont. As gracious as the letter may have sounded to its listeners, the railroad was hardly engaging in corporate charity. The men in the audience were leaders in their communities and, by 1867, the West Virginia public was increasingly critical of the B&O for its special tax privileges and its discriminatory freight rates.[26]

After relaying the good news from the railroad, Reeves faced an awkward request from one of his fellow Fairmont physicians, James Lazzell. Lazzell asked Reeves to add another doctor, John Berkebile, to the convention. Reeves responded that he had deliberately omitted Berkebile from the invitation list because he was not well-assured of Berkebile's regularity. Reeves wanted a committee to investigate Berkebile's qualifications for membership as well as the qualifications of a several others who had arrived at the meeting without an invitation. Lazzell said that he would vouch for Berkebile and brushed aside Reeves' suggestion for a committee. The other physicians agreed with Lazzell and chose to accept Berkebile. Then they went about forming a state medical society.

The group selected Reeves and six others, including Hupp and Preston County's William Dent, the father of the future plaintiff in *Dent v West Virginia,* to draft a constitution and bylaws. Once this work was completed, it accepted three more uninvited attendees and elected Wheeling's John Frissell and John Hupp as president and treasurer. The new delegates also chose Reeves as the organization's secretary. The group decided that the next meeting, the first one of the new state medical society, would be held at Wheeling in six months.

Subsequent events set the stage for Reeves' feud with fellow founder Hupp and his disillusionment with the organization. Hupp assumed the chair of the committee on arrangements for the Wheeling meeting and, at the last minute, announced its members would include six Wheeling physicians who not had attended the Fairmont meeting and had not yet been elected members of the new society. One of these committee members was his father-in-law, A.S. Todd. Hupp's effort to slip Todd into the workings of the new medical society was incompatible with Reeves' vision of an organization where "none but the worthy will be allowed to enter its lofty portals." Reeves had emphasized his vision by asking the group to consider Dr. Berkebile's admissibility, even if his fellow physicians did not see an issue.

Berkebile's situation was far less problematic than Todd's. Berkebile was a regular graduate of Jefferson Medical College who specialized in eye and ear surgery. His specialization was probably the issue that Reeves wanted to consider, as the AMA had considered specialization the year before. Berkebile proved to be a solid member of the Medical Society of West Virginia, recognized by his peers by being elected to the Society's Board of Censors from 1870 until he moved to Illinois in 1875.[27] If, to Reeves, the minimally controversial Berkebile merited discussion, then the chief prescriber, owner, and proponent of Todd's Pills certainly required scrutiny.

Another unexpected episode involving Hupp followed the society's choice of delegates for the upcoming AMA meeting in Cincinnati. The group decided that three of their number, Drs. Brock, Campbell, and Ramsey, would be the new society's official delegates. However, when it came time for the AMA meeting, somehow Hupp replaced Brock. Hupp benefited in more ways than one. On May 14, 1867, the *Wheeling Intelligencer* reported that local physicians John C. Hupp, John Frissell, and E.A. Hildreth: "three prominent members of the Association," attended the AMA meeting in Cincinnati. Two other West Virginia delegates were also mentioned in the article, but did not merit the adjective "prominent."[28]

With its formative meeting behind it, the Medical Society of West Virginia held its first regular meeting on October 2, 1867, in Wheeling. The delegates convened in the State Capitol and were greeted by Mayor Sweeny and West Virginia Governor Boreman. Following the dignitaries' welcome, Society President Frissell set forth the mission and character of the society for the thirty-two attendees. In his lengthy presidential address Frissell described the wonders of the new transatlantic telegraph and the railroad, tying medicine's present and future to these examples of modern science. He assured everyone that the Society would set high membership standards, emphasizing the role of honor which, to him, meant professional loyalty: "We do not propose to admit into this Society, those with whom you cannot consistently and honorably act or hold professional intercourse."[29]

Frissell made the difference between professional honor and Reeves' Methodist morality clear as he presented a tour of medical history, during which he touched on the bombastic Swiss physician, Paracelsus (1493–1541). Instead of using Paracelsus' well-known vanity as an example of improper professional behavior, he criticized the critics. Jumping to the present, Frissell told his audience that he had heard of Society members who had similarly been charged with unprofessional and undignified conduct. His answer, probably directed at Reeves: "I suggest that it is better to get along, if possible, without having such cases come before the Society for investigation." To Frissell, it was more important for the young society to encourage harmony than to become a temple to anything.[30]

The delegates next considered the constitution that Reeves had drafted six months earlier. William Bates and his Wheeling friends were not comfortable with Reeves' plans for the Society, but they did not challenge him directly. Instead, Bates requested a number of procedural adjustments, for example the meetings should be annual rather than semi-annual and the size of a quorum should be increased. Bates agreed to report on a revised constitution at the next meeting.

Only eleven of the thirty two attendees had been present in Fairmont and, once again, Lazzell presented Secretary Reeves with a difficult moment. Given the constitutional requirement for the election of members, Lazzell asked why there were so many new faces. Reeves responded that he had sent out many circulars, but only a few physicians had responded. In consultation with President Frissell he had notified the original invitees that they could become members if they were willing to pay the membership fee. The delegates quickly approved his actions. As before, all of the new members were from northwestern West Virginia.

Although Reeves helped form the Medical Society of West Virginia, he was an outsider who did not have much say in its membership or its character. The initial mailing list represented the interests of Wheeling Republicans. Hupp, in particular, had chaired the Union (Republican) Party's state meeting in November 1866.[31] The Society's founders did not invite West Virginia physicians with secessionist histories, no matter how well-qualified they were. Among the physicians not invited in 1867, who later joined, were Confederate sympathizer Thomas Camden, Reeves' 1850 Sutton housemate, and Confederate soldier William Bland, Reeves' good friend from Weston who helped him with his 1859 typhoid book.

If Reeves was bothered by the Medical Society's sectional politics, Frissell's open willingness to relax ethical requirements against boasting, and Hupp's backroom pressure to admit Todd, he did not let it show. He was extraordinarily active during the meeting's program, describing several of his own experiences and discussing those of others. He gave a speech as the meeting concluded lauding the character and contributions of Wheeling's physicians. From all appearances he was an energetic and committed founder of the Medical Society of West Virginia.

Reeves told his colleagues that theirs was the last state to form a state medical society, but he was usually more in front of a medical trend than behind it. Despite West Virginia's isolation and its tumultuous postwar environment, Reeves organized a state medical society more quickly than physicians in many other states. West Virginia's state medical society preceded eight of the other thirty-six existing states, including five that pre-dated the Civil War.[32]

Reeves' complimentary remarks to Wheeling's physicians at the conclusion of the 1867 Medical Society meeting may have been more than organizational pleasantries. He intended to move to Wheeling and it made sense to shore up his relationships. Right after the meeting he sold his Fairmont house, again at a loss. The property that he had purchased before the war for a thousand dollars only brought him nine hundred.[33]

⼁⽊ 10 ⽊⼁

His Lucid and Graceful Pen

Instead of issuing a printed announcement when he arrived in Wheeling in November 1867, Reeves made a personal call on the city's largest newspaper, the *Intelligencer.* The paper published a two-paragraph notice of his arrival the next day, favorably commenting on his reputation as a skillful practitioner and reporting that his 1859 typhoid fever book: "is spoken of as possessing more than a little merit."[1] This flattering mention met ethical guidelines because it was an editor's reporting of community opinion. It also showed that Reeves understood how newspapers worked.

Reeves and Mary joined Wheeling's Fourth Street Methodist Church and he was quietly busy. His name appeared in the paper on November 26, 1867, because he and Frissell treated a B&O fireman whose left foot was crushed between two cars. The report simply stated that the "injuries were attended to by Drs. Frissell and Reeves." As other young doctors did, he supplemented his income by doing examinations for a life insurance company.[2]

The small city was a sanitation disaster. Ten percent of Wheeling's 20,000 inhabitants worked in the iron mills and the city's air was filled with soot. The municipal water supply flowed through iron pipes that pumped unfiltered water from the upstream Ohio River. Wheeling's waste system emptied raw sewage into the downstream Ohio River. Most residences and shops relied on privies that owners were supposed to empty into the sewer system or the river. When owners did not care for their privies, they overflowed into the public streets. Wheeling Creek, running through town to the Ohio River, carried the drainage of mills, tanneries, and slaughterhouses.

Wheeling's doctors recognized the connection between decaying substances and illness, later called the filth theory of disease, even if they did not understand the bacteriologic connections. They assumed that the problem was foul gasses, a miasm. If it smelled bad, it was bad.[3] They protested the city's malodorous condition during the war and in 1865 the city council formed a board of health in response to their demands. When the cholera scare arrived in 1866 the council created a temporary physician position and elected Richard Blum Wheeling's first temporary health officer. Blum created a scavenger force to clean Wheeling's public areas and began fining those who disobeyed city health ordinances. Health Officer Blum removed almost two hundred tons of accumulated refuse in a matter of months.[4]

Wheeling did not experience a cholera outbreak in 1866, as did nearby Cincinnati, but not everyone appreciated Blum's efforts. Several members of the city council objected to his vigorous enforcement actions and questioned whether the city really needed him. Proposing to save money, the council suspended Blum's position in November 1866. The *Intelligencer's* editor disagreed with the council's action. He commended his city's good fortune in escaping cholera and supported the health officer. He wrote, "It is plain to even a careless observer that there are still places that need the supervision of the Health Officer or somebody else."[5]

The council's issues with Blum ran deeper than city budgets. As elsewhere, Wheeling's regular physicians attacked the public's gullibility for using unscientific sectarian practitioners and denigrated less well-educated and slow-moving city politicians. Mayor Sweeney sensed the council's hostility and sent it a lengthy letter in February 1867 commending Blum's work and urging council members to reinstate the position of city health officer.[6]

The council grudgingly acceded to the mayor's request, as well as public concerns about the ongoing cholera threat, but not without thumbing its nose at Wheeling's regular physicians. The members decided that they needed to re-open the selection process. In a confused meeting on March 6, 1867, Wheeling's city council elected Ebenezer McCoy health officer. McCoy was a Wheeling botanic doctor who had voted for secession in 1861 and been jailed in 1863. He could not have been more offensive to Wheeling's regulars, who vigorously attacked the city's new health officer and the council.[7]

The *Intelligencer* joined in, often asking whether McCoy was doing his job and, when he did, deriding his performance. In November 1867 the council again suspended the health officer's position. It did not re-open the position until July 1868, well past the onset of summer epidemics.[8]

Reeves' transition to public health was pushed along by events at the April 1868 Grafton medical society meeting. President Frissell began by urging the group to revisit Reeves' original constitution. He followed with a lengthy discourse praising the benefits of anatomical knowledge, deriding homeopathy and cancer treatment quacks, and once again encouraging organizational harmony.[9]

The group considered several constitutional revisions and accepted all of them. It discussed the need for a statewide fee table and selected two essayists for the following annual meeting, one of whom was Reeves. But when it came time to choose officers for next year, Reeves did not stand for re-election as secretary. Instead, he left before the second day, asking the newly elected secretary to assume his meeting duties.

Reeves was disenchanted with the group he had helped found. The most extensive record of his struggle with the Medical Society of West Virginia was an anonymous 1879 pamphlet, "A Plain Statement of Facts: Dr. John C. Hupp Before the 'Medical Society of Wheeling and County of Ohio' at the Last Moment He Confesses, before the Board of Censors a Heinous Offence." Only Reeves could have known all of the information it contains. Today there are few privately-held copies of this document. The one contemporary mention of it was by Frissell in his personal notes from 1879.[10]

According to this pamphlet the troubles began shortly before the Grafton meeting. In April 1868 Reeves decided not to continue as secretary and presented Treasurer Hupp with a final bill of $6.63 for his expenses. Reminding Reeves of his station, Hupp said that he needed President Frissell's approval before he could reimburse him. Reeves told Hupp that he had collected five dollars from a new member and he wanted Hupp to credit him $1.63 toward his annual dues. Reeves saw Hupp make a notation in the treasurer's book and he left the meeting believing the matter was settled. However, after the Grafton meeting began, the newly elected secretary sent Reeves a note saying that Reeves still owed the Society $5. Reeves sent him back to Hupp for an explanation. The matter lay dormant until the following year.

The contrast between the goals Reeves wanted for the Medical Society and those that most others preferred was apparent in the original and revised 1868 constitutions. Reeves planned to set a high bar for membership that would facilitate a claim to public legitimacy. In his version of the constitution, new members needed to: 1) be graduates of a respectable school of medicine with grounding in medical ethics and "without stain of charlatanism," or 2) have completed one full course of medical school lectures and been in "respectable practice" for five years, or 3) have ten years of "respectable practice" and pass an examination administered by the Society.[11]

The Society's leaders spoke of high standards, but moved the organization away from Reeves' publicly-accountable vision and closer to a fraternal organization. They weakened Reeves' requirements and increased their own flexibility. The pathway of graduation from a respectable medical school remained in the new constitution; however the other options were changed to examination by the Society's Board of Censors and a minimum of five years' experience, with the proviso that the experience requirement could be waived for a candidate possessing special merit.[12]

A frustrated Reeves maintained relationships with the other Wheeling physicians after April 1868. When the city council selected a health officer in July 1868 he offered his name for consideration, with endorsements by four prominent local physicians, including Frissell and Hupp. The council did not choose Reeves to be temporary city health officer in 1868, instead selecting an affable young regular physician, Henry Weisel, over Reeves and the two previous office holders.[13]

Led by Hupp, Wheeling's physicians rejuvenated two dormant local medical societies in August 1868, creating the Medical Society of Wheeling and Ohio County, with Todd as the group's first president and Hupp its treasurer. Reeves did not join the organization until 1880, after Hupp and Todd were gone. However, in 1868 he gave the group a lengthy address on his favorite topic, typhoid (enteric) fever. He made frequent reference to Wheeling's sanitation problems: "What is Wheeling Creek for the distance of a mile above its junction with the Ohio, but an open cess-pool?"[14]

But Reeves was disenchanted with medical organizing. He wanted to take his ambitions for preventive medicine directly to the public. When the city council decided in 1869 that the health officer's position should be permanent, it was Reeves' doing. As he later described his role: "Witnessing the situation, a physician of the city busied himself about the matter and prepared an ordinance, and exerted his influence to have that ordinance passed by the Council, establishing a permanent health office, with a salary of $800 a year for the health officer." His friend and biographer, Louis Wilson, also wrote that Reeves drafted and secured passage of the city health ordinance. Neither account mentioned the job's requirements, but the ordinance stipulated that only physicians could occupy the new position.[15]

The city council selected a new health officer in March 1869 and, having helped write the ordinance, Reeves was ready. There were five nominees, including former Wheeling mayor George Baird, former health officers Weisel and McCoy, and a new arrival in town, D.J. McGinnis. It was hardly a contest. The city council gave Reeves sixteen of twenty-eight votes on the first ballot and appointed him Wheeling's first permanent health officer on March 16. The ordinance allowed the health officer to "order or contract for the immediate cleansing or disinfecting" of private property within city limits. The city also required Reeves to attend to all city prisoners and vaccinate all persons in the city who were unable to pay for vaccination.[16]

Within two weeks of his appointment Reeves examined almost 2,000 school children, determining that 163 had not been vaccinated for smallpox and that 61 of those would require vaccination by him. He also notified Wheeling residents that he would begin inspecting property on April 2 and that owners would be fined twenty dollars if their premises were not free of standing waste.[17]

The council tasked Reeves with disinfecting property even before the principles of bacterial infection were known. The AMA's Committee on Disinfectants wrote in 1866, "A large number of diseases are produced by infection." This may seem odd to twenty-first century eyes, but the scaffolding of the germ theory existed well before the bacteriological revolution filled in the details.

To the AMA Committee, an infection was an organic poison that existed in nature, was incapable of reproduction in the human body, and could not be directly transmitted. In contrast a contagion was an organic poison that was capable of reproduction in the body and therefore could be conveyed from human to human. Yellow fever was an infection and smallpox was a contagion. The first was managed by disinfection, the second by quarantine. It was no coincidence that the Committee's Chairman, Ezra Hunt, later a public health leader in New Jersey, had been a Union Army surgeon assigned to a Baltimore Army hospital in 1863. The Civil War introduced disinfection to thousands of physicians and millions of Americans.[18]

Mid nineteenth-century techniques for dealing with infection included waste removal, cleansing with water, white-washing, heat, burial, and antisepsis (decay prevention) with chemical agents, such as carbolic acid, sodium chlorite, and bromine. Physicians and the public could see that these techniques provided health benefits, even if they had no idea that microscopic organisms living within the waste were the true source of infections and contagions.

Reeves did not attend the June 1869 meeting of the Medical Society of West Virginia in Clarksburg, but President Brock commended the group on bringing Society membership close to one hundred. Then, in what to Reeves would have been an ironic, if not hypocritical moment of self-congratulation, Brock told the gathering that the membership could have been "still more greatly increased but for the fact of our Society's having, very properly, excluded all applicants for admission except such whose attainments and character could conform to the standards it had erected."[19]

The points of irony were that Todd, the proprietor of Todd's Antibilious Pills, who should have been ineligible for membership, was active at the meeting and also attended as president of the newly formed Medical Society of Wheeling and Ohio County. In contrast, former secessionists, some of whom were Reeves' friends and otherwise would have met the membership standards, were never invited. Reeves' concerns were not yet openly visible, even though he did not attend and did not meet his obligation as an essayist. The president, still assuming Reeves' interest and loyalty, appointed him to the committee on necrology for the following year.

The matter of Reeves' debt to the Medical Society surfaced again following the 1869 meeting. The newly elected secretary sent Reeves a dunning notice for the five dollars he had collected from a member and never submitted. Reeves responded with a pointed letter to the secretary, replying as he had a year earlier, that he had squared the matter with Hupp and seen Hupp's entry in the Society's books. The secretary shared Reeves' reply with Hupp and, in Reeves' words, "from that date [1869] Dr. Reeves and Dr. Hupp ... had no friendly relations with each other."[20]

When the feud began, Hupp clearly held the upper hand in Wheeling. He had graduated from Philadelphia's Jefferson Medical College in 1847 and moved from Pennsylvania to Wheeling to open his practice the same year. He married Carolene Todd in 1853, the daughter of Wheeling's best-known physician, a man who had already made a name and soon would make a modest fortune with his proprietary liver pills.[21]

Hupp and his family were members of Wheeling's Presbyterian Church, the Christian denomination favored by wealthy Southerners, and Hupp frequently appeared in the local newspapers for his social, political, and medical activities. Hupp also promoted his pioneer roots. He made the deaths of his grandfather and granduncle at the hands of Indians a constant part of his biography and, in 1864, front page reading for Wheeling's citizens.[22]

Hupp was a well esteemed community fixture by 1869. Yet, despite his secure position, Reeves seemed to be more than Hupp could take. For one, the newcomer had better medical credentials. Hupp could say that he had been a permanent AMA member since 1858, was state vaccine agent beginning 1863, and had authored several small medical papers.[23] However, Reeves was also an AMA permanent member who had graduated from a more prestigious medical college, published national medical papers and a respected book, and was a member of the Pathological Society of Philadelphia. Worse yet, Reeves had objectionable Confederate sympathies, including friendship with Redeemer Samuel Woods

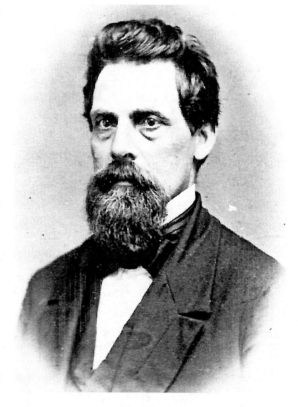

John Cox Hupp (1819–1905), date unknown. Hupp was a socially prominent Wheeling regular physician and fellow founder of the Medical Society of West Virginia whose personal feud with Reeves from 1869 to 1879 almost destroyed the medical society (courtesy Caroline Hoag).

Professional experiences could have brought the two men together, but their personality and political differences fostered competitive friction. Hupp was a staunch Republican in reconstruction West Virginia and Reeves was an unapologetic Democrat. Hupp was a well-to-do, socially-connected Presbyterian while outsider Reeves was the son of a stern Methodist preacher. At the most basic level Reeves' inclination to responded when his moral values were offended challenged Hupp's go-along, get-along existence.

Hupp was not the only one who found Reeves difficult. The Society's first president, John Frissell, clearly resented Reeves' energetic self-righteousness. Many years later, Samuel Jepson, who followed Reeves as City Health Officer and knew him well, scorned what he felt was Reeves' misdirected criticism of Todd for a mere "technical breach of the code of ethics."[24]

Nevertheless, the Medical Society had more pressing matters than founding members' personal differences and its former secretary's small debt. The organization faced a political crisis in 1869 that stemmed from its Republican roots. Regular physicians who had been excluded by the Medical Society's Wheeling organizers met in Point Pleasant, near Charleston, on November 24, 1869, to organize a competing state medical society. Wheeling's newspapers reported the threat.[25]

Learning of the uprising, the Medical Society dispatched three non–Wheeling physicians to make amends and, although he had no official capacity, Reeves also forwarded a letter to the group.[26] The assembled physicians accepted the Medical Society's assurances and next year the West Virginia Medical Society sent membership invitations to an additional 108 West Virginia regulars. The excluded physicians' furor may have had more to do with wounded pride than interest in a medical society. After the fuss subsided, only thirteen new regulars joined.[27]

The Medical Society of West Virginia claimed sixty-two regular physician members in its first year, all from northern and western West Virginia. Twenty-five of these members attended the Society's 1868 meeting in Grafton, where Reeves assumed his duties as secretary. At most, the new society represented 15 percent of the state's physicians, with perhaps 7 percent making its policy. This unrepresentative situation was the national norm, and it did not change over the following years. Only 20 percent of the West Virginia's physicians belonged to the state medical society in 1901, and just 5 percent attended its annual meeting. Garceau observed in 1961 that even as participation increased, medical societies and associations remained the work of a small group of sometimes noble, sometimes venal actors who had various reasons for their participation.[28]

Reeves had the political instincts and affinity for the city health officer position. Wheeling's politicians and newspapers supported his efforts to force property owners to clean their premises. His first year as health officer was notable for its lack of confrontation. There were no epidemics and, at the end of 1869, the council was pleased enough with his work to authorize him to spend $150 in preparing a sanitary history of Wheeling for public distribution.

He was a visibly busy Wheeling doctor in 1870. Reeves managed workplace and public accidents. He was physician to the county jail and the City Council again elected him to the $800 per year post of City Health Officer. He ignored medical society work and did not join local fraternal organizations, civic groups, or business boards in his off hours. Instead, he used his free time to write about medicine and public health.[29]

Reeves' contemporary biographer, Louis Wilson, praised his writing skills: "His pen was lucid and graceful and he possessed a felicity of expression and fluency of style which but few could hope to emulate." After the city council authorized him to prepare a report on Wheeling's sanitary history, Reeves used his pen to share his knowledge with Wheeling's citizens. He dedicated his 1870 report on *The Physical and Medical Topography of Wheeling* to the mayor and city council.[30]

The fifty-page pamphlet described the geology, commerce, demographics, and public hygiene of Wheeling. It was part civic boosterism and part introduction to sanitary science. The council distributed 1,500 copies and Reeves shared it with medical and scientific journals. Five well-respected publications praised him and Wheeling for the effort. The editor of *The New York Medical Journal* wrote, "Dr. Reeves for his own city and vicinity has done this work most admirably, and the City Council have displayed a wise liberality in making public the results of his labors."[31]

As other nineteenth-century leaders often did, Reeves used Biblical and mythological references to bring home his messages. He wrote, " a community ignorant of properly collated facts concerning its vital history, is, indeed but feebly defended against 'the pestilence that walketh in darkness, and the destruction that wasteth at noon-day.'" To the church-goers in his audience the quotation from Psalm 91 ("the pestilence...") illustrated the secret perils from which God protected the faithful, but Reeves borrowed the Old Testament's phrasing to glorify vital statistics. He embellished religious imagery with classical humanism, reminding readers that in ancient Greece health was personified by the goddess Hygeia, who presided over feats of exercise and whose temples were marked by flowers, not the blood of sacrifices.[32]

This 1870 pamphlet was the first time Reeves publicly used the term "the true church in medicine," an image he may have borrowed from New York's Stephen Smith who had, in turn, appropriated it from an eighteenth-century German physician.[33] Reeves incorporated the metaphor as it had been originally intended, not as a religious reference but a vision of human community. He paid homage to the recognized lights of the healing arts, scientist physicians such as Sydenham, Blane, Jenner, Laennec, and their companion worshippers and ministers "in the true church in medicine." He lauded these careful observers for building the foundation from which sanitary science and sanitary tools had "markedly increased the average duration of human life, notwithstanding the many unfavorable hygienic conditions and influences that result from a dense and constantly increasing population."[34]

Sanitarians believed that there had been general increases in human longevity due to hygienic improvements, but this was more wishful thinking in 1870 than actuarial fact. Smith and the other New York reformers repeatedly presented improved mortality data from European cities as they lobbied for the Metropolitan Health Act in 1865 and 1866. German physician Rudolph Virchow appreciated the logic as he argued for improvements in Berlin's sewer system, but he was a better scientist than most. In looking at the oft-cited British data, he cautiously warned in 1868: "It is difficult to say how much the improvement in the state of health is attributable to one or another factor."[35]

English and American life expectancies hardly changed between 1800 and 1870 and, depending on the period, were sometimes shorter than what had gone before. It was unlikely that human mortality was under mankind's control until about 1880.[36]

Reeves was eager to share his science with the Wheeling public and his public experiences with the medical profession. He sent a descriptive "Letter from Wheeling" to the *Medical Times* of Philadelphia in October. This was a new journal emphasizing the rapid communication of medical information. He talked up his home town and the work of the city health officer. He exemplified the contemporary understanding that human disease was caused by organic poisons spread from decaying matter, not from man-made inorganic environmental toxins, by boasting that Wheeling's sulfurous smoke and soot showed its industrial prosperity, and "were not in anywise detrimental to health."[37]

Reeves promoted his and Wheeling's visibility by sending five more articles to the *Medical Times* within the year. One was a report of an unusual seizure patient and four were related to his observations on the management of dysentery, diphtheria, scarlet fever, and enteric (typhoid) fever. The journal was the work of Pennsylvania's medical elite, including Samuel Gross, Weir Mitchell, Alfred Stillé, and William Pepper. Their association was helpful for Reeves' national aspirations and he took full advantage of the new journal's need for material. None of the illustrious authors supplied more papers to the first volume of the *Medical Times* than Reeves, nor did any other West Virginian contribute a single article.[38]

Reeves' medical papers showed that he remained in step with changes in therapy. The theories and treatments of heroic medicine had run their course by 1870 and were considered relics of a less advanced time. Still, up-to-date physicians did not totally abandon depletive therapies; instead they reduced their use of them. For major illnesses they often switched to less dangerous stimulative agents, such as alcohol. Reeves used relatively gentle, supportive treatments for self-limited diseases, including bismuth for dysentery, stimulants for diphtheria, and gargles for scarlet fever, but his overall plan was: "Feed the patient and, thus 'keep him alive until he recovers.'"[39] For more serious illnesses, such as pneumonia, he favored stimulants and denigrated the outdated physicians who still tortured their patients with bleeding, blisters, and calomel.

While Reeves was building a national reputation, sharing his knowledge with Wheeling's citizenry, and flattering the city council, his quarrel with Hupp and the state medical society simmered. The Medical Society of West Virginia met in the Ohio River town of Parkersburg in 1870, a short rail trip from Wheeling. Reeves had been appointed to the committee on necrology a year earlier, but he did not attend the meeting. Continuing to protest his treatment, he did not pay his dues.[40]

Medical politics marred the Society's 1870 gatherings and presentations. The assembled delegates hasty accepted thirteen invited physicians whom they had previously excluded, adding Reeves' secessionist friends Thomas Camden and William Bland to the membership rolls. The enlarged group then chose former Confederate physician Bland to be Society president for the coming year. Camden's brother, rising industrialist and Democratic power-broker, Johnson Newlon Camden, hosted the physicians in his Parkersburg home. Bland's presidency marked a gradual move toward the Democratic resurgence of West Virginia's reconstruction, which favored men like Bland, Camden, and Reeves, and away from the Medical Society's Wheeling Republicans who had founded and dominated the organization.[41]

In the Society's haste to reconcile with disaffected secessionists, it invited and accepted an eclectic physician, J.C. Sidebottom, to membership. As botanically-oriented successors to Thomsonians, eclectic physicians had their own medical colleges, some of which taught anatomy and other regular medical courses, but regulars considered them quacks.

One of the members caught this problem late in the evening of the second day. The delegates immediately removed Sidebottom from the Society and censured the Cabell County Medical Society, which he represented, for sending him. They admonished the county society to remove all irregulars from its ranks and to rigorously enforce the letter and spirit of the AMA's *Code of Medical Ethics*. Similarly, a month earlier the AMA threatened to expel the Massachusetts Medical Society for tolerating irregulars in violation of its *Code*.[42] The Sidebottom episode emphasized the national association's efforts to influence local membership decisions and made Todd's continued involvement increasingly problematic, even if Hupp and his fellow Wheeling Republicans wanted to ignore the inconsistency.

Reeves tried to mend relationships even though he did not participate in the meeting. He sent a private letter to the Society detailing his complaint and asking that his account be settled. Rather than reconcile a minor financial matter on the spot, the delegates acknowledged the letter and appointed a committee to investigate and report its findings the following year.

Reeves was outraged when his quiet diplomacy soon surfaced in the Wheeling press. Two days after the Parkersburg meeting, the *Intelligencer* printed a lengthy report of the event, supplied to the paper by an anonymous source, ironically named "Adolescentulus."[43] Reeves was sure this was Hupp. The report gave an accurate summary of the events, but devoted a paragraph to the matter of Reeves' confidential letter, referring to Reeves by name and "the moneys received by *this* ex–Secretary"[44] (italics in original).

Reeves' ire was justified by the public airing of his letter and the italicized "*this*." Looking from the outside, there was circumstantial evidence incriminating Hupp. One indication was that Hupp's name appeared more than any other in the *Intelligencer's* report. Another was that Hupp was a frequent and sometimes anonymous contributor of medical news to the *Intelligencer*. The paper published another summary of the same meeting later that year, based on a printed copy of the Medical Society's *Transactions*, but not mentioning Reeves. The *Transactions* had arrived unannounced at the paper's door and the editor surmised, based on his past experience, that it was furnished "through the courtesy ... of Dr. John C. Hupp."[45] Despite his anger, Reeves let the matter lie while he pursued his interest in sanitary science.

⑈ 11 ⑈

A Particularly
Challenging Year

Reeves soon added his ideas to the growing American public health movement. He expanded his 1870 pamphlet on Wheeling's medical topography into his second book in January 1871. He printed *The Health and Wealth of the City of Wheeling* at his own expense in Baltimore. Like his 1859 treatise on typhoid fever, this 158-page book was also a practical guide, but intended for Wheeling's better-educated citizens. He dedicated the work to Wheeling's mayor and city council.[1]

Reeves also sought to preserve relations with the Wheeling medical community. In the book he acknowledged assistance from his "excellent friend," Robert Cummins, President of the Wheeling and Ohio County Medical Society. He complimented the city medical society and expressed his debt to Archibald Todd for sharing information on Wheeling obstetrical practices.[2]

The book began with a short homily on the importance of sanitary science. Reeves again used the phrase, "the pestilence that walketh in darkness," to reinforce the need for vital statistics. He made the same arguments about the life-saving accomplishments of public hygiene and he repeated his reference to the true church in medicine. He expanded his use of the term preventive medicine, and encouraged laws to protect public health and exterminate pestilential diseases. He predicted the day when "*sanitary sciences* may prove omnipotent against epidemics" (italics in original). He told the Wheeling public that enlightened physicians already recognized the subordination of pharmaceutic agents and formula to hygienic influences. Reeves saw medicine and public health as the same thing, unified by sanitary science.[3]

Proselytizing to the public about the benefits of prevention and hygiene was hardly new territory for a Methodist preacher's son, but it was an unusual activity for a regular physician. The few regulars who had any interest in public health saw their duty, as Henry Bowditch described it in 1876, as organization—improving their science and using the messages of science to change the regulatory landscape.[4] It was not until the next century that the public health establishment accepted public education and persuasion as part of its mission.

Reeves' 1871 book was his first effort to change the prevailing public health dialogue. Rather than arguing that a paternalistic government had an obligation to promote public welfare or that better-off citizens had a moral duty to improve the lives of the poor, Reeves enlisted the self-interests of Wheeling's citizens by framing public sanitation in economic terms.

It was not just that epidemics wrongly took the lives of Wheeling's inhabitants or that poor sanitation led to moral degradation, what hurt most was that public health failures stole the sources of Wheeling's prosperity, the "laborers and mechanics to whom a healthful and vigorous frame is the greatest wealth." He used numbers to make his point, estimating the societal investment in an unskilled laborer as $1,500, an investment lost by the community if the laborer emigrated or died.[5]

This logic had occasionally been used elsewhere, but it fell on deaf ears in 1871, even in more sophisticated settings than Wheeling. Virchow argued for sanitary improvements in Berlin in 1868 by stating "State and town acquire their value only through human beings and their work." Virchow wrote, "Unfortunately, this mode of consideration is so new to most people that during the last session of the house of representatives I was ridiculed by a very well-known political economist."[6] Reeves helped bring these arguments into American public health by repeating and refining them.

Reeves ended his book's economic discourse with the aphorism that Elisha Harris had used in his 1865 Introduction to the New York City Council of Hygiene and Public Health Report: "public health is public wealth," but he did not attribute it to Ben Franklin as Harris had done. Professional sanitarians found the phrase "public health is public wealth" increasingly useful and they almost always tied it to Franklin, even in Europe. Dublin physician Edward Mapother said in his 1867 lectures to the Irish Royal College of Surgeons, "the truth of Benjamin Franklin's opinion that 'public health is public wealth' is generally felt."[7] The American journal *The Sanitarian* added it to its masthead in 1876.[8] Public health advocates have used the phrase and credited it to Franklin to the present day.[9]

Reeves' failure to attribute the maxim to Franklin shows how meticulous he was. There is no record of "public health is public wealth" in Franklin's writings and, according to a contemporary Franklin scholar, it is too modern to be Franklin's.[10] Franklin may have favored the sentiment, but he likely never uttered the words. The most reasonable hypothesis is that it began with a nineteenth-century public health activist who enhanced its legitimacy by adding a famous name. Reeves liked the aphorism, but he seemed to know that it wasn't Franklin's.

Reeves also enlisted his readers' self-interests by linking public and personal health. He provided a brief overview of the history, topography, and climate of Wheeling and presented a description of Wheeling's civic infrastructure. This information might interest any educated citizen. Then he made it relevant by adding details about Wheeling's private dwellings and their ventilation, the city water supply, the manufacture and use of coal gas and kerosene for lighting, slaughterhouses, soap factories, and nail manufactories.

He connected Wheeling's infrastructure and its commercial activities to individual well-being. In the case of kerosene, for example, he reported his study of kerosene samples throughout the city, finding an adulteration with benzene leading to dangerously low flash points. This was a well-known danger that the New York City Health Department had also uncovered two years earlier. Reeves described the kerosene threat to Wheeling's citizens in vivid prose: "A keg of gunpowder would be safer in a family as a chimney corner stool and convenience than such oil, because it is so volatile that *it seeks* the flame to accomplish its mission of horrid death!" (italics in original). He recommended a law regulating kerosene purity, as some states already had. He depicted the vile state of the city's slaughterhouses and concluded, "Every city should have a meat inspector."[11]

The book offered practical advice that people could use in their homes. Reeves devoted twenty-seven pages to describing how and why to build an earth closet, a recently invented indoor toilet that, instead of sending its water-laden waste into an overflowing sewer system or nearby street, covered its discharge with a layer of dry dirt in a subterranean vault or removable box. Recognizing that his likely reader could well be the lady of the house, he also spoke about the city's food supply, infant feeding and the city milk supply. But he did not spare Victorian sensibilities or resist his urges to moralize. As he wrote favorably about the city's medical facilities, he also told readers of the pestilence of prostitution and the criminality of abortion.[12]

Reeves sent a copy of *Health and Wealth* to the *Intelligencer* and other publishers. The Wheeling paper loved the work. Its editor devoted three columns, outlining Reeves' advice and urging readers to buy the book. The editor of the New York *World* was also impressed, even if the book was meant for Wheeling's residents. He lauded Reeves' intelligent and practical guidance and concluded, "Dr. Reeves must be an exceptionally active and clear-headed public officer." The *Intelligencer* happily shared this big-city accolade with Wheeling's citizens.[13]

Several medical publications applauded him. The *Boston Medical and Surgical Journal* appreciated the novelty of Reeves' direct approach: "We wish every city in the land had a health officer as earnest as Dr. Reeves to inspire his fellow citizens with a desire to be healthy, wealthy and wise, and to show them how to do it." Philadelphia's *Medical Times,* where Reeves had submitted a half dozen articles, could not have been more positive: "Let the health officers of cities peopled with their hundreds of thousands imitate his good example!" The *Intelligencer* passed along Philadelphia's praise of the Wheeling City Health Officer to its readers as well.[14]

Reeves cited the country's most common cause of death to highlight Wheeling's healthy environment. The disease was pulmonary phthisis, which he also called consumption, and which many others increasingly referred to as tuberculosis. Wheeling's death rate from the disease was just one in 550 while New York's was one in 253 and London's was one in 369. He wrote in *Health and Wealth*: "Notwithstanding the smoky, sulphurous atmosphere which constantly envelopes the city, the mortality from consumption is even less than occurs in the most salubrious country districts of the State."[15]

On a personal level Reeves' civic optimism was tragically misplaced. Mary Reeves died abruptly from tuberculosis on January 2, 1872. Reeves printed four brief letters for his children during her last weeks. Dated Christmas Day, 1871, the notes described a small endearment from Mary to each child. They were titled "Mamma's Last Gift" and ended with a prayer that Mary would one day see the children again in God's Home.[16] Reeves was again a widower raising four children, ages thirteen to twenty.

Reeves occupied himself with medical work and his health officer duties after Mary's death. In April, he managed problems that had arrived with a circus troupe. A train worker suffered a hand injury and, of more concern to Wheeling's health officer, one of the passengers on the train had smallpox. The sick man was taken to the city hospital and the circus owner was fined fifty dollars for bringing a smallpox case into Wheeling.[17]

He attended the annual meeting of the Medical Society of West Virginia in June 1872. He could hardly avoid the Wheeling event, but he did not participate in the presentations. He gave no talks and he did not contribute to the medical discussions. He was there to resolve his long-brewing financial disagreement and feud with fellow founder Hupp.

William Bates, who had watered down Reeves' original constitution for the sake of organizational harmony, was chairman of the Society's Arrangements Committee. Bates made a point of acknowledging the Society's internal bickering in his welcoming address. He encouraged the delegates to avoid contention and wrangling.

The Medical Society wanted no part of a public spat between members. The committee that had been tasked a year earlier to investigate Reeves' dispute presented its report at the close of the first day and recommended that the question was a personal matter between two physicians, one that should not concern the Society. Wheeling's Robert Cummins quickly moved to accept the report as disposing of the issue.[18]

But Hupp was furious that Reeves had answered the committee's inquiry with another letter, one more pointed than the letter that had fractured their relationship in 1869. He relished the spotlight and demanded that Reeves' angry correspondence be read aloud. Reeves moved for the society to do so, but Cummins interrupted, saying that the language was not proper for the Society. So Hupp attacked the committee's report. He gave a detailed list of his objections and charged that the issue was not a simple personal problem between the two men, but an unresolved financial matter between Reeves and the Society. He demanded that Reeves' harsh words be brought to the Society's Board of Censors. The exhausted delegates agreed to send the matter to their censors for a final resolution.[19]

Hupp had one more reason to attack Reeves that he did not mention. Earlier in 1872 Reeves had provided evidence of his father-in-law's nostrum business to the AMA and Todd resigned his membership in the Medical Society of West Virginia. Even though Reeves showed public respect to Todd and stated that he admired Todd as a Christian, he insisted that his pill adventure was a violation of the *Code of Medical Ethics*. Hupp had a family score to settle with the self-righteous Reeves.

The Society's Board of Censors presented its report at the end of the final day. The Board addressed the financial question by agreeing that the Society owed Reeves for his 1868 expenses and, he, in turn, owed the Society the fee he had collected in 1868 and his unpaid dues. Reeves paid the difference, which settled his account.

The Board next considered Reeves' heated letter, finding it so offensive that, unless Reeves apologized, he should be expelled from the Society. Reeves offered a verbal apology, which the members rejected. He then provided a written apology, saying that he had claimed the original entry on Hupp's books must have been erased, but he was clearly mistaken and he regretted any unkind allusions. The members accepted his apology and reinstated Reeves' membership.

This was not enough for Hupp. After the meeting's conclusion, the Society, as usual, memorialized the proceedings in its *Transactions*. Society treasurer Hupp controlled the printing of this document. Although the Society never published Reeves' allegations, all of Hupp's assertions, many in italics, found their way into the official record, as did Reeves' admission of error and apology. Likewise, the discussion of Reeves' debt to the Society, along with his full apology, appeared on page three of the *Intelligencer* one day after the event occurred. The war between the two doctors continued for another seven years and Reeves did not fully return to the Medical Society of West Virginia until it ended.[20]

Reeves married for the third time in October 1872 to Frances Starrett of Cumberland Maryland. Frances was a year younger than Reeves and had never wed. She may have brought a considerable dowry. Six months after the ceremony the couple purchased an $11,500 lot on Chapline Street with two houses in her name. For the next seven years Reeves and his family lived at 2227 Chapline Street, which was also his office. They rented out the neighboring house at 2225 Chapline.[21]

To complete a particularly challenging year, Reeves got into a public fistfight with another prominent doctor in December 1872. His antagonist was George Baird, former mayor, a city council member, and one of the Wheeling physicians he had run against for health officer in 1869. Baird was a regular medical graduate of the University of Pennsylvania who had practiced in Wheeling for twenty years. An early member of the Medical Society of West Virginia, Baird was not a typical Wheeling Republican. He had been the Democratic mayor of Wheeling in 1863. Baird was strongly opposed to separation from Virginia and the entry of free blacks into the area. After the war, he remained active on the city council and showed an interest in public health.[22]

Reeves and Baird traded blows for unknown reasons in the Wheeling Recorder's office on December 19, 1872. The battle was a draw and both men were charged with assault. Baird was declared guilty and received the maximum fine while the court dismissed the charges against Reeves.[23] Reeves got into several public scrapes during his Wheeling years, and, as in this case, he usually emerged with his dignity and criminal record intact. Reeves and Baird later found common ground and became friends and political allies.

While Reeves was tending to his many problems in 1872 New York City's Stephen Smith began building an organizational home for America's public health professionals. Other cities, including Wheeling, had begun creating health boards modeled after the one he fashioned for New York and Smith believed the country was ready for a national public health association.

Smith asked six friends to meet at his New York Board of Health office on April 18, 1872, to discuss the idea. As he described the event, it was "entirely informal, and the discussion was limited to the question of the contemplated organization of a National Sanitary Association." Judging by those present, the meeting hardly occurred by happenstance. Three of the attendees were from other states and all were particularly qualified for the task Smith envisioned.[24]

Those who met with Smith on the afternoon of April 18 were: John Ordronaux, Professor of Law at Columbia University in New York, also a physician and perhaps the country's pre-eminent medical-legal expert, Edward Janes, one of Smith's most energetic physician sanitary inspectors for his 1865 survey and an Assistant Sanitary Superintendent for the New York Metropolitan Board of Health, Christopher Cox, a physician, former Lieutenant Governor of Maryland, and professor of medical jurisprudence at Georgetown University in Washington, D.C., Carl Pfeiffer, a New York architect noted for his expertise in designing heating and ventilation systems, John Rauch, a Chicago physician who had helped organize his city's health board on New York's model and was then serving on the Chicago Board of Health, and Edwin Snow, a Providence, Rhode Island physician and health officer who was one of the organizers of the prewar sanitary conventions and America's foremost leader in vital statistics. After favorably considering Smith's idea, the group decided that it should hold another meeting that evening at a nearby hotel.[25]

The second meeting added three more New York physicians, Elisha Harris, Moreau Morris, and Heber Smith. This small assembly declared itself a temporary committee for the purpose of creating a permanent association for promoting public health interests and named a committee to arrange an appropriate national meeting. The Organization Committee consisted of five of those in attendance: Smith, Harris, Rauch, Cox, and Jane, and thirteen other nationally prominent sanitarians, one of whom was James Reeves. There is no evidence that Reeves participated in the Organization Committee's work, but, whether he knew it at the time or not, he was a founding member of the new organization.

Like Reeves, most of the physician sanitarians who met in New York in April did not attend the AMA's annual meeting in nearby Philadelphia the following month. The absence of public health advocates such as Smith, Rauch, and Snow was understandable as the AMA relegated their interests to the small Section on Medical Jurisprudence, Hygiene, and Physiology. However, they missed a landmark presentation by one of their own, sixty-four-year-old Thomas Logan, the permanent secretary of the newly formed California State Board of Health. Logan's remarks carried extra weight because he was due to become AMA president the following year.[26]

Logan was chairman of a Committee on a National Health Council and in his committee report he made recommendations that would have appealed to Smith and his fellow sanitarians. Without advocating for a specific approach, he urged governments to protect the populace from the health dangers of industrialization. He made it clear that the state should use medical science to do so: "For while private enterprise is hastening after the acquisition of wealth, and applying all the resources of science in its production, so also should recourse be had to science by the State for protection against the evils which the hurtful, because selfish, spirit of enterprise is continually engendering."[27]

Logan subtly challenged his profession's long-standing isolation from politics, as well as its guardianship of medical science. But knowing when to quit, he ended the presentation with a modest request that his committee be continued as a new section on State Medicine and Public Hygiene. Another Californian offered a resolution that the federal government should establish a national sanitary bureau, but the resolution was voted down. After that Logan got his wish for the new AMA section, a barely noticed testimony to the increasing visibility of public health.

Smith's Committee on Permanent Organization moved ahead; calling for an organizational meeting on September 12, 1872, in Long Branch, New Jersey. When the day arrived there were only fifteen attendees and Reeves was not among them. This group, most of whom had also been present at the April meeting in New York, decided that the new organization would be called The American Public Health Association and optimistically adopted a Constitution requiring a quorum of twenty-five members to conduct business. The attendees chose Stephen Smith as the Association's first president. They decided that the initial meeting of the APHA would be in Cincinnati in May 1873.[28]

Shortly after his fight with Baird in December 1872 Reeves resigned his position as Wheeling Health Officer. He submitted his final report in February 1873, pronouncing the city in good shape, and thanking the council for its kindness. However, he continued to discreetly advocate for his city's health interests. The *Intelligencer* issued a call in March 1873 for a law to ensure the purity of kerosene, using the information from his 1871 book, *Health and Wealth.* The West Virginia Legislature, which was dominated by oil and coal interests, took no action and the *Intelligencer* dropped the cause.[29]

Reeves attended the first APHA meeting in Cincinnati on May 1, 1873. He was part of a small group of seventeen physicians who made the trip. The presentations generally dealt with statistics, disease registration, and quarantine laws, the kinds of organizational matters that the country's sanitarians saw as their mission. In contrast to the AMA, the newly-formed APHA favored government involvement at all levels. A year earlier AMA members had voted down a resolution calling for a national sanitary bureau, one that the small group of APHA doctors in Cincinnati enthusiastically endorsed.[30]

Reeves met two men at the APHA meeting who became friends and sources of professional inspiration. One was John Rauch, the Chicago health board member who also had an interest in medical education and licensure. Another was Joseph Woodward, an Army officer and a new member to the group. Woodward, who had helped Hammond establish the Army Medical Museum, had an interest in medical microscopy, later Reeves' passion.[31]

AMA members assembled for their association's annual conference in St. Louis three days after the APHA meeting ended. This was just an overnight train ride from Cincinnati, but, despite the proximity, only six of the seventeen APHA physicians continued westward to St. Louis. Chicago's Rauch and Wheeling's Reeves were not among them. Those who did go heard AMA President Thomas Logan describe the new laboratory science that troubled American medicine.[32]

Logan began his presidential address by paying compliments to the delegates and acknowledging the country's persisting problems with medical education. However, unlike many of his predecessors, he did not comfort his countrymen by demeaning Europe's medical laboratories. AMA President David Yandell had praised German science a year earlier, acknowledging the country's visible contributions in histology, microscopy, and animal chemistry, but followed his compliments with the standard American takedown: "And what, let me ask in a spirit of perfect candor, has it all amounted to?" Yandell's answer was that medical education should not waste a student's time with laboratory science, but emphasize practical, bedside skills, presumably derived through individual clinical observation and trial and error.[33]

Logan took an opposing position to Yandell. Science was taking a new path and medicine should follow the path, the same message Bartlett delivered about an earlier scientific path in 1844. Logan called German laboratory science: "the crowning glory of modern medicine.... Imbued with the conviction that the beginning of wisdom is the knowledge of ignorance, and conscious of the difficulties which, on every hand, beset him, the scientific physician explores cautiously, doubts judiciously, and determines slowly." Medical science, in particular laboratory science, must serve the public by removing causes of human disease, a concept Logan summed up in two words, "preventive medicine."[34]

Logan turned his attention to the AMA's historic resistance to public cooperation. Here too he challenged professional orthodoxy. He noted how a request for public engagement a year earlier had been "disposed of by the conservative element of this body." Although he had not attended the APHA's meetings he offered "the recent formation of a Public Health Association" as an example of the changing times. He concluded with a call for the AMA to shift its perspective from detachment to public collaboration: "I believe the time has come when we must place ourselves in a more intimate relationship with the people than has hitherto ruled; in other words, the people are looking to us to utilize the capacity which this Association actually possesses, for the general welfare."[35]

Logan again framed the choice facing American physicians: whether they should acknowledge and follow the scientific discoveries coming from European laboratories, such as the breakthroughs of France's Claude Bernard and Louis Pasteur, and Germany's Rudolph Virchow, even if they had no visible application to daily medical practice, or remain aloof, claiming to be scientists on their own terms.

Even as Logan sensed that European laboratory science was pushing public health away from its sanitation origins, the movement remained small and undefined, lacking a true scientific identity. The key that would open the door for public health's scientific ascendency was present at the AMA's 1873 meeting, but not in Logan's new section on State Medicine and Public Hygiene. Instead, it lay almost unnoticed within the sections on materia medica and surgery. With little clear understanding of how it worked, American doctors were trying carbolic acid on almost everything, from smallpox and malaria to surgical antisepsis and abscess management.[36]

They were encouraged by Scottish physician Joseph Lister's 1867 papers extolling the virtues of carbolic acid in surgery. Lister cited French scientist Louis Pasteur's laboratory demonstration that small airborne living beings caused putrefaction and stated that this work provided proof of the controversial germ theory of disease. Lister concluded that the appropriate treatment was to destroy germs where they were present in the body and prevent new ones from entering. He found carbolic acid to be the best agent for this purpose. A few American physicians, including former AMA president Yandell, were familiar with Lister's work. While they were not willing to accept Lister's laboratory-based premise that living particles were the problem, they were adequately impressed by Lister's results to experiment with carbolic acid.[37]

⚡ 12 ⚡

The Moral High Ground

As cholera moved up the Mississippi River in June 1873, the Wheeling *Intelligencer* published two editorials dealing with cholera prevention. The first included a memorandum published by the Executive Committee of the new APHA. The article did not mention any Wheeling officials, thus Reeves was most likely the guiding influence if not the source for the paper's recommendations. The second editorial, two days later, reiterated the need for prevention and concluded with: "Let us be taxed heavily if need be to secure the public health, without which there can be no business prosperity." A sentiment that was pure Reeves.[1]

There were just twenty-five physicians, one attorney, and a few invited dignitaries in the room when President Stephen Smith opened the second APHA annual meeting in New York City on November 11, 1873. Shortly after noon, Reeves presented his paper, "Physical and Moral Causes of Bad Health in American Women."[2]

Reeves' presentation was one of three that week on individual health and hygiene. When the APHA published the meeting's reports, it omitted two of these papers, Reeves' talk on American women and Edward Jarvis' on the power of the housekeeper. These communications were not the community-oriented, observational studies that fit with the APHA's vision of science-based public health. The presentations that APHA Secretary Elisha Harris selected for the *Reports* focused, instead, on cholera, yellow fever, quarantine, public sanitation, and sanitary laws.[3]

Without the perspective that Reeves campaigned for the next dozen years to broaden public health's mission, it's easy to dismiss his 1873 talk as what twentieth-century historian Carroll Smith-Rosenberg called the standard product of a would-be physiological reformer. Smith-Rosenberg saw Reeves as a typical progressive male physician who was interested in upgrading women's maternal capacities rather than freeing middle-class women for other responsibilities.[4]

The essence of Reeves' paper was that American women, formerly hardy frontier wives and mothers, had become soft and frail. They needed new proficiencies for a modern, industrializing world. Reeves advised against sending girls to boarding and finishing schools because the mental tasks sacrificed physical challenges, leaving girls unfit for the serious duties of life. He generally held that the work of women was to be wives and mothers, but he denied that this meant servitude. He advocated for girls acquiring the practical skills that, in the next century, would be taught in home economics classes. He urged women to escape the follies of frivolous, confining fashion and argued that that women and men should be held to the same standards of virtue.[5]

Hardly a feminist manifesto, Reeves' sentiment was still a far cry from the misogyny of many nineteenth-century male physicians, particularly those who led the AMA. Reeves encouraged women to take the domestic road most of them would follow, but, he also promoted later marriages, smaller families, and less restraining apparel, all items that the small number of aspiring professional women said they needed. Reeves could have spoken about sanitation problems, the health officer's role, or other issues better suited to the APHA's agenda, but, he wanted his public health audience to think about the practical advice a doctor gave to his female patients. To Reeves, the obligations of medicine and public health were the same.

Two other events occurred at the APHA's 1873 meeting that shed light on the times. One arose as the roll was called on the second day. To the delegates' chagrin, the constitutional quorum of twenty-five members was not present. Worse, someone observed that this number had never been met at any meeting. Army surgeon Joseph Woodward successfully moved to dissolve the APHA and adjourn the meeting.[6]

The next step was to reorganize the group, with a different requirement for a quorum. Reeves, Woodward, and three others quickly prepared a new constitution defining a quorum as nine members. Those present adopted the revised constitution, named the new organization the American Public Health Association, and assumed all assets and liabilities of the former association by the same name. The small band of sanitarians had resolved the APHA's constitutional crisis.

APHA attendance problems persisted throughout the decade, even though the organization managed to reshape legislative and professional discussions. In 1879 John Shaw Billings, who would become the APHA's president the following year, remarked that with more than four hundred physician members, it was rare to see fifty physicians present at an APHA meeting.[7] The reality was that most physicians were even less interested in organized public health than they were in organized medicine.

Another meeting event that framed contemporary issues, while setting a path for the future, was a perceptive talk by a layman, Frederick Barnard, the aging and deaf president of Columbia University. His academic work was in mathematics, physics, and chemistry, but Barnard chose to address his listeners on the evolving germ theory. The small audience may have had trouble understanding Barnard because his deafness made speaking difficult, but his paper, which the APHA published in 1875, became a public health landmark. In 1921 APHA President Mazÿck Ravenel called it "a beacon to guide the young organization ... in advance of much of the medical opinion of the day."[8]

Barnard began his talk with a broad overview of scientific principles, stating that human health was ruled by such principles, even if they were difficult to understand. There was no room for Divine displeasure as an explanation of disease. He reminded the group that the germ theory, in various forms, had existed for at least two hundred years. Now, he said, arriving laboratory evidence showed that this theory provided a sensible explanation for the origins of infectious and contagious diseases. The most logical alternative, and the one which most physicians still accepted, was what he called the chemical theory. The difference between the two theories, which both presumed that sources of infection and contagion arose in decaying or diseased matter, was whether the agent was a chemical entity or a microscopic living organism.

Barnard masterfully summarized European evidence for the presence of living, airborne organisms as causes of decay and fermentation, but he was astute enough to sense the emotional and spiritual consequences of these findings. He spoke about their implications, including the frightening one that, if all living matter originated solely from other living matter, as Pasteur proposed, then death was final. If death was final, then there was no immortal soul. Barnard was also a man of religion and he did not welcome this conclusion: "If this, after all, is the best that science can give me, give me then, I pray, no more science. Let me live on, in my simple ignorance, as my fathers lived before me."[9]

However, Barnard quickly returned from spiritual musings to the scientific questions. He drew on Lister to provide clinical relevance. Lister's surgical experience and English physicist John Tyndall's experiments clearly showed that airborne "parasitic vegetation" caused certain types of human illness. For Barnard the conclusion was that the germ theory of disease was at least partially correct. The only remaining question was whether some diseases were caused by living organisms, while others were caused by chemical agents.[10]

Barnard ended the talk by suggesting how his public health audience should deal with the controversies surrounding the germ theory. The solution to the quandary about which disease theory was correct was that the answer did not really matter: "The necessary measures of precaution or of extirpation will be substantially the same, whatever may be the theoretic views entertained as to the nature and the origin of the evil to be met." In short, everything that the audience already wanted: pure air, pure water, wholesome food, removal of noxious effluvia, and prevention of overcrowding, was the right answer. Having prepared a masterful summary of the available scientific evidence, Barnard brought his listeners to the comfortable conclusion that they were already doing the right thing.[11]

Barnard's presentation exemplified issues that had important ramifications. The growing acceptance of airborne parasitic vegetation in the 1870s created unintentional problems for medicine and public health. This interpretation of the germ theory encouraged physicians to protect wounds from airborne contamination, which was beneficial, but it did not encourage them to protect wounds from other sources of contamination, including their own hands. The unfortunate consequence was vividly apparent at the autopsy of James Garfield in 1881. The assassin's bullet, which had entered the president's body eleven weeks earlier, did not kill Garfield. He died from extensive infection caused by numerous physician examinations.[12] From a public health perspective, the airborne version of the germ theory retarded appreciation of the spread of bacterial diseases by other means, such as human contact.

Secondly, Barnard made it clear that there were impediments to acceptance of the germ theory beyond ignorance of the information or a disregard for the relevance of laboratory science. Twentieth-century research in human cognition would describe Barnard's theological concern as a source of biased assimilation, a propensity to be sharply critical of facts that threaten one's identity.[13]

Former AMA president Alfred Stillé, in his 1874 text on medical therapeutics, denigrated Lister's use of carbolic acid and his "purely hypothetical idea" of septic organisms floating in the atmosphere. Stillé had to be aware, as Barnard noted in his talk and Austin Flint wrote in his 1873 textbook, that the idea of airborne septic organisms was well supported, but he could not bring himself to consider the evidence. In the setting of biased assimilation, almost no amount of proof is enough.[14]

Lastly, Barnard's keen observations demonstrated that non-physicians of the time appreciated medicine's emerging discoveries more than many doctors. Scientists such as Barnard, as well as the educated public, were fascinated by the exciting news from Europe's laboratories. Soon enough this created a path for public health that took it into the laboratory and away from social issues.

Reeves lost interest in medical organizing and made a daring move. Although a busy practitioner, he took his medical curiosity, his evangelical spirit, his love of medical writing, and his family's forbearance into the competitive world of medical journal publishing. The country had little medical science to claim for its own, but the United States had forty-four regular medical journals in 1873, published from Oregon to Georgia. Considering dental, eclectic, and homeopathic journals, the total was closer to seventy-five. This number not only exceeded any other country, it probably exceeded all of Europe.[15] Still, West Virginia did not have a medical journal. In February 1874 he purchased paper, type and, shortly thereafter, a foot-powered rotary printing press. Probably taxing Frances' expectations, he set up a printing shop in their house.[16]

Reeves launched his printing business with his APHA monograph on "The Physical and Moral Causes of Bad Health in American Women," which he offered for fifty cents in July 1875. The Wheeling *Intelligencer* gave the piece front-page coverage and pronounced it "in all respects a useful paper." *The Virginia Medical Monthly* lauded the printer's handiwork and Reeves' advice, describing his product as: "a beautifully printed pamphlet of 44 pages ... the lessons attempted to be inculcated so valuable that we would be glad to know this pamphlet was read by every mother and adult daughter in the land."[17]

Reeves launched West Virginia's first medical journal, *The West Virginia Medical Student*, in November 1875. As with his typhoid writings, he wanted to encourage his colleagues to reflect and report on their experiences: "no man is so busy in practice, either in country or city, that he cannot find time to make a brief daily record of his most important cases." But now he went a step further. He announced his intention to foster "a stricter observance of the reasonable demands of the National Code of Medical Ethics."[18]

Moses Hall, past president of the Medical Society of West Virginia, wrote Reeves praising his effort: "The truly first-class original matter which you have furnished in the first number fully deserves the fine paper and beautiful typography in which the work is presented.... Put me down for two copies." The editor of the influential Cincinnati *Lancet and Observer* pronounced: "Its contents are of a high character. Its typographical appearance is excellent." Reeves was pleased with praise for his home-based typography because his seventeen-year-old son, Charles, was the pressman.[19]

The first volume of the *Medical Student* documented the changing times and Reeves' Methodist-influenced medical ethics. The infectious disease papers illustrated physicians' evolving understanding of the germ theory. Samuel Jepson, Reeves' successor as Wheeling Health Officer, wrote an article on the origin and propagation of typhoid fever. Jepson presented the accepted formulation that infectious poisons emanated from filth and decay and caused typhoid. However, he admitted that new evidence, masterfully organized by English physician William Budd and confirmed by others, showed that typhoid poisons could be transmitted via water contaminated by human excrement. Jepson and his fellow health officers assumed that contaminated water caused disease by releasing infectious gasses, but their knowledge of how to prevent illness by addressing the water supply had improved during the seventeen years since Reeves wrote his *Practical Treatise* on the disease.[20]

Two other papers showed that many regular physicians accepted botanic remedies, even as Reeves and his colleagues attacked eclectics for their self-promotion and "unscientific" dogmas. In January 1876 a professor from a prestigious regular medical college wrote about a "valuable but neglected medicine," the folk cure, Cimicifuga racemosa, now known as *Actaea racemosa* or black cohosh. Four months later, another regular physician thanked the previous author for reminding the profession of Cimicifuga racemosa, adding his own testimony in favor of black cohosh.[21]

This was all standard medical journal fare, but Reeves had grown up with Wesley's admonitions to call out backsliders and reprove neighbors who had strayed from the righteous path and he followed Wesley's advice from his journal's editorial pages in a way that few other editors dared. He announced his intention to reprint any newspaper article that mentioned the name of a physician who had provided professional service. This was an unprecedented proposal. When another medical journal heard of it, the editor remarked tongue-in-cheek: "A good idea, but if followed by all medical journals, some would contain nothing else than these records."[22]

Reeves wrote, "All such covert worming before the public is entirely beneath the dignity of the regular profession and does great injustice to the acknowledged charlatan, who is compelled to pay, at advertising rates, for every line of his self-puffs." He never carried out this amazing threat, except against his nemesis, J.C. Hupp. In the second issue of the *Medical Student* Reeves reprinted, "for what they are worth," three newspaper notices reporting that Hupp had been appointed a member of the 1876 Centennial Medical Commission. Several other Wheeling physicians, including Reeves, had also been nominated to be members of this commission, but only Hupp had announced it in the papers.[23]

He attacked the poor quality of The Medical Society of West Virginia's *Transactions* in 1875. He noted that his old friend, Matthew Campbell's, 1875 presidential address was "not undeserving of criticism." He sniped at a Wheeling surgeon's paper for its author's self-promotion: "If the merits and value of this case are to be measured by the amount of newspaper puffing it has received, then, assuredly, it is the most important contribution made to the present volume of *Transactions* [author's italics]."[24]

As he publicized the Society's annual meeting in Wheeling in 1876, he could not resist disparaging its "local and bitter political prejudices, which, even to this day, embarrass its progress, notwithstanding the well-known fact that the author of the Society [i.e., Reeves] was a so-called 'Rebel sympathizer.'" Nor could he pass up another dig at its *Transactions*: "The few really valuable papers which it contains are so outraged by bad proof-reading that their interest is almost entirely destroyed."[25]

If Reeves wanted medical society members and their friends to buy his journal and take the time to write articles for it, this type of sermonizing was not the way to go. In the final issue of the first year he acknowledged his disappointment that so few West Virginia physicians had contributed material and then told his delinquent subscribers that he planned to publish their names as free readers in the next issue.[26]

He also told readers that the *Medical Student* had succeeded his business expectations and that he planned to continue the journal, increasing its size from thirty-two to forty-eight pages per issue. But he never did. The *Medical Student* ended after one year, as did his printing business. Samuel Jepson later proposed that Reeves was simply ahead of his time, but Reeves' *ad hominem* confrontations could not have been comfortable reading to West Virginia's stubborn and often isolated physicians.[27]

Forty years later Jepson became the first editor of *The West Virginia Medical Journal,* the publication of the State Medical Association and the second medical journal published in the state. In his welcoming editorial Jepson showed his appreciation of the fraternal nature of physician organizations. Rather than chiding his colleagues, Jepson comforted them: "Knowing that no one is infallible, we shall exercise the largest charity towards all with whom we may have dealings, whenever they appear to be striving to act fairly and honestly."[28]

Regulars' disdain for quackery and false promotion did not apply to his own choice of therapies, which left him and his journal with a long-persisting ethical blind spot. *The West Virginia Medical Student* sought drug company advertising, as did most medical journals. Some of the *Student's* ads, such as the W.R. Warner Company's glossy promotion of its sugar-coated quinine pills, were not controversial. However, the *Medical Student* also promoted proprietary compounds such as Lactopeptine, a mixture of digestive enzymes and hydrochloric acid that claimed to be "the most important remedy for Dyspepsia that has ever been produced." Reeves' Lactopeptine advertisements included eight pages of testimonials from doctors in their official capacities. *The Boston Medical and Surgical Journal* advertised the same product. Lactopeptine's proprietary formulation and overdone praise were unethical at the time and if similar ads had run in a lay publication, Reeves and other regulars would have accused its editor of abetting quackery.[29]

But this inconsistency was built into the medical journal business. The AMA's first Committee on Medical Literature observed in 1848, "The advertising portion of the journals seems to be considered by some editors as beyond the jurisdiction of medical ethics." Medical journals accepted advertisements and endorsements for proprietary drugs with inflated claims and regular physicians prescribed these drugs well into the twentieth century. Physician editors justified their advertising fees and opposition to lay promotion of the same compounds by arguing that, as scientists, doctors could discern the truth or falsehoods of drug advertisements, whereas laymen could not.[30]

If Reeves saw a moral opportunity in the medical information market of the 1870s, the medical publisher who best exploited the era's financial prospects was eclectic physician Joseph Joshua Lawrence. Lawrence started his business about the same time as Reeves, but he created a lasting medical publishing model and the country's most famous medical nostrum. Lawrence never crossed personal paths with Reeves, but his successful example and his creations played a role in Reeves' last professional battle.

Lawrence graduated from Cincinnati's Eclectic Medical Institute in 1858 and returned home to North Carolina where he practiced medicine and served intermittently in the Confederate Army. Following the Civil War he turned to nostrum manufacturing in Virginia and Maryland. He began with "The best blood purifier in the world—Lawrence's Compound Extract of Rosadalis" in 1867 and then "Dr. Lawrence's Celebrated Woman's Friend" and Koskoo in 1869. He filed the first of several bankruptcies in 1869 and again returned to North Carolina where he continued pushing Koskoo and Woman's Friend until 1872.[31]

Lawrence then moved into medical publishing, which worked beyond his dreams. He announced *The Medical Brief* in 1873, a new monthly devoted to "Practical Medicine, Chemistry, Pharmacy, and Hygiene." The *Brief* was a bargain, "the *largest, handsomest* (and we hope *the best*) Dollar magazine published in the United States. *Just think of it!* 600 pages for 'a dollar'" (punctuation in original).[32]

The typical medical journal publisher charged three to five dollars per year and was thrilled if he attracted a thousand paying subscribers. When Reeves launched *The West Virginia Medical Student* in 1875 he sold it for two dollars per annum and he couldn't make it work. The *Philadelphia Medical Times,* where Reeves had published several articles, charged five dollars annually and had 960 subscribers. The prestigious *New York Medical Journal* charged four dollars and claimed 1,400 subscribers. The influential *Cincinnati Lancet and Observer* charged three dollars and had 1,500 subscribers.[33]

If Lawrence was going to succeed in selling a monthly medical journal at the rock-bottom price of one dollar, he had to fill his six hundred pages and gather far more subscribers than his most successful competitors. Adding to his task Lawrence promised that he would avoid commercial or organizational sponsors. He was not interested, he told readers, "in the manufacture or sale of any Medicines or the advancement of any medical school or 'pathy."[34]

After starting *The Medical Brief* in 1873 Lawrence moved his family and his journal from Wilson, North Carolina to St. Louis, Missouri, where he obtained a professorship at a new eclectic medical school. Unlike the state of North Carolina, which had no medical journals, his new city already had two medical monthlies, both charging three dollars per year: *The St. Louis Medical and Surgical Journal,* with a circulation of 750, and *The St. Louis Medical Archives,* with approximately 960 subscribers.[35]

But Lawrence was not concerned with the competition in St. Louis. He had a novel approach to medical journalism that reduced his costs and expanded his appeal. Instead of printing lengthy communications, medical lectures, commentaries, detailed book reviews, and medical society minutes, he presented terse summaries, one or two per page, of material previously printed by his competitors. His publication's motto was, "Multum in parvo," Latin for "much in little."[36]

Lawrence's journal differed from publications such as Reeves,' which were fashioned on scholarly European standards. He promulgated no ethical or scientific ideals, and, by sticking to clinical practice, tapped into all medical sects. Regular medicine, eclecticism, and homeopathy still challenged each other's dogmatic legacies and social failings, but most doctors managed their patients in similar fashion. With his focus on everyday medicine, the *Brief* provided information to physicians of all stripes.[37]

Lawrence's real genius lay in the low-cost and self-promoting way he obtained his content. He kept his costs down by borrowing whatever work that caught his eye and he printed any experience that a reader sent him, so long as it was limited to five hundred words. Sprinkled among Lawrence's' abstracted articles were numerous reports, all carefully indexed, such as the following one on morning sickness from 1876:

> Editor, Medical Brief:
>
> Dear Sir: About fifteen days ago, a pregnant lady applied to me for something to cure or relieve sick-stomach. For ten days, I tried everything I could think of, without giving relief; at last, I cut the end of a lemon, stuffed it with fine sugar, and gave it to the patient to suck. It gave immediate relief; and she has had no return of the sick-stomach since.
>
> Yours truly, E. M. Baldwin, M. D.[38]

It was not serious medical science, but it worked. Subscribers got to sift through buckets of advice and an opportunity to see their names in print for a dollar. Lawrence claimed a staggering readership of 10,000 in 1877. By 1880 his paid circulation, still at one dollar per year, exceeded 21,000, allowing Lawrence to brag that *The Medical Brief* had the largest circulation of any medical journal in the world. He boasted to his readers about the journal's independence and its commercial purpose. It was "run on business principles, *in the interest of its editor*, TO MAKE MONEY" (punctuation in original). Lawrence's personal and personalized approach to medical science and medical journalism was an essential contributor to the success of his next medical nostrum, Listerine.[39]

⚡ 13 ⚡

Going It Alone

Reeves attended the state medical society's annual meeting in Wheeling in June 1876 and, as in 1872, he listened but did not participate. The Wheeling old guard still dominated the Medical Society of West Virginia and Reeves thought they were running it into the ground. He had vented his frustrations from the pages of *The Medical Student*, where he wrote that the organization's selfish motives were "permitted to control its action and thus oppose the very objects for which it was created."[1]

He stayed away from the APHA's 1876 gathering in Boston and the AMA's 1876 meeting in Philadelphia. However, he did find time for another 1876 event in Philadelphia, the United States' first International Medical Congress. The September Congress was one of the celebratory events of the Centennial year and 375 of the country's medical luminaries, as well as seventy-one distinguished foreign physicians, participated. The surgery section was chaired by the leading advocate of antiseptic surgery, Scotland's Joseph Lister.[2]

Reeves heard speaker after speaker recount the changes that had occurred in American medicine, many of whom referred to its bright future in terms of its recently dark past. Congress President Samuel Gross told the delegates, "The science of medicine has been completely revolutionized within our day.... 'Old things are passed away; behold all things are become new,' has literally been fulfilled." Other speakers, such as Austin Flint, saw a longer scientific continuum, but this event helped establish the premise that modern, scientific medicine began during Samuel Gross' lifetime.[3]

The Philadelphia spotlight shone most brightly on Gross, Flint, and Lister; however, Reeves received his due. Lunsford Yandell described the state of America's medical literature and mentioned Reeves for his 1859 book on typhoid and for his *West Virginia Medical Student*. Gross, with whom Reeves had first corresponded in 1859, considered West Virginia delegate Reeves an old friend.[4]

Reeves returned home thoroughly energized. He devoted twenty pages of *The West Virginia Medical Student* to the meeting, describing it a feast of reason: "Never on this continent," he wrote, " was there such a large congregation of representative men, so many distinguished teachers and leaders, so many of the good and truly great in the profession."[5]

Reeves had not lost his professional ideals, but his efforts to uplift his West Virginia colleagues were not succeeding. His journal was failing and the medical society he founded was a long way from its potential. He left medical soul-saving for others in 1876 and entered the more mundane worlds of civic service and local politics.

Reeves had always been a Democrat, but in post-reconstruction West Virginia party names did not provide political and philosophical distinctions. The bigger differences were between Regular Democrats, who along with Republicans, favored industrialization and monopolies, and Redeemer Democrats, who opposed the industrialists and sought to restore ante-bellum relationships.

Reeves was a Redeemer but Wheeling, like the state, was increasingly run by the Regular Democrat successors to the Republican Party. The city's two newspapers, the *Intelligencer* and the *Register,* Republican and Democratic, respectively, bitterly feuded over state and national politics, but generally saw eye to eye on important city matters. Both papers supported public health and both favored industrialization and the interests of industrialists. The *Intelligencer,* for example, mistrusted Democratic Mayor Andrew Sweeney when Wheeling was under Republican control during the Civil War. But, in the 1870s, it willingly supported industrialist Mayor Sweeney.[6]

While the *Intelligencer* tolerated or sometimes accepted the state's Regular Democrats, like Johnson Camden, Andrew Sweeney, and many ex-Confederates, it loathed Redeemers, such as Barbour County's Samuel Woods. Woods was active in state politics and, importantly for Reeves, would soon serve on the state's Supreme Court of Appeals. The *Intelligencer* called the church-going Woods a Judas Iscariot-level traitor in 1868 and heaped vitriol onto his wartime record into the 1880s.[7]

Unlike Woods Reeves did not wear his Redeemer leanings on his sleeve and, except for his Know-Nothing orations in 1855, he avoided political controversy. He was a nationally-recognized physician with a civic record focused on public health. He cautiously entered city affairs by speaking at a local Democratic club in September 1876. The *Register* covered this event and politely called his remarks interesting and appropriate, with no further details.[8]

In the November 1876 gubernatorial elections voters elected Henry Matthews, a moderate Redeemer and former Confederate, to succeed Independent John Jacob. Matthews was West Virginia's first Bourbon Democrat governor. At the same time the state legislature moved the capital back to Wheeling from Charleston, where it had been transferred in 1870. In anticipation the city erected a handsome capitol building and included a copy of Reeves' *Health and Wealth of the City of Wheeling* in its cornerstone.[9] Reeves felt encouraged to enter local politics.

The voters in Wheeling's fifth ward chose him as their delegate to the city's Democratic Convention on January 8, 1877. The next day Convention delegates chose Reeves chairman and president of the Wheeling Democratic Executive Committee, putting him in the capital city's power structure. Following the organizational necessities the Convention selected the Democratic slate for the upcoming city officer elections, nominating Mayor Sweeney for re-election.[10]

Reeves ran in this election as a candidate for one of the three fifth ward positions on the Wheeling City Council's Second Branch, the Council section that controlled city appropriations. On January 25, 1877, the voters elected him to the council and chose Democrats for four of the six city offices, including mayor. He focused his considerable energies on the Wheeling city council for the next four years.[11]

Reeves made a partisan move shortly after joining the council that was appropriate for a new Democratic politician, but uncharacteristic for him. He tried to use a procedural tactic to give James Sweeney, the mayor's cousin, a position he had lost in the election. Reeves joined a small group of council members who sought to overturn the election for city sergeant by claiming that Sweeney's opponent's bond was invalid. Reeves' political intrigue was quashed by the council, which voted to reject his group's procedural diversion and accept the Republican candidate as city sergeant.[12]

This type of backroom dealing was not Reeves' style. When it came to furthering goals that resisted orderly debate, he preferred direct confrontation, often in a gentlemanly manner reminiscent of dueling. As Samuel Woods put it, he could be "severe without being unparliamentary." During one council meeting Reeves accused another member of spreading falsehoods and then replied to the outraged gentleman when he threatened to pull Reeves' beard that he did not mean to say he lied, only that he spoke incorrectly.[13]

During his time on the council Reeves generally avoided political maneuvering and heated arguments, assuming the role of a thrifty public servant instead. He managed several issues of financial malfeasance, such as a case of fraud by the operators of the city's gas works. When James Sweeney was eventually elected city sergeant in 1879, Reeves opposed Sweeney's proposal to increase the size of the police force. Reeves objected to the idea because of the costs and the potential for graft and political patronage, in his words: "a political ring around the office of City Sergeant." Reeves increasingly demonstrated anti-monopolistic Redeemer leanings as he became more comfortable in his council position.[14]

The council met monthly and on an *ad hoc* basis to settle minor crises; it was tedious civic work. The *Intelligencer* titled the report of one typical nighttime assembly that discussed bills, reports, and lamp posts, "City Council—Regular Monthly Meeting—The Usual Monotony." During his tenure Reeves participated in at least seventy-two Wheeling City Council meetings.[15]

Reeves took his council duties seriously, although few of them included public health or sanitation. He got involved when there was a smallpox outbreak in 1877 and he offered advice to the health committee in 1879, but he avoided pressing his public health agenda on the council. He was comfortably re-elected in 1879 and retired from the council in 1881. An anonymous observer wrote to the *Register* in 1882, "There is no man in our city, perhaps, that is better posted on city affairs than Dr. Reeves."[16]

During his city council years Reeves confronted two personal challenges that re-energized his public health mission. The first was a family tragedy that sharpened the messages of preventive medicine and personalized his hopes for medical science. The second was the dramatic conclusion of his ten-year battle with the medical society he helped found.

Reeves' twenty-one-year-old son, Joseph Cullen, was known in Wheeling as young Joe Reeves who ran the Twelfth Street candy store. Joe was engaged to be married in March 1878, but he fell ill. Reeves knew the characteristic symptoms of typhoid fever and must have been encouraged when his son seemed to improve. Unfortunately, a month later, Joe died. He was buried in his wedding suit with a Methodist preacher presiding. At age forty-nine, the Wheeling councilman had lost a wife and a son to infectious diseases that he was sure were preventable. Even if he did not know their secrets, Reeves believed medical science would find them.[17]

A month after his son's death in 1878 Reeves sent the only anti-quackery admonition to the papers that he posted during his four years of council service. It was an article from a medical journal reporting that the Arkansas State Medical Society had expelled two doctors for self-promotion. The *Intelligencer* summarized the article and thanked Reeves for reminding its readers that physician self-promotion was unethical. On the following page there were advertisements for a Wheeling homeopathic physician, Dr. Ricord's Essence of Life, Dr. Olin's private hospital, and Dr. Ayer's cathartic pills.[18] *Caveat emptor.*

Reeves had pushed Hupp's father-in-law, Archibald Todd, out of the Medical Society of West Virginia in 1872 and he travelled to Buffalo in June 1878 to ask the AMA to censure the Medical Society of Wheeling and Ohio County for its ongoing tolerance of Todd's nostrum-pushing. According to Reeves' anonymous pamphlet, several AMA members told him to take the matter up with his state medical society and bring it back if the state society did not act. There is no official record that Reeves attended the Buffalo AMA meet-

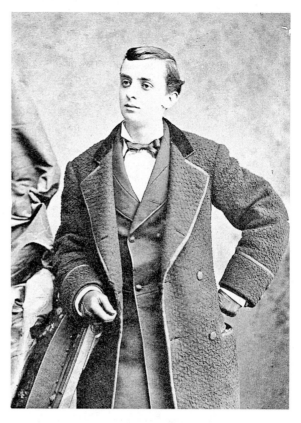

Reeves' older son, Joseph Cullen Reeves (1856–1878), date unknown. Recognized in Wheeling as young Joe Reeves who ran the Twelfth Street candy store, he died of typhoid fever in 1878, just before his wedding. In addition to Joe, Reeves lost his second wife, Mary, in 1872 to consumption (tuberculosis), another disease that he was sure could be prevented (courtesy Joan Webb).

ing, evidence that would help verify the information in his pamphlet, but the public firestorm that arose in 1879 suggests that the story it told was accurate.[19]

The story Reeves recounted was that Hupp's antipathy led him to send out copies of the Society's 1872 *Transactions,* vividly marked with Reeves' admission of wrongdoing and apology. Hupp sent this material to APHA President Stephen Smith in 1873, then to various Wheeling citizens, and in 1877, to the president of the Wheeling City Council's Second Branch. But he went too far in 1878. Hupp had seen Reeves in conversation with his fellow sanitarian, Joseph Cabell, at the 1878 AMA meeting in Buffalo and sent Cabell a copy of the 1872 *Transactions,* calling attention to Reeves' admission of error and apology, but signing the copy in another physician's name, "with compliments of W.J. Bates."[20]

Cabell was affronted by the document's lame and time-worn impeachment of Reeves and wrote Bates demanding an explanation. Bates was hardly one of Reeves' close friends, but Hupp had besmirched his name. Bates immediately responded that he had not sent the materials to Cabell. Bates thought the handwriting was Hupp's and in 1879 he charged Hupp in front of the Medical Society of Wheeling and Ohio County with severe misconduct. Hupp denied the charges, and then confessed that he had sent the 1872 *Transactions* to Cabell, but meant no harm. Hupp's longtime friends, particularly local society president Frissell, brushed Bates' charges aside. But, with Reeves' forceful urging, the members agreed to consider Hupp's expulsion. The *Intelligencer* did not mention any of this, but the Democratic Wheeling *Register* shared the spicy details with Wheeling's citizens, suspensefully concluding: "How the matter will end yet remains to be seen." The affair was now in the open.[21]

Reeves had the evidence he needed and he was not about to let the Medical Society of Wheeling and Ohio County paint Hupp's prolonged misdeeds as an innocent and "technical" violation of the Code of Ethics. Before the next meeting of the Medical Society of Wheeling and Ohio County, he took his cause to the annual meeting of the Medical Society of West Virginia in Martinsburg, a railroad town several hundred miles east of Wheeling.

By now Reeves had an adequate number of like-minded colleagues and enemies of Hupp to make a run at Hupp and his medical society cronies. He had traded fisticuffs with fellow councilman George Baird in 1872, but Baird backed Reeves in 1879. Likewise Morgantown's Hugh Brock, a society founder, former president, and professor at the newly established University of West Virginia, was Reeves' supporter. Whether Reeves knew it or not, Louis Wilson, a young Wheeling doctor who had not yet joined the Medical Society of West Virginia also admired and supported him. Wilson was a West Virginia native who had taken his medical training at the University of Pennsylvania and he was elected secretary of the Medical Society of Wheeling and Ohio County in April 1879. West Virginia's political tides now favored Reeves and several younger physicians shared his concerns over the Society's ethical transgressions.[22]

Only eighteen members attended the Martinsburg meeting, including Reeves and his key supporters, Baird and Brock. This time Reeves was more than willing to participate in the deliberations. He submitted a written grievance, charging Hupp with gross misconduct and prostitution of his official duties, the wording the society's constitution used as grounds for expulsion.[23]

Reeves' accusation split the society's board of censors along predetermined lines. Hupp's allies sought to preserve societal unity and handled the touchy matter the same way the AMA dealt with black and women physicians, by avoiding hard decisions and recommending that the problem go back to the local society. Reeves' friends, led by Brock, demanded resolution. They submitted a minority report accusing their colleagues in the Medical Society of Wheeling and Ohio County of affiliating with quackery. They recommended that Hupp's conduct be evaluated by the state society and that relations with the Wheeling society be suspended until that organization: "purged itself of all complicity and connection with quackery."[24]

Reeves' actions threatened the society's organizational principles and its existence. Former state society president Frissell moved to accept the Board's recommendation to send the matter back to Wheeling, but the members rejected his motion. Eventually, the group decided to consider all matters at the following annual meeting and adjourned until 1880.

Reeves did not wait. He confronted the Medical Society of Wheeling and Ohio County at its next meeting, just one week after the state conclave. He offered a resolution calling for Treasurer Hupp's expulsion. Frissell, then the local society president, left the event's only record in his personal notes. According to Frissell, there were two motions offered, one by Reeves for Hupp's expulsion and another for Hupp's censure. Both motions failed and Frissell announced that the matter was settled. Frissell then had to leave the meeting and Samuel Jepson presided.[25]

At the next meeting, a week later, Frissell was appalled to find that the society's new secretary, Louis Wilson, had neglected to record the vote on the two motions. After a heated debate, Frissell had to ask Wilson to separately poll the members who were not present at the earlier meeting. Frissell's exasperation boiled over and, according to him, he made a clear commitment to Hupp, no matter what the subsequent polling might show: "I beg to say that the decision announced from this chair at the meeting of June 13th 1879 relative to the resolutions of expulsion and Censure of Dr. Hupp must be maintained while I am president."

Frissell's notes showed how differently he viewed the two transgressions of Hupp's prolonged unethical conduct and someone's (i.e., Reeves') anonymous tract that aired the society's laundry. He agreed that Hupp deserved censure, but nothing more: "Would that all of us would keep more in mind the words of the Enshrined Master 'let him that is without [sin] throw out the first stone.'" However, distributing a public pamphlet that recounted Hupp's acts was professional treason: "The authors of it have perpetrated an outrage that will deserve expulsion from a respectable medical society." Frissell was in the professional mainstream. Medical societies, including the AMA, fought well into the next century to keep their linen from public inspection.

There are no subsequent society minutes or other sources that document whether Hupp's Wheeling colleagues voted to censure or expel him, but the answer was soon visible. The *Intelligencer* reported on October 3, 1879, that the local society's members elected a new president and for the first time since the re-organized society began in 1868, a new treasurer. The members also re-elected Louis Wilson secretary. When the Medical Society of Wheeling and Ohio County selected delegates to the upcoming AMA meeting, they did not choose Hupp. Instead, they selected Reeves to represent them.[26] Reeves had won and Hupp and Frissell had finally lost.

Reeves attended his first AMA meeting in June 1880 as an official delegate from an organized medical society. The AMA recorded him as rejoining that year, probably because he finally paid his dues. He may have enjoyed his small triumph, but professionally, the meeting did not offer much. In particular the newly amalgamated and hydra-headed Section on Medical Jurisprudence, Psychology, Chemistry, State Medicine, and Public Hygiene accomplished nothing. This small group of men like Reeves could not even agree on the necessity of state health boards; D.B. Whitney of New York called them an unnecessary expense.[27]

After returning from the AMA meeting, Reeves travelled down the Ohio River to Parkersburg for the 1880 meeting the Medical Society of West Virginia. This was a much bigger group than the year before, with thirty members present and society co-founder William Dent in the chair. Before dealing with Hupp, the Board of Censors had to address two diversionary efforts by Hupp against Reeves' supporter Brock. The Board found nothing to justify Hupp's allegations of impropriety and then turned its attention to the list of charges against Hupp by Reeves.[28]

The Medical Society's Board of Censors found Hupp guilty of gross misconduct and forgery. The members unanimously accepted the Board's decision and decided that Hupp needed to produce a satisfactory written apology or be expelled. The members did not consider the tabled motion to sanction the Medical Society of Wheeling and Ohio County, most likely because the Society's leadership change made it unnecessary.

Wheeling's newspapers covered the episode along partisan lines. The Republican *Intelligencer*, where Hupp had been and probably still was the chief source of medical society information, gave front page coverage to the meeting's attendees, papers, and social events, while never mentioning the unprecedented actions against the Society's treasurer. In contrast the Democratic *Register* devoted several paragraphs to the celebrated case of Dr. Hupp, his crimes, and his sentence.[29]

The Society's official records and the newspapers did not record the organization's final actions, but the outcome was clear. Hupp remained socially visible and continued to practice in Wheeling, but he disappeared from the membership rolls of the Medical Society of West Virginia and he never attend another AMA meeting. Clearly he was expelled. Reeves never referred to the affair again. Having completed his time as a city councilman and cleared his path of Hupp, he was ready to return to the work of medicine's true church.[30]

Reeves saw Hupp's original sin as self-promotion, although Hupp added years of dishonest harassment to the bill. But most physicians did not see self-promotion the way Reeves did. A few, like his fellow sanitarian Henry Bowditch, found medical societies' imbroglios over physician advertising useless distractions from their real task of improving medical science. Many more physicians tolerated modest self-promotion and redefined their ethics in light of changing market circumstances.

The entrepreneurial New York gynecologist J. Marion Sims made this point in his 1876 AMA President's Address. It was time to relax the AMA's standards for self-promotion: "Twenty years ago it was considered disreputable for a physician to put on his door, or in his window, a plate giving his office hours. Now, every one does it, greatly to the convenience of both physician and public."[31]

Reeves' Methodism was not so flexible. Wesley counseled personal humility, with no prospects for situational adjustment based on personal needs. Reeves and a few other physicians opposed medicine's changing standards, typically with silent resistance. Sometimes they were more outspoken. This happened in 1878 when the AMA's Permanent Secretary, William Atkinson, printed a directory of *The Physicians and Surgeons of the United States*. This book was the fourth compendium of medical biographies published in the United States, but, in a remarkable break with tradition, Atkinson printed the biographies of living doctors.[32]

Atkinson confined his directory "to those who by their work had brought themselves more or less prominently to notice" and he invited selected physicians to send him their biographies. His directory contained 788 pages of self-reported profiles from 2,661 of the country's 85,000 physicians. It was the first listing of America's best (living) doctors.

Almost no one objected to Atkinson's book, which was an open invitation for physicians to violate the AMA's *Code of Medical Ethics* and, in the *Code's* words, "boast of cures and remedies, to adduce certificates of skill and success, or to perform any other similar acts." Moreover, even if every respondent was scrupulously humble, Atkinson's directory was still a promotion of the skill and success of the men he chose to include. Not only did the AMA not oppose its secretary's enterprise, Atkinson published an enlarged edition two years later.[33]

The Wheeling doctors who replied to Atkinson's invitation included Baird, Frissell, Hupp, Jepson, and three others, the city's most prominent physicians save one, city councilman, author, and former city health officer, James Reeves. The directory was a national Who's Who of medicine, with Samuel Gross and Austin Flint being the first two names. The keeper of the AMA's ethical flame, Nathan Smith Davis, supplied a lengthy personal sketch and an engraved portrait. His biography was written in the third person and stated, among a long list of accomplishments, that the American Medical Association "owes its existence to him."[34]

Atkinson supplied the reason Reeves and probably Morgantown's Hugh Brock were not listed. He wrote in the book's introduction, "There were a very few who blindly adhered to a prejudice against the publication of biographies of the living."[35] There is little question that Reeves held a prejudice against biographies of the living, particularly if they consisted of unverified statements supplied by the subject. This was the definition of self-promotion.

Reeves did not publicly criticize Atkinson's directory; he just refused to participate. However, a few physicians were openly hostile. James F. Baldwin, a twenty-nine-year-old surgeon, who later became one of Reeves' closest friends, was one. Writing as the editor of *The Ohio Medical Recorder,* he began his review of Atkinson's directory: "We cannot say that the book before us is valuable, though we have found it interesting, amusing, and, as showing the vanities, weaknesses and baser motives of men, instructive." Following this stinging introductory, Baldwin pointed out numerous falsehoods and misrepresentations in the biographies. He blasted the directory as a useless ode to vanity, filled with puffery and lies from men who were often "country bumpkins, city snobs, and provincial 'professors.'"[36]

Reeves sometimes had a following to the moral high ground, as he eventually did in his fight with Hupp. But, most of the time, he trudged the slopes alone. He was beginning to accept that physicians were not well-suited to self-policing. If he wanted to improve his profession and help his community, he would turn to the political lessons he learned on the Wheeling city council.

⑃ 14 ⑃

Medical Licensure Becomes
a Public Health Problem

Reeves was a member of the Wheeling Democratic Executive Committee at the end of his second city council term in 1881. He had political stature in his state's capital and was ready to use it to advance his public health goals. Two separate health care movements had gathered national momentum while he was handling civic matters between 1877 and 1881 and he wanted to bring them together for West Virginia.

One movement was the creation of state health boards. Massachusetts had created the first state board in 1869, following a nineteen-year effort launched by a layman and supported by the state medical society. Its board was composed of three physicians and four laymen. Boston physician Henry Bowditch, the board's first chairman, welcomed the non-physician members. He proudly wrote in 1874, "The natural good sense of lay-members has greatly assisted the medical portion of the Board." The Massachusetts law focused on data collection, but was amended in 1871 to allow the board to regulate public nuisances, like slaughterhouses. The law made no mention of physician licensure.[1]

Following the formation of the American Public Health Association in 1872 a cadre of physician sanitarians, notably Bowditch, Stephen Smith, and Elisha Harris, campaigned for state boards of health. The APHA developed draft legislation for physicians to offer to their legislators in 1875. The APHA's model state board act only considered information-gathering and dissemination. The APHA did not advocate for powers to quarantine or regulate nuisances, much less control medical practice.[2]

State health board growth proceeded sporadically, overcoming inertia when there was a favorable confluence of physician advocacy, a sympathetic legislature, and public receptivity, usually prompted by a cholera, smallpox, or yellow fever outbreak. The physician sanitarians who led the movement welcomed outside participation and favored a mixed board of physicians and laymen, as in Massachusetts. There were a few within the AMA who wanted the organization to advocate for a national government health board to oversee and stimulate state efforts, but APHA leaders Harris, Bowditch, and John Shaw Billings discouraged such activity. Billings told his fellow AMA delegates, "I do not think it is the part of the American Medical Association to lay out a plan of legislation."[3]

The AMA adopted the role of scorekeeper more than advocate. It reported that there were ten state health boards in 1876 and sixteen in 1877. Some boards were active, such as in Massachusetts and Michigan, while others, including Virginia, were unfunded and essentially powerless. The functioning boards devoted their efforts to data collection. No state health board of the time dealt with physician licensure.[4]

Most physicians and state politicians did not care about public health. They saw little reward in gathering vital statistics and advocating for disease prevention. Ezra Hunt, the physician secretary of New Jersey's newly-created state board of health, summed up the situation in 1877: "No one who has been in any wise identified with Boards of Health will not testify that the apathy of average practitioners and the activity of average politicians have been the two trying elements with which to contend."[5]

The other national health care movement that had emerged was a push to reestablish physician licensure. Regular physicians had more interest in legislative issues related to their medical practice, such as licensure, but these interests were divided. Some doctors fought for licensure while many opposed it. Recognizing the country's fifty years of legislative indifference, the AMA's position was that state medical societies should establish their own boards of medical examiners, independent of state governments, but only Wisconsin made the effort.[6] Reeves wanted this power for the Medical Society of West Virginia in 1868, but he never got it. As with state boards of public health, the AMA watched medical licensure reform from the sidelines.

New York was one of the first states to bring back physician licensure and its experience exemplified the day's legislative realities and conflicting physician agendas. The progressive Medico-Legal Society of the City of New York sent a proposed "Act to Protect the People against Quackery and Crime," to the legislature in 1872. The Act's benefits to regular physicians could not have been more explicit. It would have given local medical societies complete power to license physicians in their district. Yet, the Medical Society of the State of New York opposed this legislative windfall.[7]

The state medical society resisted protecting New Yorkers "against quackery and crime" for two reasons. First was the inclusion, and apparent legitimization, of homeopaths and eclectics. The proposed act allowed each sect's local society to control licensure for its practitioners. As objectionable as this may have been to regular physicians, it was the admission price for legislation. Politicians were not about to disenfranchise their voters' doctors.

The state medical society's second and more serious concern was its distrust of *any* oversight. Some physicians feared the baser instincts of their colleagues more than their market competitors. As one member complained, "Now, it seems to me this may be the means of petty persecutions, and not for protection against incompetency."[8]

In a soon to be common scenario, the 1872 New York licensing act failed and the eventual resolution was a much weaker, "Act to Regulate the Practice of Medicine and Surgery," which passed in 1874. The new law kept some of the original language, but permitted a practitioner to use almost any kind of diploma or certificate to satisfy state licensure requirements. Regular physicians gained nothing.

West Virginia's multiple failures, eventually overcome by Reeves, provide another look at the twin tracks of public health and medical licensure legislation, demonstrating the AMA's non-involvement in the process.[9] The first visible steps had occurred in 1872 when West Virginia Medical Society President Lazzell delivered his presidential address.

As several preceding presidents, plus Reeves, had done, Lazzell roused Society members by assaulting regulars' sectarian competitors and quackery. But his polemic took a new turn when he suggested that sectarianism and quackery were public health issues that required a political response. There was a need to protect the public *"against a hurtful class of men"* (his italics). Lazzell's solution rejected the AMA's longstanding refusal of government participation. He told his fellow regulars legislation was coming, no matter what: "The times clearly and unmistakably indicate that some legislation on the subject *will* transpire in our State, not very remote in the future, *whether the profession will it or not"* (italics in original). Lazzell erroneously assured his listeners that New York's legislature had passed a stringent physician licensing law just a week before.[10]

A West Virginia House of Delegates representative introduced a licensure bill to protect the citizens of the State and to elevate the standing of the medical profession seven months later. Society President Moses Hall described the bill's welcome: "it was received with jeers, misrepresentations and back-handed compliments until it was defeated." Hall then ran for the West Virginia House of Delegates and made a personal attempt to pass a licensure law. Representative Hall presented another "bill to provide for Boards of Medical Examiners and to guard against the evils resulting from the practice of quacks," in January 1875. Hall had little help from his fellow physicians and this bill also failed.[11]

After two unsuccessful tries, and despite the urging of the Medical Society president to continue the fight, Hall and his few supporters in the Medical Society of West Virginia gave up on licensure. Acknowledging that many physicians never wanted a licensure law in the first place, the Society's leaders switched gears and, in 1875, decided to encourage a board of health act. This was a complete change from medical licensure to sanitation and public health.[12]

This new proposal caught Reeves and the state's physicians by surprise. Reeves heard of an initiative to establish a state board of health and endorsed it from the pages of *The West Virginia Medical Student*, but he thought it was a licensure act. Before he knew what the Medical Society intended, one of its members asked him to publish a copy of the "California Bill" in his journal. California already had a state health board, so Reeves assumed that the member wanted to see California's current (1875) medical licensure bill, which he printed. An anonymous letter-writer quickly corrected him, pointing out that the State Medical Society was finished with licensing laws: "This proposition to restrict the Practice of Medicine by law has already been before the State Medical Society and there defeated." Reeves apologized for the misunderstanding.[13]

Moses Hall wanted to get something done, so he introduced the APHA's model state board of public health bill as West Virginia House Bill 86 in the winter of 1875. The motion to consider the bill was tabled and Hall moved to have it reconsidered in the 1877 biennial session. Hall and his colleagues were better prepared this time. Outgoing Governor Jacob commended the idea in his opening remarks and the bill had the AMA's public endorsement.[14]

The AMA's 1877 endorsement of West Virginia's board of health bill shows how the AMA got credit for fostering legislation where it played no role. In January 1877, state society treasurer Hupp sent a letter to the legislature signed by him and two other state society members, supposedly a special committee appointed at the 1876 AMA meeting, "to memorialize your honorable bodies on the subject of the establishment of a State Board of Health."[15]

The 1876 AMA *Transactions* recorded Hupp's attendance and mentioned him several times without referring to the special committee he described. Moreover, there was no record in the *Transactions* or the local papers that the two other members of Hupp's special committee even attended the AMA meeting. Given Hupp's propensity for embellishment he and Hall likely prepared the letter to help the bill, with no connection to the AMA at all.[16]

An official-sounding letter was all it took for the West Virginia legislature to associate the state medical society's proposal with the AMA. In January 1877 the state senator whose committee was considering the bill reported that it was "expedient to legislate upon the petition of the American Medical Association for the establishment of a State Board of Health." Throughout the session the legislature referred to Hall's bill as the petition from the American Medical Association.[17] Anyone who read the legislature's official journal would have to assume that the AMA developed and endorsed West Virginia's proposed board of health bill, when it did neither.

Hall's efforts to get some kind of helpful legislation, first a licensing act and then a board of health act, failed again. His fellow physicians did little to help him and he finally accepted that West Virginia wasn't ready: "Upon reflection I now feel that in doing what I did I exercised more zeal than sense. This question had never been agitated in this State, and but few knew little or nothing of State Medicine."[18]

Hall's dismal record was hardly unique. Only eight states had functioning licensure laws in 1877: California, Kentucky, Missouri, Nevada, New Hampshire, New York, Pennsylvania, Texas, and Vermont, and they provided the same ineffective solutions. They treated all medical sects equally and handed a license to anyone with a diploma from a medical college, with no mechanism for separating bogus certificates from legitimate medical diplomas. Several other states, such as Ohio, had licensure laws on the books that had never been enforced. California was the only state with both a licensure law and a separate state board of health, created six years before its licensure law.[19]

Sanitation and licensure tides began shifting at the time Reeves assumed his city council position in 1877. Two organizational models that dominated the next century emerged in vastly different cultural settings. In Alabama an energetic Southern sanitarian and former Confederate medical officer created a militaristic physician guild that controlled public health and medical licensure. In Illinois a Union Army medical hero founded a state board of health that also brought medical licensure and medical education reform under public control.

Jerome Cochran was an ex-Confederate Army physician who was Mobile Alabama's health officer in 1871, 1872, and 1875. Reconstruction Alabama was destitute and overrun with yellow fever, as well as Union soldiers and paramilitary civilian groups. Seeing a legislative vacuum and no viable public alternatives, Cochran remade the moribund Medical Association of the State of Alabama into a military-inspired physician organization for addressing Alabama's public health problems, which, to him, included sanitation, quarantine, and medical licensure.[20]

Cochran was not interested in scientific advancement or moral improvement for his fellow physicians. Seeing the devastation around him, he wanted organizational discipline. He stated this in 1875: "We will appreciate most adequately the real character of the Association if we regard it as a Medical Legislature, having for its highest function the governmental direction of the Medical Profession of the State; while its other functions, important as they may be in themselves, are, in comparison with this, of quite subordinate rank."[21]

Cochran created a management hierarchy fashioned on a Roman legion that directed the Association's members and all local societies. For him the state society president was not an honorific position, but the Association's commanding general. He promoted the election of physicians to the Alabama legislature and the legislature made the Medical Association a de facto government branch in 1875, giving it authority over state and local health boards. The legislature granted the society control of medical licensure within the state in 1877. Cementing the Association's internal power structure, the legislature awarded county medical associations control of public health and licensure in their jurisdictions.[22]

The Alabama model of medical society delegation was remarkably effective in encouraging professional discipline, removing poorly-educated competitors, and creating the appearance of public health action. However, it was only mildly successful in meeting Alabama's needs. Cochran was State Health Officer from 1879 until his death in 1896 and a strong advocate of strict quarantine to manage yellow fever, but not of vaccination to prevent smallpox. The legislature intermittently funded and resisted his work. During Cochran's tenure Alabama's delegated public health approach fell short of its aims and promises. Alabama proved to be a unique legislative experiment, as no other state formally granted such public power to an independent physician organization.[23]

The AMA did not aid or influence Cochran. If anything, it was the other way around. Cochran attended very few AMA meetings and the AMA never mentioned his activities until they had been accomplished. However, when the AMA reorganized in the early twentieth century it touted the Medical Association of the State of Alabama as an exemplary organizational model. Cochran's society held genuine power within the state and had remarkable physician discipline and participation. The state medical association claimed forty-four percent physician membership in 1873 and twenty years later it had an astounding two-thirds of the state's physicians.[24]

The economic, social, and professional realities could hardly have been more different in Illinois. Between 1860 and 1870 Alabama's population barely changed from 960,000, including 44 per cent slaves, to 996,000, 48 percent poorly-prepared "coloreds." Over the same Civil War decade, Illinois grew from 1,700,000, virtually 100 percent white, to 2,500,000. The value of personal property in Alabama fell from $516 per capita in 1860 to $293 in 1870, while it rose in Illinois, from $513 to $835. Alabama's literacy rate in 1870 was 65 percent, versus 97 percent in Illinois.[25]

Alabama's physicians were a small, elite group of well-educated white males, with 703 Alabama residents per physician in 1870 versus a national average of 618. It is not surprising that they banded together or that Alabama welcomed their efforts. In contrast, physicians of all sorts poured into the west's wide-open medical marketplace. There were 523 Illinois residents per physician in 1870, one of the lowest ratios of any major state. The Illinois State Medical Society had just 253 members in 1877 out of a regular physician population of at least 5,000, and less than half of those members paid their dues. With no physician loyalty or political power, the Illinois society's leaders looked to their state government to deal with public health problems, which, to them, included too many poorly trained physicians.[26]

What Illinois had that many other states lacked in 1877 was favorable experience with a government-run board of health. Facing a cholera scare, the state legislature created a Chicago Board of Health in 1867, modeled after New York City's board. Illinois State Medical Society member and APHA founder, John Rauch, helped write this legislation. Rauch served as chief sanitary officer of the Chicago health board from 1867 until 1873 and played a visible role in sanitation, smallpox prevention, and disaster relief following the Chicago fire of 1871. His board's work was demonstrably effective. With aggressive vaccination the number of smallpox cases in Chicago fell from 2,382 in 1872 to thirty-nine in 1875.[27]

Rauch was a year older than Reeves, born in Pennsylvania in 1828. He received his M.D. degree from the University of Pennsylvania in 1849 and moved to Iowa, where he entered medical practice. Rauch showed early interests in sanitation, natural sciences, and medical organizing. In 1855–1856 he spent time in Louis Agassiz's zoology laboratory at Harvard. The Iowa State Medical Society elected him its president in 1858, but before he could assume the position, he moved to Chicago to accept a faculty appointment at Rush Medical College. During the Civil War Rauch served with distinction in the Union Army Medical Corps, including evacuating the wounded after Antietam (1862) and serving as medical director during the lengthy siege of Port Hudson (1863).

Rauch became a public health ambassador after returning from his wartime service. He helped create the Chicago Board of Health in 1867 and served as its key officer until 1873. He helped organize the APHA in 1872 and served as its secretary until becoming vice president in 1875 and president in 1876. During the APHA's early development, from 1873–1875, he did not practice medicine, devoting his time to public health with little compensation.

Rauch had to know Chicago's other national medical organizer because of their common interests in public health and medical education. AMA founder Nathan Smith Davis moved from New York to Chicago in 1849 and he and Rauch were on the faculty of Rush Medical College in 1858. The two men were also members of the Illinois State Medical Society, where Davis was the Society's Permanent Secretary, although, after the war, neither man was particularly active in state society affairs. Rauch was busy with public health and Davis, who virtually always participated in national AMA events, was otherwise occupied with one of the largest medical practices in Chicago.[28]

Given Davis' position as the Illinois Medical Society's Permanent Secretary, one would assume that his state society rigorously followed the AMA's lead. But when Illinois passed its State Board of Health Act and its Medical Practice Act in 1877, the members of the Illinois State Medical Society were in open rebellion against the AMA. As Society President Thomas Fitch explained to his membership in 1877: "Our relation to the A.M.A. has always been of the most pleasant character till the past year, and I am quite sure that no cause of disturbance has ever been given, until the Illinois State

Medical Society through its executive became the leader in a revolution which I hope and believe will be heartily sustained by the Society."[29]

The revolution that separated the Illinois Medical Society from the AMA in 1877 was Illinois' answer to the woman question. The national organization, with Davis' guidance, sought to exclude women and blacks by changing its constitution in 1874 so that it only recognized delegates from state medical societies, local societies in good standing within the state, and branches of the military. By no longer seating delegates from medical colleges, hospitals, or any other non-medical society organizations, the AMA resolved the challenge from women's colleges and hospitals. "The woman question" and also the "colored" question were settled by referring them to local medical societies, where Davis knew they would quietly die.[30]

But Davis' Illinois colleagues saw the matter differently. The Illinois State Medical Society was one of eleven state societies that admitted women physicians (doctresses). The Society invited one of its new women members, Sarah Hackett Stevenson from the Women's Medical College in Chicago, to present a report on physiology at its 1876 annual meeting. Shortly thereafter, a delegate to the upcoming 1876 AMA annual meeting fell ill and asked that Stevenson be appointed in his place. After considerable controversy, which Stevenson sought to avoid, but her fellow Illinois delegates confronted on her behalf, the AMA agreed to seat her. The AMA reluctantly seated its first woman delegate in June 1876, during the country's Centennial celebration. When Illinois physicians began lobbying for state public health and medical licensing legislation in 1877, the state society was the national organization's black sheep cousin, not its dutiful offspring.[31]

Rauch, Davis and the state society's leaders launched a two-pronged legislative initiative in the 1877 Illinois General Assembly. The first bill, HB 485, sought to establish a state health board based on the Massachusetts model, the second, SB 196, was designed to institute medical licensure. Neither bill was identified with the AMA.[32]

The Chicago *Tribune* publicly opposed both measures, calling the board of health act "[an] expensive superfluity" and the medical licensure act, "the Doctors' Monopoly bill." The board of health act did not face serious legislative opposition, but the state's medical schools introduced an alternative licensing act that afforded certain colleges the right to examine and grant diplomas to practicing physicians not already possessing one. Rauch, Davis, and a few others pressed both causes, working the Assembly and, in opposition to the medical colleges' licensure bill, writing articles in the *Tribune* over the pseudonyms, "Judicium," and "S.S." (perhaps Sarah Stevenson).[33]

The two proposals moved easily through the Illinois Assembly, although their authors did not take success for granted. The Medical Practice Act stipulated that local medical societies would administer the licensing law unless the legislature created a state board of health, which would then oversee enactment of the licensing law. The successful passage of the State Board of Health Act in 1877 put Illinois in the business of medical licensure and, for the first time anywhere, brought licensure under a publicly-controlled state health board. The new health board would be appointed by the governor, with no mention of a requirement for physician members, and the licensure law applied to all physicians, regardless of sect.[34]

Illinois Governor Cullom appointed three regular physicians, including Rauch, one homeopathic physician, one eclectic physician, and two attorneys as the board's initial members. They quickly selected Rauch as Board President. Later, as its Secretary, Rauch dominated the Illinois State Board of Health until he was forced to resign in 1891.[35]

The new Illinois Board of Health contended with a yellow fever outbreak and began the tedious work of collecting vital statistics, but it devoted most of its energies to physician licensure. In his 1879 report to the Assembly, commenting on the Board's accomplishments, Governor Cullom acknowledged: "Owing to the pressure of the work imposed by the Medical Practice act, the Board has not done much in the way of sanitary investigation."[36]

The Medical Practice Act required the Board to register all Illinois physicians and issue licenses to those who: possessed a diploma or license from legally chartered medical institutions in good standing, passed an examination administered by the Board, or could document ten years' practice in good standing. In its first six months, the Board issued license certificates to 4,950 physicians and 424 midwives. It failed 221 out of 371 physician examinees and rejected about 400 inadequate or fraudulent diplomas.[37]

There is no evidence that Rauch and his fellow regulars initially used the Medical Practice Act to discriminate against irregulars. Starr estimated that approximately 80 percent of practicing physicians during this period were regulars and during its first year 76 percent of the physician licenses issued by the Illinois Board went to regular physicians, 18 percent to eclectics and homeopaths, and most of the remainder did not specify a branch of medicine. Likewise, eclectics and homeopaths could skip the section on therapeutics on the Board's examination and request examination by a Board member from their branch of medicine.[38]

The Illinois Board's initial emphasis on physician licensure and medical education was an understandable public health effort for the times. Regular physicians had an economic interest in reducing competition, but they also saw the consequences of poorly-trained and fraudulent practitioners, for example itinerant bone-setters with no knowledge of anatomy. The major medical sects publicly, if grudgingly, allied against dogma and ignorance. Illinois Medical Society President Washburn said in 1876: "But let us discriminate between the true and false, even in Eclecticism. I do not say all are guilty. Many are as innocent as any of the best who claim the strictest orthodoxy ... they have fair ability, study hard, and are devoted to their patients and profession.... Let us have wise and impartial legislation, so that every meritorious, well educated man shall be recognized, but every ignoramus debarred, whether he be regular or irregular."[39]

Arguments about medical ineptitude not only played off public fears, but, before the age of bacteriology and genuine disease abatement, produced an appearance of results. These efforts could be quantified and morally justified, whereas the consequences of other health activities, such as vaccination, sanitation, and quarantine, were often immeasurable and visibly disruptive. At the close of its first six months, the Illinois State Health Board's proudest accomplishment was that Iowa was overrun with Illinois doctors who could not comply with the new licensure law.[40]

Rauch saw the root of the practitioner problem as poor medical education, the same concern that had spawned the AMA thirty years earlier, but which the AMA had not solved. Rauch used state power to refuse diplomas from medical schools that did not meet the Board's standards. This unprecedented action was bolstered by the Illinois Attorney General's ruling that the Board could interpret the medical institutions in good standing language of the Medical Practice Act to exclude diplomas from any medical college that, in the Board's sole judgment, did not offer a course of study that would be generally regarded by the medical profession as sufficient to entitle a student to graduate and receive a diploma as Doctor of Medicine.[41]

Rauch launched an ambitious project to document the quality of American medical colleges. His Board asked a number of respected medical educators to specify the minimum curricular requirements for a diploma in 1880 and the following year it published a list of 119 active regular, eclectic, and homeopathic medical colleges in the United States and Canada, rejecting eighteen as either clearly fraudulent or failing to meet minimal education standards. The next year it added to the list and included new information on numbers of students.[42] Rauch's board was the first to tie physician licensing to educational specifics, which, in the next century, became the regulatory cudgel that closed dozens of marginal medical schools.

The Illinois Board vigorously enforced its licensure laws, imprisoning nine individuals in 1880 for violating the Medical Practice Act. In the short run, the Illinois Board's licensure actions had the desired effect, reducing the number of medical practitioners in the state from 7,400 in 1877 to 6,000 in 1885. In the longer run, Rauch's detailed review of medical colleges was the forerunner of the AMA's 1902 Council on Medical Education which, in turn, launched Abraham Flexner's landmark 1910 report for the Carnegie Foundation, *Medical Education in the United States and Canada.*[43]

Rauch's efforts had mixed results within Illinois. His Board implemented smallpox vaccination, collected data, published reports, and intermittently enforced yellow fever and diphtheria quarantines, but until the development of laboratory-based infection control in the next century, it lacked strong public support. Rauch later harassed alternative practitioners such as midwives, osteopaths, and opticians, and persecuted physicians who sought to advertise their services. Ultimately, Rauch created enough influential enemies that the legislature forced him to resign in 1891.[44]

Rauch's path-breaking educational efforts were not enough to deter shady educators seeking to profit from Illinois' gilded-age prosperity. He expressed his concerns about the influx anticipating Chicago's 1893 Columbian Exposition: "And never before in the same length of time has [sic] there been so many professional frauds attempting to obtain a foot-hold in that city."[45] But Rauch could not stop it. The AMA's Council on Medical Education concluded in 1906 that Illinois had some of the worst medical schools in the country.[46]

The legislative events in Alabama and Illinois marked the end of the Jacksonian approach to American medical regulation. Alabama created an American version of a British medical guild, and by including public health, granted greater powers to its medical organizations than the English did to theirs. Illinois followed a typically American route by bringing medical professionals inside government-run regulatory agencies. The growing role of governments in all levels of society and modest advances in medical and sanitary science fostered the rise of public health activism throughout the country.[47]

Reeves followed all of this and was ready to bring Illinois' public health ideas to West Virginia, but he needed a sympathetic state government. West Virginians obliged in 1880 by electing Jacob Jackson governor. The son of a jurist and a classic Redeemer, Jackson was a reformer with a particular interest in education. Reeves looked to the legislative session of 1881 and sought the assistance of a shrewd lawmaker many called West Virginia's Daniel Webster.

15

Reeves' Legislative Triumph

The state medical society could not bring preventive medicine to the public and secure the foundations of medical practice, so Reeves asked sixty-three-year-old James Ferguson to help him write a law that would improve on the Illinois model. Judge Ferguson, who had briefly served on the circuit court, was the Democratic leader of the West Virginia House of Delegates and a conduit to Charleston's business interests. Some West Virginians called Ferguson the state's Daniel Webster. Others referred to him as the alleged evil genius of the West Virginia Democratic Party.[1]

Reeves and Ferguson prepared a board of health bill for the 1881 legislative session. Ferguson was quickly tied up defending challenges to his authority and getting Johnson Camden elected U.S. senator, so Reeves turned to Wheeling attorney and state senator, Joseph Woods, to guide the bill's passage. Reeves chose well. Woods was an energetic twenty-eight-year-old graduate of Princeton law school, unrelated to Samuel Woods, who was serving his first term in the West Virginia legislature. He was a talented politician who later became Speaker of the West Virginia House of Delegates.[2]

After Woods introduced SB 35, An Act to Establish a State Board of Health and Vital Statistics and Regulating the Practice of Medicine and Surgery, Reeves went to work. He ignored his practice and spent his time answering questions, giving presentations, and meeting with legislators. When he was not lobbying for the bill, he built relationships. A month after Woods introduced the bill, he and Frances entertained legislators in their Chapline Street home.[3]

The three major components of the bill were the evaluation and control of disease outbreaks in humans and animals, the collection of vital statistics, and the regulation of the practice of medicine and surgery. Reeves used the same arguments he had repeated many times. He spoke to the State Senate's Judiciary Committee, contending that public health was important to a community's economic well-being and that three-fourths of diseases could be prevented by observing the laws of health. He claimed that physician regulation made overdue sense. A teacher must pass an examination before entering a classroom and a river pilot must know every shoal and bend before being permitted at the wheel: "But any man calling himself a doctor can swing his shingle and without any sort of restraint prey upon the lives and property of the people." Unlike the Chicago *Tribune*, which had resisted Rauch, the Wheeling *Intelligencer* endorsed his case, writing: "No man has a right to practice medicine who has not qualified himself for his duties by a reasonable course of study."[4]

Reeves' Democratic relationships brought political support and his medical society connections added six physician members of the West Virginia Legislature to the cause: former society president and state senator Andrew Barbee, and delegates Isaiah Bee, B.F. Irons, J.B. Crumrine, D.Q. Steere, and W.H. Wayt. The state's regular physicians supported the measure as did its newspapers. When an anonymous sectarian physician complained that the bill was a power-grab by regulars, the *Intelligencer's* editor responded that the small difficulties noted by the writer "have already been obviated."[5]

Reeves got most of what he wanted when the law passed in March 1881. The West Virginia Board of Health would be composed of six "reputable" physicians, two from each of the state's three Congressional districts, and no one else. The act did not specify regular physicians, but Reeves had the governor's ear. West Virginia would be the first state with a powerful health board run by regular physicians. County health boards, comprised of three persons, one of whom had to be a practicing physician, would implement the board's authority locally. These health boards were charged with monitoring disease threats to people and animals and empowered to "take such action, and adopt such rules, as they may in the exercise of their discretion deem efficient in preventing the introduction and spread of such disease or diseases."[6]

The new law included a physician licensure section, similar to Illinois' licensure law, which required that physicians needed to present a diploma from a reputable medical college, an affidavit that they had practiced in West Virginia more than ten years as of the date of the act, or pass an examination administered by the state board or a local board in order to practice medicine in West Virginia. As in Illinois, the penalty for non-compliance was a fine of not less than fifty or more than five hundred dollars and/or imprisonment in the county jail for not less than thirty days or more than one year.

There were two shortcomings to the act. The first was that the legislature removed vital statistics collection. This occurred because there was already a law requiring undertakers and burial ground sextons to report deaths to the county court.[7] The second issue was that the new state board was funded from one-time licensing fees, which would evaporate once the physician licensure process was completed. Reeves could live with the first problem because the law allowed for data gathering, but he knew that the second one had to be remedied.

Governor Jackson filled the Board with six regular physicians, including Reeves, on June 6, 1881. Two weeks later Board's members chose Reeves for secretary, the Board's executive officer. Reeves announced that on July 20 he would hold his first public session in Wheeling to begin issuing medical licensing certificates. The *Intelligencer* reported, "Hunt up your sheep skins gentlemen and be prepared to present them."[8]

Reeves represented the Medical Society of West Virginia at the AMA's annual meeting in Richmond shortly after the law passed. He attended the section on surgery but did not participate in or even attend the Section on State Medicine, the group that should have had the most relevance for him. This body was one of the AMA's six permanent sections, comprised of one member from each state plus the Army and Navy and representing the state boards of health.[9]

The most likely explanation for his lack of participation in an AMA section seemingly tailored for him was that the national physician organization was not interested in public health. The 1881 Section on State Medicine had barely enough participants to warrant the reading of two papers and its secretary recommended that if attendance did not improve in 1882, the group should disband.[10]

Reeves paid more attention to the annual meeting of the Medical Society of West Virginia, which he attended as an honored statesman in Wheeling on May 18 and 19, 1881. George Baird welcomed the forty-two delegates by praising the new law and singling out Reeves as the framer and guiding spirit of the new State Board of Health. President William van Kirk saw the law as the beginning of a new era of professional pride: "Never in the history of the Society, was there a more auspicious time than the present for turning over a new leaf in our government."[11]

Van Kirk was the nephew of Reeves' old friend Matthew Campbell and, like Louis Wilson of the Medical Society of Wheeling and Ohio County, a young Reeves admirer. He made clear who his model was, the man who had founded the Medical Society and created the State Board of Health: "Gentlemen, for those two most notable steps of medical progress in West Virginia, we are principally indebted to Dr. James E. Reeves, whose energies and self-sacrifices for legitimate medicine within our borders, will never be forgotten."[12]

Van Kirk signaled his moral kinship with Reeves by breaking with the post–Civil War medical society presidents who had preached organizational harmony. He reminded his peers that there were higher values than professional loyalty: "To say that a physician should do nothing derogatory to his profession, is not all that is demanded to complete the description of a perfect character, in which there must be the happy consummation of professional skill, refined tastes, unsullied honor, unimpeachable integrity, and the spirit of the humble and devout christian [sic]. What is learning, what is professional skill, without the quickening power which springs from a high moral character?"[13]

Reeves played a visibly supportive role. He participated in Society discussions and hosted members at his home. As the meeting ended, the grateful delegates elected Reeves the Society's next president. A month later the Ohio State Medical Society invited him to talk about West Virginia's new law at its annual meeting in Columbus.[14]

The Ohio invitation probably originated with the Ohio society's secretary, James Baldwin, the physician-editor who had harshly attacked AMA secretary Atkinson's self-serving *Physicians and Surgeons of the United States* in 1878. Baldwin was the well-educated scion of a scholarly family. His uncle was president of Oberlin College, where Baldwin graduated Phi Beta Kappa in 1870. The thirty-one-year-old Baldwin was beginning a fifty-year surgical career that would generate numerous technical innovations, more than two hundred papers, and a major textbook.[15]

Reeves and Baldwin were from different generations and backgrounds, but cut from the same cloth in their view of professional duties. Baldwin never took a vacation or went to the theater; medicine was all Baldwin knew. He fought for high professional standards and he vigorously opposed the era's abuses, such as diploma mills, fee-splitting, and nostrum-pushing. He confronted his peers even more than Reeves. His biographer, George Paulson, wrote, "He was ahead of his time, that is sure, but we cannot dissociate his strengths and weaknesses from his willingness to offend his colleagues."[16]

Baldwin sought Reeves' help because Ohio had no functioning medical licensure law and no state health board. Shortly after the Ohio meeting he asked Reeves to be West Virginia's correspondent for his new *Ohio Medical Journal.* Reeves obliged by reporting on the West Virginia Medical Society's recent meeting. He praised van Kirk's speech, noting that it afforded much pleasure to the members of the Society. He described the new state health law, downplaying its licensing provisions and summarizing its intent: "public health is public wealth."[17]

Nevertheless, physician licensing was the first order of business for the new West Virginia Board of Health, just as it had been for Rauch's board in Illinois. The process began with two contentious moments. Ten days after holding his first licensing session on July 20 in Wheeling, Reeves issued arrest warrants for two Wheeling doctors, M.J. Rhees and S.M. Hopkins, for violating the law. Rhees was a homeopathic physician who had missed his licensing appointment, but he quickly presented his diploma and received a license. In a sign of the changing times, Rhees wrote in the newspaper that the matter could have been quietly settled if Reeves had just called him on the telephone.[18]

Hopkins was another matter. He had not been in practice for ten years, did not have a diploma, and, on July 26, failed an examination administered by Reeves. Hopkins chose to appeal but he heard that Reeves would preside over his appeal and tracked Reeves down at his office. He verbally assaulted Reeves in the street and then challenged him to a brawl in front of a growing crowd. Reeves declined to fight. Instead he drove his buggy to the local magistrate and had Hopkins arrested for abusing him and disturbing the peace. Hopkins was fined five dollars and released on three hundred dollars bail. Shortly thereafter he failed to attend his licensure appeal and the matter, along with his right to practice medicine in West Virginia, was dismissed. The combative Hopkins threatened to challenge the law's constitutionality, but he never did.[19]

Reeves and the Board went about licensing physicians and setting up the administrative apparatus necessary for its sanitary duties. Given the newness of physician licensing and its troublesome record elsewhere, things went well for West Virginia. Hopkins proved to be the year's only serious incident. The Board issued certificates to 843 physicians during 1881. Most certificates were based on reputable diplomas or ten years of practice. Only ninety-four resulted from the Board's examination, which had an overall success rate of 80 percent.[20] According to the 1880 census, the state had 939 physicians.[21] Since the census likely inflated the total of practicing doctors, Reeves' Board licensed almost every practicing West Virginia physician in its first six months, rejecting very few, and getting only one threatening complaint. Reeves reported that his licensure work was well in hand at year's end and the board was ready to begin its sanitary duties.

In contrast to many states, the West Virginia press supported its Board's mandates. The Point Pleasant *Weekly Register*, near the Ohio River, wanted the Board to get down to work removing nuisances and investigating contagions. The Charles Town *Spirit of Jefferson*, on the opposite side of the state, asked the Board to prevent the introduction and spread of smallpox. In Wheeling, the *Intelligencer* ran a front-page article on a disreputable Ohio doctor to remind citizens of the need for professional regulation: "The territory of every State in the Union ought to be made hot for all such imposters."[22]

Reeves travelled to Savannah, Georgia, to attend the APHA's annual meeting in November 1881. This was more to his liking than the earlier AMA event. He was elected a member of the association's executive committee and entered into an intense debate over the future of the National Board of Health, which had been created in 1879 and was destined to die from lack of funding in 1883. Reeves' position was that the National Board should remain a freestanding entity and not a representative body of state health boards. He differed in this with the APHA's incoming second vice-president, Albert Gihon, Medical Director of the U.S. Navy. Reeves' sentiment carried the day, but he added future APHA president Gihon to his circle of friends. Reeves was so impressed with Gihon's presentation on the nobility of health that he asked Gihon to repeat his talk to West Virginia's physicians.[23]

The busy Board Secretary sent a three-page letter to West Virginia's physicians on Christmas Eve, 1881, listing the Board's accomplishments and seeking his fellow doctors' help in securing funding from the legislature. The Wheeling *Register* congratulated the State Board a few days later and encouraged local health boards to warn the populace against the scourges of domiciliary filth, bad air, bad whisky, and bad cooking.[24]

The hectic year included a personal watershed for Reeves. He left the Fourth Street Methodist Church in February 1881 and transferred his religious affiliation to St. Matthews Episcopal Church. From then on he was a regular member of St. Matthews, where his Wheeling funeral services were held in 1896. Those who knew him in later years saw him only as a sincere Episcopalian, despite his having been a devout Methodist for fifty-two years.[25]

Reeves did not leave an explanation for this important change. Everything about him stayed consistent with the teachings and practices of early nineteenth-century Methodism and his family, particularly his sister Ann, remained close to the Methodist Church. Reeves' wife Frances had been baptized in the Episcopal Church, so perhaps he switched to accommodate her wishes. Alternatively, Methodism was no longer the evangelical country religion that Reeves knew as a boy. Rural Methodist institutions, such as classes and itinerant preachers, could not exist in urban areas. Reeves may have felt, as Methodism sought to broaden its urban reach, that it had lost its identity. Perhaps he appreciated the more traditional doctrines of Frances' Episcopal Church. Consistent with a turn to religious formalism, he became longtime friends with John Kain, the popular Bishop of Wheeling's Catholic diocese.[26]

As 1882 began Reeves asked Governor Jackson and the Wheeling press to help prevent the board's fiscal death. The governor opened the 1882 special session of the legislature by encouraging delegates to provide a regular appropriation. The *Intelligencer* published a lengthy article praising Reeves and the new State Board of Health.[27]

The *Intelligencer* simultaneously reported that a steamer from Pittsburgh had arrived in Wheeling bearing a patient with smallpox. The reporter noted that the diligent board secretary, Dr. Reeves, quickly issued a quarantine order for all transportation entering West Virginia from Pittsburgh. The Wheeling papers used Pittsburgh's smallpox scare to highlight the board's work and Reeves literally made the point by personally vaccinating state senators.[28]

Reeves' funding campaign met little resistance and the legislature passed a revised Board of Health Act on March 15, 1882, which guaranteed the board's expenses up to $1,500 per year. The board's secretary could receive as much as $500 in annual salary, well below the $800 Reeves had received as Wheeling's health officer in 1869. The appropriation was hardly generous, but during the State Board's first two and one-half years, the thrifty Reeves spent an average of $1,300 per year.[29]

Reeves pushed the board's sanitation work forward in 1882, but events of his own making brought him into public confrontation with the extended medical clan of his long-time associate, William Dent. William's father, eighty-one-year-old Marmaduke Dent, was the first physician in northwestern Virginia's Preston County. William's brother, George was also an original member of the Medical Society of West Virginia. William's son, Frank, practiced with his father in Newburg. Another of William's brothers, Marshall, was a well-known newspaper man who had been an anti-secessionist delegate to the 1863 Richmond Convention. Marshall's son, Arthur Dent, was a physician who was a Medical Society member and secretary of the board of directors of the state insane asylum at Weston.[30]

Troubles began when Reeves made his Presidential Address to the Medical Society of West Virginia in May 1882. Most of the speech was a rallying call for the virtues of scientific medicine and public health. He highlighted France's Louis Pasteur and the young German, Robert Koch. He praised the work of West Virginia's physician legislators in securing the benefits of preventive medicine and sanitation for its citizenry.[31]

Near the talk's conclusion he turned to the problem of "cheap diplomas." Reeves used the case of an unnamed West Virginia physician who could not pass West Virginia's licensing examination in January 1882 to illustrate the bad faith of many medical colleges. After failing his examination this West Virginia doctor travelled to Columbus (Ohio) Medical College, where, without completing any courses, he paid his fees, passed the school's examinations, and a month later, received a diploma. Reeves continued by describing another 1882 Columbus medical graduate who was so ignorant that he did not know where the iris or pupil were located. He castigated medical colleges that relaxed their rules and named Ohio as the worst state for diploma mills.

The medical society audience did not know that Reeves was assisting his Ohio friend James Baldwin. Baldwin had helped found Columbus Medical College six years earlier, but he had been fired following the college's February graduation ceremonies. According to Baldwin, this was because he had objected to the school's awarding a degree to a student who didn't deserve to graduate. Reeves used his talk to buttress Baldwin's argument.[32]

Reeves' supportive medical society address had the desired effect. It soon appeared in Baldwin's *Columbus Medical Journal.* Several other medical publications attacked Columbus Medical College. William Wile, the editor of *The New England Medical Monthly*, wrote, "We join heartily with Dr. Reeves in the fight for higher medical education." The *Intelligencer* reprinted Wile's comments, complimenting Reeves' work to improve medical education and linking Columbus Medical College to "Ohio cheap diplomas."[33]

However, if the men in the speaker's audience knew nothing of Reeves' intentions to support Baldwin, many of them had to know the anonymous West Virginia physician he called out. Public records showed that Weston's Arthur Melville Dent was the only West Virginian in Columbus' 1882 graduating class.[34]

Dent and Columbus surgeon John W. Hamilton, the college's owner, were furious. Dent claimed that Reeves had acted out of deliberate malice and was a fraud. Hamilton placed a notice in the Wheeling papers that he would send the written component of Dent's final examination to anyone requesting a copy. Baldwin fought back in his Ohio journal. He accused Hamilton of attempting to "crush out a young man [Baldwin] who had the manhood to stand up for his own rights as a physician and surgeon and to oppose schemes that he regarded as dishonorable."[35]

And Arthur Dent was trapped in the middle, caught between the way things had always been and where they were going. His story exemplified the medical society machinations that Reeves wanted to end. Dent worked in a pharmacy and attended only one course of medical lectures before he began practicing in Weston in 1875. The Medical Society of West Virginia used its flexible standards to admit Dent to membership in 1878, even though he did not meet the diploma nor five years' practice requirements required by its constitution.[36]

Outside issues also dragged Dent into the West Virginia health board's spotlight. During the legislature's 1882 session, a special committee investigating problems at Weston's insane asylum reported that asylum board member Dent had repeatedly been publicly intoxicated. This would certainly have added to Reeves' concerns. Worse for Dent, Reeves' fellow health board member, West Virginia State Senator Andrew Barbee, was also leader in the state's temperance movement.[37]

The state board had to respond to Dent's seemingly legitimate but questionable diploma. Reeves encouraged board members, who had previously relied on Rauch's Illinois standards, to establish their own criteria for a reputable medical college. The group agreed, and the board's new criteria issued in July 1882 included course requirements similar to those mandated by Illinois, but with a stipulation that students must attend at least 80 percent of all required lectures. In adopting the attendance criteria the Board of Health determined that the Columbus Medical College did not meet them and refused to recognize its diplomas after 1881. The Board's retroactive actions affected only one West Virginian, Arthur Dent.[38]

Rather than retaking his West Virginia licensing examination or enrolling in a regular course of medical instruction, Dent followed the path used by many marginal physicians. He moved to a state where there were less effective licensure laws. Dent lived a comfortable medical life in Coshocton, Ohio, and died in 1900 at age fifty-one.[39]

Reeves' licensure net also caught Arthur's cousin, Frank. Frank Mortimer Dent had helped his uncle William in his Newburg medical practice and drug store as a teenager. He began calling himself "Dr. Dent" in 1876 and seeing patients on his own. When William applied for his medical license in August 1881, claiming the ten-year exemption rather than presenting a diploma, he also applied for a license for M. Dent based on thirty years practice, with the licenses to be sent to his office. Reeves forwarded the certificates to Newburg as William requested.[40]

After almost all of West Virginia's physicians were licensed in July 1882 Thomas Lanham, a prominent Newberg regular physician, wrote the board secretary asking the class of physicians from which Frank M. Dent was registered. Reeves was perplexed because his records only contained certificates for William and M. Dent. He wondered if he had made a mistake with M. Dent's certificate, omitting the letter "F." He had no personal knowledge of William's father Marmaduke or his son Frank, so he sent a letter to Dr. F. M. Dent in Newberg asking about the presumed error in his certificate.[41]

William returned a sorrowful letter, stating that his son Frank was too ill to practice and confined to a sanatorium. William had searched for the missing certificate, but could not find it. Would Reeves be kind enough to send a replacement to F.M. Dent and William would return the original when it was discovered? Reeves was about to forward a duplicate in the name of F.M. Dent when Lanham sent him another letter, advising that M. Dent, the physician grandfather, was bed-ridden with a stroke while his grandson, F.M. Dent, was seeing patients in town.

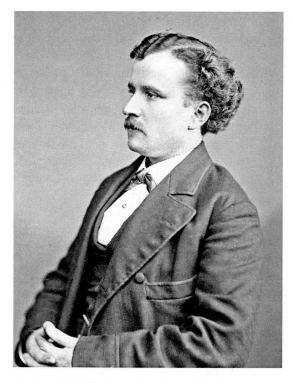

Arthur Melville Dent (1848–1900), approximately 1882. Arthur practiced medicine in Weston, WV, where he was a board member of the state's insane asylum. He never completed formal medical training and ran afoul of Reeves' licensure law when he passed final exams at Columbus (OH) Medical College in 1882 and received a diploma without attending classes. The West Virginia Board of Health rejected his diploma and Dent left the state (West Virginia and Regional History Center, WVU Libraries).

Seemingly arisen from his sanatorium bed, Frank Dent quickly sent Reeves an explanatory letter on his father's stationery. According to Frank, his father had made an error, confusing his grandfather's certificate with his own. Despite his poor health Frank had obtained a diploma earlier that year from a Cincinnati medical college, which he had sent to the Board. He said he had never received a reply, but he had. Not yet known to Reeves, the local board had rejected Frank's certificate as coming from an unrecognized eclectic institution.[42]

When these facts came to light, Reeves felt that his overly protective colleague, William, had attempted to dupe him and that Frank had broken the law. Frank was not institutionalized, as his father had stated, he was actively practicing medicine without a license. Reeves had Frank arrested and he was indicted in November 1882 for violating West Virginia's Board of Health Act. Frank replied in the local paper that while he was so ill he was confined to his room, he had still completed two full courses from a medical college "whose curriculum is not excelled."[43] He intended to fight the charges and, if necessary, the law. His trial was set for April 1883.

The Dent family saw a personal vendetta in Reeves' persecutions of Arthur and Frank and turned to Frank's cousin, Marmaduke H. Dent to fight their cause. Arthur's half-brother was a young Grafton attorney who was the initial graduate of the University of West Virginia (1870) and the recipient of the school's first graduate degree (1873).[44] M.H. Dent was also a stubborn country lawyer and Frank's arrest was the kind of underdog battle that he loved. A later biographer described him as, "a mountaineer Don Quixote."[45] M.H. Dent and Samuel Woods attended a Democratic convention in August 1882 where Dent vigorously took one side of a difficult issue and Woods quietly took the other. Woods pronounced Dent's efforts: "an apple of discord."[46]

M.H. Dent moved to overturn his cousin's indictment, claiming that Reeves' law was unconstitutional. This request was quashed and the Dents entered a plea of not guilty. Frank half-heartedly claimed that his diploma from the American Eclectic Medical College in Cincinnati satisfied the Board's requirements, but at his April 1883 trial the judge sided with the Board's rejection and found him guilty, fining him fifty dollars and costs. M.H. Dent promptly filed an appeal.

The deck was stacked against the Dents, but they probably did not know it. Governor Jackson had appointed Woods to the state's Supreme Court in January 1883. If the fervent Grafton attorney hoped to challenge the constitutionality of Reeves' law, he had to go through Reeves' lifelong friend, Justice Samuel Woods. Woods received the case for the West Virginia Court of Appeals and issued a stay of proceeding, pending the appeal.[47]

The Dents never again argued for the legitimacy of Frank's diploma. Instead they maintained that West Virginia had no authority to interfere with his constitutional right to practice medicine. But, in hindsight, was Dent's diploma valid, suggesting that Reeves and the board may have pursued him because he was not a regularly-trained physician?[48]

The local board relied on Illinois' determination that the American Eclectic Medical College was not a reputable medical college when it ruled on Dent's diploma. According to Reeves, anyone could buy a diploma from the American Eclectic Medical College for thirty dollars. The AMA reiterated in 1906 that the defunct American Eclectic Medical College had been a fraudulent diploma mill, whereas Cincinnati's Eclectic Medical Institute was, and remained, a legitimate institution. Although the West Virginia Board denied Dent's diploma, it accepted twenty graduates from the Eclectic Medical Institute during the same period. The evidence suggests that Dent's diploma was fraudulent and that Reeves' board accepted eclectic physicians who met reasonable training standards.[49]

Before the West Virginia Supreme Court ruled on Dent's appeal, the family circulated a petition to overturn the state's Board of Health Act. According to the petition, the law's only purpose was "to furnish the 'charlatan' who lobbied it through the legislature [a] means of subsistence." The most specific objection, harking to Dent's constitutional claim and having nothing to do with sanitation, disease prevention, or Frank's diploma, was that the law penalized a man for an act that was not punishable at the time it was committed.[50]

M.H. Dent's formal appeal to the West Virginia Supreme Court was a legal broadside directed at the act's licensing language, claiming that it violated long-standing concepts of justice and multiple sections of the West Virginia and United States Constitutions. Calling on the Magna Carta, Dent claimed that no government can interfere with the right of a citizen to pursue his lawful trade.[51]

Woods delivered the Court's unanimous decision to Frank and M. H. Dent on November 1, 1884. Chief Justice Green, writing for the four-member Court, rejected all of Dent's arguments. Green began by refuting Dent's assertion that the Court should consider principles of natural justice. He noted that legislatures may do whatever they want, so long as they act constitutionally. He pointed out that states had legitimate police powers and regulated all manner of commerce. Where other laws regulating physicians had been challenged, state courts had upheld them. Green observed that states had an interest in protecting citizens from untrained physicians and that laws accomplishing this goal need not be wise, but they must be fair and constitutional. He found no evidence that West Virginia's statute violated these requirements, even as he acknowledged that the law's enforcers might act capriciously. The Court affirmed the circuit court's judgment against Frank Dent.[52]

M.H. Dent was not done. Medical licensure had not been challenged under the U.S. Constitution and the Mountaineer lawyer wanted to prove that West Virginia's legislation violated the Fourteenth Amendment. A month after losing in West Virginia, he notified Woods that he intended to appeal the court's decision to the U.S. Supreme Court. He filed in time for the October 1885 session; however, the Supreme Court was backlogged. It did not hear his case for another four years.[53]

M.H. Dent's public insults affronted Reeves and the Board of Health. When the Court of Appeals ruled against Frank Dent, Reeves reprinted Justice Green's decision in his annual report to the governor. He called attorney Dent, "an obscure lawyer—but with large pretensions [who] had the temerity to read a lesson in Constitutional law to the Supreme Court of the State."[54]

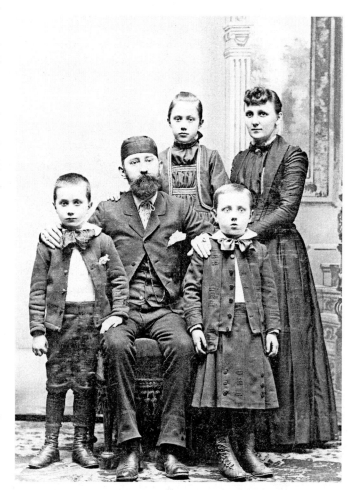

Frank Mortimer Dent (1854–1900) and family in 1890. Left to right: Francis Dent, Frank Dent, Nellie Dent, Gaylord Dent, and Ida (Frazier) Dent. He lived in Newburg, WV, as did his father and grandfather, also physicians. He fought his 1882 arrest for practicing medicine without a valid license and was the plaintiff in the landmark U.S. Supreme Court case, *Dent v. West Virginia* (1889). Frank was Arthur M. Dent's cousin (courtesy Sue Hersman).

Despite their assertions, the Dents did not have popular support. The Wheeling *Intelligencer* reported on the Dent decision as, "A Doctor's Diploma and What His Deceit Cost Him." In contrast to the petition's claim that the populace wanted nothing to do with the law, the paper told its readers that Reeves' law was well-received by physicians and the public and that the Dent family was unlikely to achieve its goal of repeal: "in light of the threatened invasion by the Asiatic cholera."[55]

Frank Dent did not have a medical license as his case awaited review in Washington, but, unlike his cousin Arthur, he did not leave West Virginia for a more tolerant professional location. Nor did he relinquish his claim to being a physician. Instead, he ran the family drug store in Newburg, presenting himself as "Dr. F.M. Dent—Druggist," until he died in 1900 at age 46.[56]

The flare-ups with Hopkins and the Dents were Reeves' only serious licensing altercations during his time as board secretary. He occasionally chased a travelling quack out of the state, but in 1884 he proudly reported that there were no violations of the law during the year.[57]

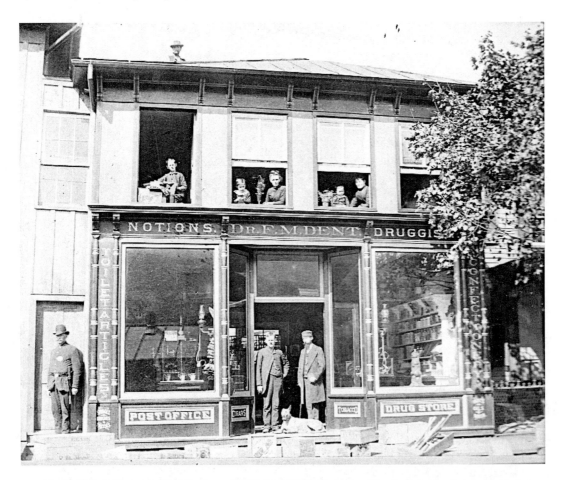

Frank Dent's drugstore in Newburg, WV, circa 1898. Dent has the skull cap and cane in center. Never licensed to practice medicine and the holder of a fraudulent eclectic diploma, Dent referred to himself as "Dr. F.M. Dent" for the remainder of his life (courtesy Sue Hersman).

Reeves' low-key approach to physician licensing generated a pivotal legal precedent even though there was far more licensing friction elsewhere. When Rauch was four years into implementing Illinois' public health laws in 1881 his board still spent much of its time dealing with licensure issues. Illinois had more than five times as many physicians as West Virginia and six medical colleges, where West Virginia had none; however, its heavy licensure workload was not due to the size of the physician population nor the evolving definition of what was considered a reputable medical institution. It resulted from the way Rauch used the law to enforce his interpretation of medical ethics.

The Illinois board undertook 350 reviews of improper behavior in 1881 and held thirty-nine formal investigations, resulting in thirteen license revocations. Most of this effort was to root out claims of specialization and other forms of unethical advertising. Rauch boasted about thinning the ranks of Illinois physicians: "As there is still an average of one physician to about every 570 inhabitants, the State can well afford to spare all of this class." Rauch's use of his government position to reduce professional competition detracted from the

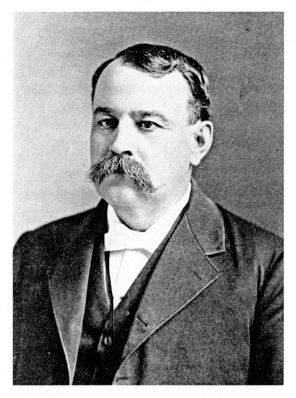

Marmaduke Herbert Dent (1849–1909), date unknown. M.H. Dent was Arthur Dent's half-brother. He received the first bachelor's (1870) and master's (1873) degrees given by the University of West Virginia. He practiced law in Grafton and represented his cousin Frank after Reeves had Frank arrested in 1882. He was later elected to the West Virginia Supreme Court of Appeals, serving from 1893 to 1905 (West Virginia and Regional History Center, WVU Libraries).

board's accomplishments, infuriated many physicians, and damaged his credibility. The Illinois Supreme Court chastised his board in 1888 for inappropriately revoking a physician's license and his enemies forced him to resign from the board in 1891.[58]

Reeves did not follow Rauch's lead, even though he deplored physician self-promotion. John E. Smith of Wheeling was a licensed regular physician who lived down the street from Reeves and regularly advertised himself in the newspaper. Smith offered numerous testimonials and claimed that: "Patients at a distance may be treated by letter and satisfaction guaranteed."[59] Smith was not a fraud, but, by AMA standards, he was unethical. Rauch would have threatened Smith with license revocation, but Reeves never bothered him.

Confederate sympathizer Reeves issued a certificate in 1882 to Boswell Stillyard, a black physician who, unlike Arthur and Frank Dent, successfully passed the Board's examination. The Wheeling *Register* applauded the action: "A Democratic Board was more than willing to give the colored brother a chance." Reeves appreciated that Wheeling's small black community needed its own physicians and Stillyard did well. He regularly served on the City Council and on his death in 1916 the *Intelligencer* praised his civic contributions, calling him, "a man of more than usual brilliancy."[60]

Perhaps the most telling example of how differently Reeves saw his responsibilities from most other physician regulators occurred in 1887, after he left the West Virginia Board of Health. Perry Millard, Secretary of Minnesota's newly formed Board of Medical Examiners and AMA First Vice President addressed the AMA on the necessity of state regulation of medical practice. Millard called for stricter educational standards, an appeal Reeves could favor, but Millard's goal was to improve his profession's economic well-being: "It is, however, ordained that in our profession, the noblest of them all, we shall be left to a competition that is intolerable to an educated man."[61]

When Millard finished his address, Reeves spoke in solitary dissent. He supported better education, but not if it reduced the public's access to medical care. He reminded the AMA, "That there are some communities where a man of first class medical qualifications could not live." He told the group that the profession had an obligation to see that poor communities were served and should exercise judgment in applying educational standards.[62]

The Dent affair had lasting national consequences, but it was a minor episode during Reeves' tenure on the West Virginia Board of Health. West Virginians wanted their health officers to prevent the spread of communicable diseases more than chase down marginal practitioners. One of Reeves' first official actions was imposing an 1882 smallpox quarantine against Pittsburgh. The next year saw a major smallpox outbreak in Baltimore, but only sporadic cases in West Virginia, to which the state and local boards responded. The newspapers followed these events closely and praised Reeves for keeping West Virginians safe.[63]

Reeves' Board did not do food inspections, but it did deal with livestock epidemics, such as an episode of cattle fever in 1882 that was called Texas cattle fever or splenic fever, probably anthrax. The solution was quarantine and culling of diseased cattle, with the belief that the disease arose in contaminated soil. Two years later the board instituted a hog quarantine in Ohio County to prevent the spread of hog cholera and the sale of contaminated meat. Reeves did microscopic examinations of hog tissues and took them to Washington, D.C., for further analysis by the Bureau of Agriculture.[64]

Reeves also requested and reviewed information from local health boards to seek potential disease connections with environmental, behavioral, and social data, including weather, geography, household hygiene, school hygiene, social habits, diet, and community moral standards. He used the same statistics to prompt communities to attend to sanitation, vaccination, work-related illnesses, and care of the sick. Reeves reminded West Virginians that diseases had financial costs in terms of care required and labor lost. He told anyone who would listen that a quarter of the annual deaths from consumption, scarlet fever, diphtheria, and typhoid fever were preventable. For Reeves, his medical science was a community good.[65]

Reeves' state board work solidified his national reputation for public health leadership. New York's Stephen Smith wrote in 1881 that Reeves' law was, "the brightest example in modern times of a state accepting, in full faith, the claims of Preventive

Medicine." Rauch told his APHA colleagues in 1882 that Reeves' law was, "better than that in any other State in this Union." Shortly after Rauch praised Reeves, the country's leading public health journal, *The Sanitarian,* repeated his comments and added accolades of its own: "West Virginia has taken position in the front rank of State health service.... This is chiefly due to the special energy and promptitude of the accomplished Secretary and executive officer of the Board, Dr. James E. Reeves and the hearty co-operation of the medical profession throughout the state."[66]

⼁ 16 ⼁

The Eminent Domain
of Sanitary Science

Reeves used his national connections to encourage public health laboratory work even if the purpose was undefined. He asked the National Board of Health to analyze Wheeling's water in 1882. The Board reported that his city's water was hazy and contained less chlorine, but about the same amounts of other measured chemicals as Washington, D.C., and Yonkers, New York. The report stated, "little can be gained from this one examination of the waters."[1]

But a Berlin speech that same year changed public health and validated Reeves' and other physicians' faith in laboratory science. Robert Koch, a thirty-eight-year-old German physician announced on March 24, 1882, that he had discovered the elusive germ that caused consumption, phthisis, and tuberculosis, all synonyms for the disease John Bunyan had called "the captain of all these men of death."[2]

Koch began his talk at the Berlin Physiological Society by reminding the assembled scientists that one in seven persons died of tuberculosis. He told the group that he had found what appeared to be the same rod-shaped micro-organism in every case of tuberculosis he studied. He had grown the bacillus in laboratory media, inoculated animals with it, where it produced the disease, and then recovered the organism from the animals. It had to be the cause.[3]

Koch's listeners were astonished. Future Nobel Prize-winner Paul Ehrlich described Koch's presentation as his greatest scientific experience. Ehrlich returned to his laboratory that evening to work on a better stain for demonstrate the bacillus. Within two months he developed a technique of heating and decolorizing with acid that made it much easier to locate the organism. Franz Ziehl and Friedrich Neeson soon improved Ehrlich's work, devising the foundation of today's acid-fast stain. By the end of 1882 any good microscopist could see the living organism that caused tuberculosis.[4]

Koch published his studies on April 10, 1882, in an eighteen-page report that was subsequently called, "One of the greatest advances in medicine recorded in one of the most concise documents of medical literature." Two weeks afterward, the London *Times* reported Koch's findings, which were sent to New York via transatlantic telegraph and reported in the New York *World* the next day. On May 3, 1882, the New York *Times* published the entire story. Three days later the *Intelligencer* broke the dramatic news to West Virginians. Given Pasteur's experiments a year earlier with an anthrax vaccine

142

in animals, the Wheeling paper wondered if a successful vaccine against consumption might not be far off?[5]

Austin Flint comprehended the meaning of Koch's discovery better than most American physicians. Flint anticipated the germ theory, but he knew it lacked a compelling archetype. He wrote in his 1881 medical textbook: "Assuming that the germ theory, as applied to all infectious diseases, will hereafter become established … it can hardly be otherwise than that great changes will be thereby wrought, not only in pathology, but in therapeutics."[6]

Following Koch's breakthrough, Flint revised his book, adding a special appendix devoted to Koch and tuberculosis. He knew that medicine had turned a corner; Koch's tubercle bacillus was the sole cause of tuberculosis and all other explanations were wrong. Physicians like Flint, who knew Elisha Bartlett's 1844 *Essay on the Philosophy of Science,* had every reason to believe that mankind might never find the causes of its major afflictions. Now here was one.[7]

Flint was equally sure that patient factors influenced susceptibility to the bacillus, but there could be no doubt that tuberculosis was a communicable disease, spread from person to person by a germ anyone could see with a microscope. Appropriately cautious, he concluded that the new information opened doors to disease prevention, but not yet to cure.

European bacteriological discoveries soon arrived in waves. Koch and Eberth described the typhoid bacillus in 1880 and Gaffky showed the connection between this organism and typhoid fever in 1884. Laveran described the malaria parasite in 1880 and American bacteriologist George Sternberg confirmed the finding in 1885. Klebs saw the diphtheria bacillus in 1883 and Löffler isolated it in 1884. Koch discovered the causative agent of cholera in 1883. Nicolaier discovered the tetanus bacillus in 1884.[8]

These stunning discoveries were hard for some scientists to duplicate. Technical problems and the lack of specific treatment for disease germs encouraged doubts about the European reports. Even if true, physicians did not know what to do with them. Historian John Harley Warner described the common physician response to the arriving bacteriologic breakthroughs as *cui bono?* For whose benefit was this new knowledge?[9]

But the germ theory provided a beacon to the struggling sanitarians who preached the messages of preventive medicine and they grasped its implications sooner than their practitioner colleagues. Reeves said in his 1882 Medical Society of West Virginia speech: "Just now the whole medical world is electrified by the light of the microscope in the hands of a young German physician—Dr. Koch of Berlin."[10] Albert Gihon addressed the AMA's sparsely-attended Section of State Medicine that year and observed that sanitation had no laboratory science behind it, perhaps, he urged: "it will be wise for us to appropriate the field in which Koch and Klebs and Fakker and Wood and Formad are gaining distinction."[11]

Reeves believed that medicine's scientific breakthroughs placed physicians at the front lines of public health. When he spoke to the APHA in 1882 he said, "If we fail in getting what we desire to carry on this great work of sanitation in America it is not because the American people are to blame. It is not the laymen, but the medical profession, whose duty it is to deal with the sick, and it is to the medical profession the people must look for their welfare." Reeves' self-imposed tasks were to expand the role of public health and ensure that physicians took the lead. At the same meeting, he campaigned to restrict APHA voting membership to professional sanitarians, which increasingly meant physicians. The APHA adopted his proposal and elected him second vice-president, behind Gihon in succession to the presidency.[12]

Reeves favored physician leadership and supported laboratory science, but he also saw a broader mission that encompassed all of his community's health needs. He presented his expanded vision of public health at the APHA's 1883 meeting: "The Eminent Domain of Sanitary Science and the Usefulness of State Boards of Health in Guarding the Public Welfare." The *Detroit Free Press*, from the meeting's host city, and the Wheeling *Intelligencer* gave the presentation extensive coverage. The APHA published the talk, as did the *Journal of the American Medical Association* and at least four other medical journals.[13]

Reeves described a future for American public health in his 1883 speech that was beyond nuisance abatement, quarantine, and data collection: "Good health, therefore, embraces *value* in the broadest sense of that term. On the individual, it confers happiness, dignity, and a thousand advantages in the struggle of life. To the state, it gives wealth, power, and freedom [author's italics]." He argued, as he had for years, for the economic benefits of a healthy workforce, that "we may have some conception of the real value of the earnings of the human machine." He stated that advances in sanitation had prolonged human life, a belief that now had actuarial legitimacy.[14]

Reeves spoke in favor of immigration, temperance, public schools, proper sewage treatment, healthy exercise, and state boards of health to oversee all of these. He argued for medical licensure: "to restrain the ignorant pretender in medical practice, who strikes at both life and purse." He advocated for women: "Woman gave Massachusetts the first state board of health in the United States, and from that beginning, in 1869, twenty-eight states have followed the example. There is yet much work for her to do, and none can do it so well as she."[15]

Reeves wanted his fellow doctors to take a view of their profession that encompassed his broad definition of public health. He invited Gihon to inspire West Virginia physicians to work for the health of their communities, which had as much, if not more to gain from medical science than individual patients. *The Intelligencer* gave Gihon's 1882 Medical Society of West Virginia address, "Health the True Nobility," wide coverage, including his criticism of physicians for "narrowing the true scope of their calling and becoming mere curers of disease."[16] Reeves invited Assistant Surgeon General John Shaw Billings to his Wheeling home in 1883 and obtained a resolution from the Medical Society urging the U.S. Congress to make appropriations necessary to protect the Army Medical Museum and the Surgeon General's library.[17]

But events foreseen by Gihon pushed American public health away from practitioners and into a narrow technical box. Reeves was APHA president-elect when the APHA met in St. Louis in October 1884. There were standard speeches on the evils of poor ventilation, decaying matter, and intemperance, but there were new presentations on disease germs. Well-known sanitarians, such as George Sternberg and Charles Smart, posed questions that required laboratory answers: did pathogenic bacteria arise from harmless predecessors? How could one detect the recently-discovered typhoid and cholera germs in drinking water? When Reeves spoke, he turned to the subject of pollution in Wheeling's water supply, and reminded his audience that clear water could carry disease. Public health was beginning its move from the streets to the medical laboratory.[18]

APHA President Gihon handed his organization's gavel to Reeves in 1884. Gihon acknowledged the incoming president's stature: "I have the pleasure of presenting to you the president-elect. I need not say anything in eulogy of him. He was present at the birth of this association, and I am sure he will be in with it at its death, if that should ever happen." Reeves thanked the group and voiced his anticipation for its upcoming meeting in the nation's capital. The Wheeling *Register* noted the events and proudly told West Virginians that their state had received a crowning honor with Reeves' election to the APHA presidency.[19]

Reeves' relationships with organized medicine during these years were supportive, if not paramount, but they were occasionally marked with friction. He had a public falling-out with Nathan Davis, AMA founder, former president, and editor of the newly launched *Journal of the American Medical Association*, over their different world views in 1884. Davis published Ohio's proposed medical licensing law in his *Journal* and called it defective for recognizing alternative medical sects. Having worked with Baldwin and other Ohio physicians to make the legislation politically acceptable, Reeves wrote back that Davis was attempting to sink something Ohio desperately needed. He suggested that Davis mind his own business.[20]

Davis countered that he was laboring to improve licensing and medical education before Reeves was old enough to know the members of one profession from another. In reality, Davis had no practical experience with passing legislation and the AMA had not changed medical education in thirty-five years; nevertheless, he encouraged Ohio to move slowly so that it might enact a law that met his version of "the correct principles on which all such legislation should be founded.."[21]

Reeves let the matter end there. He was not one to shrink from a tussle, but he had more serious difficulties to address. At the apex of his professional career, he developed serious medical problems. He was unable to work for a month in March 1884 due to an unknown illness. By May he was well enough to travel with his wife, Frances, to Washington, D.C., and later that month he participated in the West Virginia Medical Society's Clarksburg meeting. Seemingly recovered during the summer, Reeves resumed his work as Secretary of the State Health Board and played an active role in the October 1884 APHA meeting in St. Louis.[22]

But he was too sick to leave his house in January 1885. In early February he confided to Governor Jackson that he might need to step down from the state health board. The diagnosis was acute rheumatism, which, in 1885, meant a febrile sickness with pain in several joints. Among today's medical possibilities, it could have been rheumatic fever. But the more likely diagnosis, Given Reeves' handling of pathologic specimens and his later death from liver cancer, was a disease not recognized at the time, hepatitis B.[23]

Reeves resigned from the Board of Health On February 24, 1885, telling the governor, "God knows how earnestly my whole heart has been engaged in this work." Jackson appointed Reeves' kindred spirit, Louis Wilson, to succeed him. The Wheeling *Intelligencer* wrote that West Virginia had sustained a loss and the *Register* reported,

"His retirement will be deeply deplored by the members of his profession and the people of the State at large, who had long recognized his eminent fitness for the position."[24]

Baldwin wrote in his journal that Reeves' resignation was a severe loss for sanitary science. The *Maryland Medical Journal* commended West Virginia's leadership and agreed that Reeves' public health work had influenced the nation. *The Sanitarian* lauded his accomplishments and noted that sanitarians throughout the United States would regret to learn of the news.[25]

The editor of the *New England Medical Monthly* quickly asked Reeves for a personal profile for a section that sketched the lives of medical icons like Pasteur, Flint, and Gross. Reeves turned to Samuel Woods. His close friend must have feared for Reeves' health because he wrote an almost eulogistic biography. Justice Woods described Reeves as a self-made man who had successfully fought his way from the humble positions of a modest practitioner in an obscure country village to the first rank of physicians and sanitarians. After recounting Reeves' achievements, Woods turned reflective: "Would that the world, and especially the profession to which he belongs, had more of such men, that all might, truthfully say: 'The world is better— since he has lived in it.'" It was the only biography of Reeves published in his lifetime.[26]

Reeves recovered from his illness, but when Frances developed a similar episode of inflammatory rheumatism in August, he had to be concerned about the upcoming 1885 APHA meeting as well as her health. He had helped organize a forum of state health boards at the 1884 St. Louis conference, intending to provide a connection for physician regulators. He also arranged for Henry Lomb, co-founder of the Bausch and Lomb Optical Company, to offer financial prizes for scholarly papers in the social areas of public health that Reeves wanted to encourage. He needed to be in Washington in December to move these initiatives forward.[27]

Frances improved, and by November 1885 the city's press effused over Reeve's role in the approaching APHA assembly: "The reasonable expectation is that this coming meeting will be the most successful one ever held by the Association." The local newspapers talked up Reeves and West Virginia's admirable health laws.[28]

Washington's Willard Hall was filled with statistical charts when Reeves gaveled the APHA's thirteenth annual meeting to order at ten a.m. on December 8, 1885. There were no special decorations to suggest that the event was anything other than a serious affair. For the rest of the morning one hundred delegates amended the APHA's constitution, discussed incorporation, reviewed committee reports, and accepted new members, one of whom was the Wheeling *Intelligencer's* editor, Charles Hart. After several hours of tedious business, a visibly relieved Reeves announced that the time had come for the reading of papers. New Jersey's Ezra Hunt opened the scientific session with a discussion of "Sanitary and Statistical Nomenclature."[29]

Following the day's presentations the APHA reconvened at eight p.m. in public session. President Grover Cleveland sent his regrets for not being present, but invited the delegates to meet with him the next day. There were several hundred people at the evening festivities, which concluded with Reeves' presidential address.

Reeves' 1885 APHA presidential speech was more than welcoming pleasantries, but it was not the expansive discourse on sanitary science he delivered in 1883. He had people to acknowledge and the hour was late. He touched on his favorite themes: the economic value of a healthy workforce, the need for better legislation, and the elevation of the role of women. He mentioned Henry Lomb's generous offer of $2,800 in prizes for public health papers. The only specific call he made was for a national biological laboratory to be associated with the Army Medical Museum, a laboratory that was eventually funded and led to the National Institutes of Health. Reeves' remarks were mostly after-dinner commentary, but the *Intelligencer's* sympathetic editor reprinted every word.[30]

Reeves recognized Lomb and his awards several times during the daily sessions and he and John Shaw Billings saw to it that the APHA made Lomb a life member. The Lomb Prize was important to Reeves because it emphasized that public health was more than quarantine, urban sanitation, statistics, and laboratory investigation. It rewarded papers on working class nutrition and health, schoolhouse hygiene, personal management of infectious disease, and occupational illnesses. Reeves' effort was a transient success. There were numerous submissions that year, including several from foreign countries. The APHA reprinted the four winning entries in a separate, 198-page book.[31]

Reeves also wanted the APHA to nurture relationships between state health boards and the public servants, mostly physicians, who ran them. With his urging, the APHA created a standing committee on state boards and its secretary, New Hampshire's Granville Conn, read the committee's first report on December 9, 1885. Seeing the task as a mundane committee function, Conn said he had sent inquiries to all health boards requesting information, but only twelve states and two Canadian provinces had responded. He summarized the information sent to him and took his seat. APHA President Reeves was not satisfied.[32]

After Conn finished his lackluster account, Reeves went around the room, asking delegates from states that had not replied to Conn to describe their board's activities. Kentucky's J.N. McCormack summarized the dazed response of his peers: "I would say that this meeting is rather a surprise to the representatives from most of the state boards of health." Reeves politely countered that it was the chair's duty to see that all states were heard from. His audience rose to the occasion. In the end, fifteen U.S. delegates discussed the status of state boards and two Canadians commented on their provincial work. From the chair Reeves used his own example to encourage APHA members to do more: "the State Board of Health of West Virginia is merely an outgrowth of this Association."[33]

The APHA's thirteenth annual meeting concluded on December 11, 1885, and Reeves' parting homilies recounted the organization's humble origins and its considerable accomplishments: "We have grown to be a power, not only in this land, but recognized as a power and influence in sanitation wherever the English tongue is spoken." He returned to Wheeling the next day, having done his duty for public health.[34]

Reeves' APHA efforts left a bookmark on unresolved tensions within America's public health movement. Henry Lomb supported two more essay competitions over the next three years, ending in 1888 with a five hundred dollar prize that attracted seventy applications on the topic of "Practical Sanitary and Economic Cooking Adapted for Persons of Moderate and Small Means," another subject far from the public health mainstream. Once Lomb's philanthropy ended, the APHA lost interest. Well into the next century, America's public health movement could not agree that such areas were part of its mission. Likewise, the APHA and its members drifted away from organizing and improving state health boards. At the seventeenth annual meeting, in 1889, the delegates decided that the committee on state boards served no useful purpose and disbanded it.[35]

Reeves was confident that physicians had the right combination of scientific understanding and public spirit to shepherd public health and, with enough urging, they would embrace their community responsibilities. He did not grasp the conflicting issues that undermined physician-led public health.

The preacher's son saw medicine's ethics in Christian religious terms, as strictures for the faithful, not subjects for state regulation. Other physicians saw ethics as part of the regulatory bulwark that protected their profession's citadel against its competitors. Reeves sermonized against homeopathy and eclecticism as unscientific dogmas that must be confronted with better science, yet he never suggested that well-educated sectarian practitioners who advertised their services, or those who consulted with them, were criminals. Likewise, he dealt with Todd's nostrum-pushing and Hupp's duplicity within the walls of his medical society, not the courtroom.[36]

During the last years of the nineteenth century the chief function of physician-led state health boards became physician licensing, and with it came the enforcement of broadly-defined notions of professional ethical purity. It did not matter that the citizens who paid their salaries did not share physician regulators' ethical zeal. When he welcomed delegates to the 1884 APHA meeting in St. Louis, Missouri's Governor Thomas Crittenden, gave the public's view of medicine's self-serving morality: "professional ethics, so called, are as much to be dreaded as the smallpox."[37]

Nor did Reeves, who frequently spoke of the economics of public health, see the economic gulf that separated practicing physicians from the goals of preventive medicine—preventive medicine did not pay. Massachusetts physician Nathan Allen exposed the divide in 1886: "there is a direct antagonism between the interests of this profession [medicine] and sanitation. Every step in this [public health] reform diminishes more or less professional income. There is no trade or speculation in this reform. When a person has spent years in study, and made large investments to secure a livelihood, how can we expect he will sacrifice these interests?"[38]

Reeves resigned from his state health board in 1885. He left a gap his West Virginia successors could not fill, but it was not entirely a gap of their doing. The state's new governor, Emanuel Wilson, was elected on a platform of antimonopolist progressivism, based on small business and small government, which left little room for state-managed public health. Reeves commented in 1885 that sanitarians could not look to West Virginia's new governor for support. Wilson refused to approve the new board secretary's expenses in 1885; he did not name replacements for six retiring members in 1886; and he appointed a board member in 1887 whom the Wheeling and state medical societies unanimously rejected.[39]

Reeves' stature and his political skills might have bridged the divide, but he was out of the picture. Wilson replied to the medical society's objections to his 1887 Board appointment that the opinions of a few elite doctors could not sway him. The governor's disregard for the state medical society and his state health board marked the beginning of a persistent, decades-long pattern in West Virginia, with varying degrees of neglect and enmity between the executive branch and the state's organized medical profession.[40]

Like West Virginia, state health boards everywhere struggled to maintain their public health missions as the century ended. But it was not all politics. The deeper cause was that cities were always the engines of public health activism, not states. Reeves and the other founders of America's public health movement had emerged from the sanitary wreckage of urban industrialization. When public health became a laboratory-based discipline a new generation of physician leaders arose from cities with large hospitals and medical schools, such as Boston, New York, Providence, and Philadelphia. Turn-of-the-century cities with active public health movements did not need or want state oversight. State health boards were left to enforce unpopular quarantine laws and license physicians. Abandoned by sanitarians and dominated by regular practitioners, the transformation of state boards into vehicles of physician market hegemony was inevitable.[41]

⚡ 17 ⚡

Going South

Reeves moved away from his years in public health after his APHA presidency. He attended Pennsylvania's state sanitary convention in 1886 and the APHA meeting in Toronto, where he served on its Advisory Council and read two papers by Wheeling's George Baird. He travelled to the Memphis APHA gathering in 1887 and offered a few comments on typhoid fever, but in Memphis he quietly announced his new career. He invited one of the speakers, Baltimore pathologist William Councilman, to join him and a dozen other microscopists in a private demonstration of specimens and instruments. His work and his recognition were in public health, but his new passion was microscopic pathology.[1]

Reeves believed the microscope had bedside value. He praised the microscope's scientific virtues in his 1882 medical society address: "Just now the whole medical world is electrified by the light of the microscope in the hands of a young German physician—Dr. Koch of Berlin," then he went further: "[if] I were deprived of the aid afforded me in general practice by the use of this instrument, there are some diseases in the urinary and renal group I should decline to treat."[2] Again, he was ahead of the times.

In his spare moments Reeves mastered slide preparation, the newly developed microtome for making thin specimens, and the equally new technology of creating frozen histological sections. His acknowledgment of Henry Lomb at the 1885 APHA meeting and Lomb's financial support of Reeves' public health goals were hardly coincidental. Reeves bought his microscopes from Bausch and Lomb, the Rochester, New York, company that also supplied microscopes to Harvard anatomist Oliver Wendell Holmes. Reeves wrote a twenty-seven page handbook for Bausch and Lomb in 1886: "How to Work with the Bausch & Lomb Optical Co.'s Microtome and a Method of Demonstrating the Tubercle-Bacillus." Ironically, he attributed his technical success to the delicate touch he acquired during his painful time as a tailor's apprentice. Although he was a nationally-known public health advocate, the microtome handbook announced Reeves as a serious tissue pathologist, one well-acquainted with tuberculosis.[3]

Reeves attended his first meeting of the American Society of Microscopists in 1886, where he demonstrated the microtome and his methods for staining bacteria. Society members were impressed. They made Reeves a member and elected him the organization's second vice-president. However, Reeves' love was not the technology, but what the microscope could do for medicine. He only attended one other Microscopists meeting.[4]

The proper organizational home for a serious pathologist was the new Association of American Physicians. America's medical leaders, many of them young academic pathologists, established this group in 1886. At its inaugural meeting, the Association's president, Francis Delafield, made it clear that the exclusive organization, whose membership was limited to one hundred, was interested in medical science, not fraternal imperatives: "We want an association in which there will be no medical politics and no medical ethics." It was a deliberate swipe at the AMA.[5]

There were seventy-five members at the Association of American Physicians' 1886 meeting and only they could nominate new members. The group added just seven influential doctors in 1887: three from Philadelphia, one from Boston, one from New York, one from Montreal, and one from Wheeling, James Reeves. Reeves rubbed shoulders with Osler, Welch, Delafield, and the country's medical elite at five of the next eight annual meetings.[6]

Reeves quickly established himself as a pathologist. He sold his specimen slides throughout the country for a dollar each and offered examinations of biologic samples for five dollars. He published microscopic evidence in June 1887 contributing to the ongoing debate on whether the skin disease, lupus vulgaris, was cutaneous tuberculosis. In the celebrated Baker murder trial in July 1887 he travelled to New Cumberland, Pennsylvania to furnish expert testimony on whether crime scene stains were blood.[7]

Reeves' final career as a microscopic pathologist fell in the middle of a pivotal transition. Technical advances between 1880 and 1900, including the microtome, oil immersion, and better stains, joined with the conceptual revolution and tools of the germ theory to move the microscope from a gentlemanly curiosity to an indispensable implement of medical science. Reeves allied with the growing number of American medical school professors who argued that every physician should know how to use a microscope.

Reeves was ready to leave Wheeling as well. The town's harsh weather, sooty atmosphere, and his bouts of illness were taking a toll. Also, like other nineteenth-century doctors, he could not escape his patients or his community, even in retirement. When a girl was hit by a wagon in 1886 bystanders brought her to his nearby office. Two Wheeling reporters became concerned about the well-known doctor's health in October 1887 and tracked him down. They found him in his office, busy preparing microscopic slides for a New York customer. After the president of the city medical society died unexpectedly that year, Wheeling's doctors asked Reeves to take his place. If he was going to control what was left of his destiny, he needed to move. During their trip to the 1887 APHA meeting in Memphis, Reeves and his wife spent several days in Chattanooga and liked what they saw.[8]

Several medical colleges approached Reeves when they heard he was considering relocating. The University of Nebraska offered him its chair of pathology and a $2,500 annual stipend. The Kansas City Medical College also tried to attract him. But he and Frances were set on Tennessee.[9]

He sold his residence and announced plans to move to Chattanooga after returning from the APHA's Memphis meeting in November 1887. It was a noteworthy event in Southern medical circles. The *New Orleans Medical and Surgical Journal* congratulated "the people and profession of Chattanooga upon their good fortune in acquiring the services and counsel of such a physician." The *North Carolina Medical Journal* agreed, commending Chattanooga "on the accession of such an able physician."[10]

Reeves was in comfortable financial shape, but not wealthy. He sold part of his Wheeling property for five thousand dollars just before he left and the rest two years later for seven thousand, making a modest five hundred dollar profit on the property he had purchased in 1872. Shortly after arriving in Chattanooga in January 1888, he and Frances bought a home for seven thousand dollars. Over the next eight years, they purchased seven small Chattanooga properties and sold two of them for a modest profit.[11]

Chattanooga was an attractive, dynamic Southern city with better conditions than Wheeling. It was smaller, with a census of 29,000 versus 35,000, but it had more than doubled in population since 1880, while Wheeling only increased by 12 percent. Like Wheeling, Chattanooga was a railroad hub. But unlike smoke-filled Wheeling, Chattanooga was just beginning its growth as an iron center. Chattanooga's winter temperatures were ten degrees warmer than Wheeling and the surrounding mountains were pristine enough to serve as health resorts. Fifty-eight-year-old Reeves, unencumbered by harsh weather, financial worries, professional obligations, or civic expectations, fell into familiar patterns.[12]

He began by reprising his role as a civic booster. As soon as he settled in, Reeves invited two Wheeling investors to join him and a local banker on a tour of Chattanooga's financial opportunities. A few weeks later he sent copies of a chatty publication promoting Chattanooga to his friends in West Virginia. And, in April 1888, he wrote to the *Southern Hub,* a short-lived Chattanooga paper, in praise of the city's "colored" inhabitants and how this industrious, well-behaved group was favorably treated by whites: "here, in the South, the superior race wisely strives to influence the inferior race." He never publicly espoused such views in Wheeling, with its tiny black population, but in segregated Chattanooga, which was 43 percent "colored," Reeves quickly adopted the patriarchal perspectives of Tennessee's progressive white citizenry.[13]

He also promoted his pathology business. He sent microscope slides to local medical societies and the Medical Society of North Carolina pronounced them excellent, encouraging physicians with an interest in microscopy to contact him for a price list. A group of Chattanooga's physicians organized a medical college at Grant University and Reeves agreed to serve as a faculty member for no pay. If a student wanted private tutoring in histology and pathology, he offered twenty sessions for twenty-five dollars.[14]

The well-known retired sanitarian from West Virginia soon achieved statewide notoriety when a Florida yellow fever outbreak threatened his new state. On July 28, 1888, a recent arrival from Tampa died of yellow fever in Jacksonville. By August 10 a dozen persons were ill and Jacksonville was near panic. A fortnight later, there was genuine panic, with 130 cases of yellow fever in the city and twenty deaths.[15]

Jacksonville was hundreds of miles away, but its rail lines ran through Chattanooga and Tennessee's health board went on high alert. Ten years earlier, yellow fever had ravaged the Mississippi River basin and the worst-hit locale was Memphis, in western Tennessee. On August 15, 1888, the health board reported, "The whole world knows how Florida with its long-extended ocean and gulf coasts has been permeated with the seeds of a pestilence which for virulence and panic heads the list."[16]

Unsure that Florida and Georgia were taking the right precautions, the president of the Tennessee Health Board asked Reeves to travel to Georgia and report his impressions. Reeves accepted the assignment and arrived in Atlanta on August 30, 1888. He wired back that the situation had been bungled in Florida, but Atlanta seemed to be doing all one could expect.[17]

Reeves examined quarantine efforts in five Georgia cities over the next five days and Tennessee's papers published his daily dispatches. He sent his final report to the board's president on September 8 and assured him that, despite previous failures, federal agents and local governments were taking the proper steps. Jacksonville was carrying out mass fumigations. No one was allowed to enter the affected area and persons wanting to leave had to spend ten days in a federally-run camp before they could be issued a clean bill of health. Reeves was confident that Tennessee would be spared and he was right. The 1888 yellow fever epidemic did not come close to the disaster of 1878.[18]

Reeves' community work meshed well with his interest in microscopy. Shortly after submitting his final yellow fever report, Reeves headed to Washington, D.C., for the September 15 meeting of the Association of American Physicians. Baltimore's George Sternberg made a timely presentation on the etiology of yellow fever to fifty-nine of the country's elite pathologists and educators.[19]

Sternberg was a much-travelled Army field surgeon and a dogged laboratory scientist with an interest in bacteriology. He discussed the physical characteristics of bacilli reputed to cause yellow fever and their growth in various media, along with experiments in laboratory animals. His unequivocal conclusion was that "the specific infectious agent in yellow fever has not been demonstrated." Reeves asked Sternberg to send him tissues from patients who had died with yellow fever so that he could examine them microscopically.[20]

Within a few weeks Reeves found similar-appearing bacteria in the kidneys and livers of two patients who had died with yellow fever and speculated that these organisms might be the cause. He sent his slides to a fellow member of the American Society of Microscopists, Heinrich Detmer at Ohio State University. Detmer had learned microscopy in Germany and was a genuine pioneer in veterinary medicine, but he was not a bacteriologist. Detmer erroneously assured Reeves that he had found the bacterial source of yellow fever.[21]

Reeves announced that he had possibly discovered the yellow fever germ on December 20, 1888. Newspapers throughout the country made the story front page news. The reports noted that Reeves had his findings confirmed by other scientists and that he planned to consult with experts in Baltimore before making additional statements. The following day Detmer made a far less cautious proclamation, soon reported by the New York *Times* and other papers, that he had photographed Reeves' slides and that this was the first time yellow fever germs had been found in tissues. Frank Billings, the Massachusetts pathologist who had taken Nebraska's pathology chair previously offered to Reeves, told reporters that there was scarcely any doubt that the organism described by Reeves caused yellow fever.[22]

Sternberg did not stand for this nonsense. He and Reeves were close friends who shared many APHA connections. They thought well enough of each other that, when Reeves moved to Chattanooga, he represented Sternberg's interests in a local property transaction. Nevertheless, Sternberg was well-acquainted with Koch's meticulous demonstrations of disease causation and was not going to give anyone a pass on discovering the etiology of yellow fever by microscopic examination alone.[23]

Sternberg publicly disparaged Reeves' conclusions, even though they did not really belong to Reeves. He told a Baltimore paper that he had seen the organisms described in the materials he had furnished to Reeves. He had also observed these organisms in other tissues from yellow fever patients. But, Sternberg reminded readers, "The finding of bacilli in the tissues of one or more cases of an infectious disease is a long way from making the scientific demonstration that these are the specific cause of the disease." In January 1889 the *Journal of the American Medical Association* reprinted Sternberg's denial that Reeves had found the cause of yellow fever.[24]

Reeves knew that Sternberg was right, and let the matter drop. His only serious claim as a scientific investigator was made, exaggerated, denied, and done in less than a month. The embarrassing episode had little effect on his reputation as a pathologist. When W.W. Dawson lauded the country's laboratory workers in his AMA Presidential Address later in 1889, the first scientist he named was George Sternberg. Then, as he listed other well-known figures, Dawson made special mention of Reeves: "His [microscopic] technique is singularly beautiful. Many of his preparations are to be found in the National Museum."[25]

While Reeves was studying Sternberg's yellow fever specimens, Frank Dent's appeal of his 1882 arrest for violating West Virginia's licensure law finally came before the U.S. Supreme Court. As before, Mountaineer lawyer M.H. Dent represented cousin Frank.

Attorney Dent presented his arguments on December 11, 1888. He focused solely on the Fourteenth Amendment's due process clause: "No State shall deprive any person of life, liberty, or property without due process of law." He claimed that Frank was lawfully practicing medicine before the law was passed and West Virginia had unduly deprived him of his practice, which was his property. Dent cited sitting Supreme Court Justice Stephen Field, who had written an earlier decision supporting the right to practice a profession as a form of property. Dent then claimed that Reeves' board of health was incapable of due process. It was more "ministerial than judicial and wholly different than that which is meant by due process of law."[26]

Alfred Caldwell, Jr., West Virginia's Attorney General, defended Reeves' law. Caldwell made four arguments: legislatures possessed legitimate powers to ensure public health that were properly delegated to police and similar authorities such as boards; these powers included protecting the public from quacks and charlatans; West Virginia's law did not discriminate against any person or class of persons; and states had a right to pass laws to prevent objectionable practices even if persons were lawfully engaged in those practices when the law was passed. Caldwell called attention to Justice Field's prior decision about property rights, explaining how the facts of that prior case did not apply. He also cited the AMA's *Code of Medical Ethics* to support his argument that physicians should possess appropriate skills and the public should discriminate between those who had such skills and those who did not.[27]

Justice Field delivered the Court's decision in *Dent v. West Virginia* five weeks later. Field was a strong advocate of due process and his Court tended to support business interests. If Field believed that Reeves' law represented the efforts of elite physicians to suppress lawful competitors, he probably would have agreed with Dent. He had written an opinion in 1873 stating: "The granting of monopolies, or exclusive privileges to individuals or corporations is an invasion of the right of others to choose a lawful calling, and an infringement of personal liberty."[28]

However, in establishing a Constitutional precedent for all forms of professional licensure, Field rejected Dent's arguments. He began, "It is undoubtedly the right of every citizen of the United States to follow any lawful calling, business or profession he may choose" then he qualified this right, "subject only to such restrictions as are imposed upon all persons of like age, sex and condition." He wrote that states had obligations and powers to protect citizens from the ignorance of others, singling out medicine: "Few professions require more careful preparation by one who seeks to enter it than that of medicine." Field acknowledged that due process was a difficult concept, one which turned on fairness. He noted that the law provided Dent with remedies, including a licensing examination and access to the courts, which Dent had not used. The Court unanimously concluded that Reeves' law was Constitutional and appropriate: "The law of West Virginia was intended to secure such skill and learning in the profession of medicine that the community might trust with confidence those receiving a license under authority of the State."[29]

The decision was front page news in Wheeling, but other papers buried it in regular announcements of the Court's business. The medical literature mostly ignored it. The voluminous Philadelphia *Medical News,* which ran to 1,474 pages in 1889, gave it a half page under the headline, "States May Regulate Medical Practice." The editor showed no knowledge of Reeves' work or the law's history. He opined that Illinois had done well protecting its citizens and now, perhaps, West Virginia would "report that her ranks have been purified from the worst of her quackish and ignorant imposters."[30]

Regular medicine's competitors were alarmed by the monopolistic potential *Dent* represented. Irenaeus Foulon was a professor of medical jurisprudence and a licensed Illinois homeopathic physician who witnessed Rauch's expansive interpretation of ethical behavior and assaults on alternative practitioners. Foulon reported on the *Dent* decision in a homeopathic journal. He had no argument with requiring practitioners to be qualified, but he warned: "There is, however, a very real danger that iron-clad statutes might be passed through the efforts of the dominant school, that would work injury to other schools of medicine." He admonished his fellow homeopaths to maintain their guard.[31]

Legislatures and jurists saw *Dent* as a way to protect the public from quackery and fraud, but most regular physicians saw it as a vehicle to reduce unseemly and destructive competition. The decision added legitimacy to the expanding professional licensure movement; however, it did not stipulate or even suggest who should represent the public's interests when the powers of the state were applied to the medical marketplace. This problem was handed to medicine's future.[32]

Reeves paid little attention to *Dent* or to the ethical issues that often defined his earlier medical life. He moved off the public stage after the yellow fever episodes in 1888 and 1889 and settled comfortably into the local medical community. He helped the city's physicians found the Tri-State Medical Society (Tennessee, Alabama, and Georgia) in 1889 and he attended this organization's first annual meeting. He gave a talk to the Tri-State group in 1890 that reflected on what he had learned about medicine, emphasizing scholarship and humility: "The medical student who would win eminence in his profession must deny himself the glory and tinsel of society life." He became a respected and regular contributor to the Chattanooga Medical Society, where he was widely known as "Uncle Jimmy."[33]

Whenever the opportunity arose, he preached his new gospel of microscopy. At the first meeting of the Tri-State Medical Society in 1889, he gave a microscope demonstration and followed with a well-attended lecture on: "The Importance of the Microscope in the Practice of Medicine." He discussed consumption at the Chattanooga Medical Society in 1890 and related how microscopic examination could show whether a patient's symptoms were caused by tuberculosis. He spoke to the Association of American Physicians on his other favorite topic, typhoid (enteric) fever, but emphasized that his understanding of the disease had improved because his microscope now allowed him to differentiate malaria from typhoid. He reinforced this message by quoting Osler: "in the language of Dr. Osler, 'the characteristic changes in malaria are as distinctly determined in the blood as are those of tuberculosis of the lungs in the sputa.'"[34]

Reeves enjoyed his peaceful life in Chattanooga and continued promoting the town's virtues to visiting friends from Wheeling, including Catholic Bishop John Kain and physician Louis Wilson. In July 1891 he sent a series of letters to his twenty-seven-year-old niece, Anna Jarvis, who lived with his sister, Ann, in Grafton. He was sure he could find Anna a job in Chattanooga and offered to pay her way down. He wrote to Ann, encouraging the whole family to come south: "I hope that she [Anna] may be the *avant courier* of the exodus of the remainder of the family; for this is God's own country!" Anna came to Chattanooga in September 1891, although shortly afterwards she found better prospects in Philadelphia.[35]

He also befriended the local newspaper, as he had in Wheeling. He supplied a four-column article on "The Health and Wealth of the City of Chattanooga" for a December 8, 1892, souvenir edition of the Chattanooga *Times*. It was the abridged Chattanooga version of his *Health and Wealth* book from Wheeling, with topographic, meteorological, and sanitary descriptions. He again reminded readers that a community that did not understand the vital facts of its situation was feebly defended against "the pestilence that walketh in darkness, and the destruction that wasteth at noon-day."[36]

The Chattanooga *Times* had a history of positive involvement in public health, so Reeves' article was a good fit. However, the paper was not a typical small-town enterprise. It was a heavily indebted regional daily in December 1892, with its own building, the South's newest and finest newspaper headquarters. The paper's ambitious young owner, Adolph Ochs, became wealthy and achieved journalistic immortality after he purchased the *New York Times* in 1896, but in 1893 his Chattanooga publication faced a severe economic downturn and he needed to increase revenues. A few months after publishing "The Health and Wealth of the City of Chattanooga" the *Times* disturbed Reeves' quiet retirement by facilitating a frontal attack on his true church.

18

Koch's Rivals

Thoughtful physicians opposed the nationwide increase in drug use that occurred during the last fifteen years of Reeves' life. There was an explosion in medical therapies fostered by gilded age prosperity, the public's fascination with scientific breakthroughs, the growing power of America's print media, and an absence of regulation. The value of patent medicines and proprietary compounds, which were marketed to laymen and physicians, increased four hundred percent between 1880 and 1900, from $14 million to $59 million.[1]

Medical scientists had documented the body's restorative capabilities and argued for prevention since the Civil War. Chemists were isolating and standardizing the active ingredients of many botanicals and the experimental work of Claude Bernard (1813–1878) fostered a rational, physiologic approach to therapeutics. Moreover, there were only a few genuinely new compounds, such as the analgesics and antipyretics, salicylic acid, acetanilide, and phenacetin. Physician leaders, including Reeves, used and recommended fewer medications than in earlier years.[2]

Still, many practicing physicians encouraged this *fin de siècle* upsurge in drug marketing. Busy doctors had long relied on predetermined recipes, such as the joining of opium and ipecacuanha in Dover's powders. They welcomed ready-made shortcuts and encouraged pharmaceutical creativity. As one physician suggested in 1885, why couldn't some clever pharmaceutical house add different salts and create a Dover's powder for rheumatic fever, another for gout, and a third for tonsillitis?[3]

Each physician's opinion was as good as another's and the public had no way of telling the difference. The representative of a new proprietary cure, which was usually trademarked, but not often patented, approached a physician with free samples. The salesman later called back, flattering the physician and inquiring about the drug's use. If the physician was pleased, the representative added the physician's name as an endorser of the drug on the company's printed advertisements to consumers, which were everywhere. With a regulatory vacuum, there was a marketing vortex. Newspaper and periodical advertising increased two and one-half times between 1880 and 1890 and the largest single group of advertisers was the patent and proprietary medicine industry.[4]

The AMA tried to walk a fine ethical line after it recognized this advertising opportunity. It launched the *Journal of the American Medical Association* in 1883, which created an easier way to communicate the organization's messages and brought new advertising revenues to the AMA. The obvious choice for the journal's first editor was Nathan Davis, who hoped to obtain five thousand dollars in: "*legitimate* medical advertising" (author's italics) the first year.[5]

Subject to physician sniping because of its flexible interpretation of *legitimate*, the AMA's new publication gave no signs of the advertising success it would enjoy in the next century. The *Journal* had three thousand subscribers in its first year and the AMA lost seventy-seven dollars, including the *Journal's* revenues and expenses. The next year the AMA made a two thousand dollar surplus. There was little change over the following few years. The *Journal* had five thousand subscribers in 1890 and the AMA again generated a two thousand dollar surplus.[6]

The medical journal that most successfully developed the era's pharmaceutical marketing opportunities belonged to Joseph Lawrence. Lawrence claimed in 1881 that nearly one half of all practicing physicians in the United States subscribed to *The Medical Brief*. The next year he doubled the subscription price to two dollars, and, despite his original promise to avoid promoting the sale of medicines, increased his journal's advertising.[7]

In the lead-up to Koch's tuberculosis discovery, former nostrum-pusher Lawrence began marketing an antiseptic-analgesic potion he claimed was superior to Lister's carbolic acid. His distinctive blend of thymol, eucalyptol, baptisia (wild indigo), gaultheria (wintergreen), mentha arvensis (menthol), benzoic acid, and boric acid promised ten times the antiseptic strength of carbolic acid, yet was comparatively harmless. He revealed the components to his readers as well-known ingredients in a convenient form, like Dover's powders. As with many proprietary nostrums, his concoction contained twenty-six percent alcohol, enough to serve as a beverage.[8]

Lawrence transferred his formula to a St. Louis drug entrepreneur, Jordan Lambert, for a royalty of $20 per gross bottles sold in April 1881. Lambert did not patent Lawrence's formula; rather he trademarked the new product's name, "Listerine." Lambert and Lawrence marketed Listerine to physicians and its initial professional mention was in the June 1881 issue of *The Medical Brief*, where, citing no evidence, the editor noted that Listerine, combined with morphine and water, was a reliable cure for gonorrhea.[9]

Lawrence filled the *Brief* with references to Listerine, from glowing reports by individual physicians to scholarly-appearing laboratory studies. Other journals looking for content helped out. Lambert began advertising Listerine in the *Medical Brief* in 1882, providing endorsements from well-known physicians, including the secretary of the North Carolina State Board of Health. After Koch's tuberculosis announcement, Lawrence associated Listerine with consumption treatment. Given the reach of Lawrence's journal, plus constant mentions elsewhere, physicians rapidly adopted Listerine for dozens of conditions.[10]

Listerine was safe with genuine antiseptic properties, and it arrived just when antisepsis was becoming popular. An 1898 compendium of proprietary medicines described Listerine, with a lower case "L," as the prototypical antiseptic solution. Most nineteenth-century physicians consider Listerine a helpful addition, although a few raised ethical objections.[11]

Philadelphia's Solomon Solis-Cohen linked Listerine to the unprofessional use of proprietary formulations: "[the patient] deserves better treatment than to be handed over to the mercies of 'antikamnia,' or 'quickine,' or gleditschine,' or 'Frelighs's tablets,' or 'Listerine,' or any other of the unholy crew,"[12] but these arguments did not carry the day. As long as Listerine was directed to physicians, doctors were fine with it. Once Listerine's owners began advertising to the public in the twentieth century physicians took a dimmer view. In 1931 the AMA described Listerine, accepted by physicians for fifty years, as an abasement of a great name.[13]

Lambert changed his company's name to Lambert Pharmacal in 1884 and renegotiated his Listerine royalty payment to Lawrence to six dollars per gross bottles sold. The two men became rich from Listerine. Lambert died in 1889 and his sons assumed control of the business, which they eventually sold in 1955. Lawrence died in 1909, leaving an estate valued at seven to eleven million dollars.[14]

Physicians' use and endorsement of Listerine typified minor ethical transgressions, but what was unique about Listerine was its inventor's industrial-strength conflict of interest. Lawrence never mentioned his financial association with Listerine as he promoted its merits in America's most widely-read medical journal. Ten years after Listerine's invention two Cincinnati doctors sought Lawrence's publishing platform and his version of medical science to help promote a fake consumption cure. They enjoyed considerable success until they ran into Reeves.

It began in Cincinnati in 1892 where a struggling regular physician, William Riley Amick, found a novel use for his professional knowledge and the newsman's weakness for self-serving publicity. William was the younger of two physician brothers from Scipio, Indiana who had entered local practice following graduation from the Cincinnati College of Medicine and Surgery. After obtaining his degree in 1875 William acquired a faculty appointment at the medical college and represented himself as a medical ophthalmologist and otologist, a non-surgical specialist in eye and ear diseases. He published a handful of inconsequential medical articles, such as his opinion on "Snapping Noises in the Ear," but did not make much of his practice. Medical and civic biographies never mentioned him and, in 1891 when his older sibling, Marion. reported the eighth largest amount of property taxes of the 254 tax-paying physicians in Cincinnati, William paid no taxes.[15]

Seeing the success around him, Amick developed a plan to harness the publicity and disappointment surrounding Robert Koch's most recent medical announcements. Koch stated in 1890 that he had formulated a serum that could destroy human cells containing tuberculosis bacilli, allowing the patient to recover if the disease was in its early stages. His serum was popularly called "Koch's lymph" and he soon named it "tuberculin. " The medical and popular press trumpeted that Koch had found a cure for consumption.[16]

Koch was a meticulous medical scientist who knew that separating a false cure from a real one required analyzing data from large numbers of patients. He distributed his serum to other physicians and they tested it in their hospitals. In March 1891 the Prussian government summarized the results in 1,768 patients over a two-month period. The outcomes were inconclusive. American physicians likewise tried it with mixed results. The *Boston Medical and Surgical Journal* pronounced in May 1891 that tuberculin was, at best, a worthy first step: "Whilst recognizing the perils of prophesying, we are inclined to the opinion that the ultimate verdict will be that tuberculin, or some allied remedy, is serviceable in the early stages of phthisis when carefully administered under favorable conditions."[17]

A few physicians treated patients with tuberculin into the twentieth century, but, therapeutically, it turned out to be the progenitor of skin testing for tuberculosis. Koch was unimpressed with his own work. In July 1891, he decided that tuberculin was ineffective and returned to supervising the efforts of other researchers. The New York *Times* headlined its disappointment: "Lymph Called a Failure."[18]

Koch's widely-reported flop heightened excitement around consumption therapies. Virtually every newspaper advertised consumption cures, many of which contained narcotic drugs. Consumption remedy purveyors, along with some later historians, argued that their treatments were no worse than those offered by regular physicians. But the era's medical experts, who recommended fewer medicines and more fresh air for consumption patients, disagreed. They concurred with Samuel Hopkins Adams, who exposed America's patent medicine industry in his 1905 articles, "The Great American Fraud." Adams labeled false consumption cures: "the most devilish of all, in that they destroy hope where hope is struggling against bitter odds for existence."[19]

False hope was part of the consumptive's lot. Any physician who treated a meaningful number of consumption patients or read the standard medical texts knew that consumption sometimes killed rapidly, sometimes slowly, and sometimes patients recovered on their own. In the right situation, anything could look like a cure.

Amick launched his plan by manipulating the city's most prestigious medical journal, the *Lancet-Clinic,* whose editor had previously published several of his innocuous writings. Amick slipped one past him in March 1892: "A Chemical Cure for Consumption and Asthma." Eye and ear doctor Amick claimed to have made a ten-year study of the lung disease, consumption. He reminded physicians of the large number of useless consumption cures on the market, many of which contained opium or morphine. He urged doctors, as Nathan Davis had told Austin Flint in 1853, to accept that each physician should test a medicine in his own practice and decide what works best for him.[20]

Amick appealed to medicine's pseudoscientific undercurrents. In his article he attributed consumption to bodily dysharmony, which led to the formation of tubercules and collections of bacilli. Osler's well-known and widely-respected *Principles and Practice of Medicine*, first published at almost the same time, in February 1892, could not have been more at odds with Amick. Osler defined tuberculosis, which he also called phthisis and pulmonary consumption, as: "An infective disease, caused by the *bacillus tuberculosis*"[21] (author's italics).

Amick specified that to cure tuberculosis and asthma the treatment "must correct the faulty oxidation and increase or supply the wanting elements…. We have arranged our treatment to meet these indications." Amick's therapy was a combination of a liquid medicine, a tablet, and an inhaler. He presented twenty-eight cases of lung disease and twelve additional asthma patients who had used his treatment successfully. In one instance he offered a note from the *Lancet-Clinic's* editor, A.B. Richardson, that the patient was in good health after treatment. Only thirteen of the forty cases were managed by him, twenty-six were brother Marion's patients. Marion wrote that William's chemical treatment seemed to work.[22]

Amick's patients could have been genuine, but there was no way of knowing whether or not they had consumption. Proof of the disease in 1892 required microscopic evidence of the tubercle bacillus in the patient's sputum, which Amick never supplied. Plus, regular physician were well aware of its unpredictable path. A reputable scientific article of the day would have described the microbiological findings and confirmed that the cases included all patients treated, not just the success stories. It would have also disclosed the ingredients of the treatment. Amick did none of these things.[23]

An embarrassed *Lancet-Clinic* editor posted a *mea culpa* the next week. He explained to readers that the author was a physician in good standing in Cincinnati and that the editor believed Amick had furnished a preliminary communication and would soon supply the expected details. He stated that he (Richardson) had examined a patient, but he did *not* endorse the treatment. He warned Amick: "We must in all candor say to the writer of the article that if he wishes to retain the confidence and esteem of his fellow practitioners, it will be necessary for him to follow his article promptly with a full and frank statement of the treatment for which he claims such remarkable results."[24]

But Amick was not interested in the esteem of Cincinnati's elite practitioners. He intended to exploit the reality that the public, along with many physicians, lacked scientific training and got its daily medical information from newspapers and friends rather than professional journals and texts.[25]

To promote his scheme, Amick joined with Cincinnati's biggest newspaper, *The Cincinnati Post*, the flagship of Edward W. Scripps' four Midwest papers. Scripps' family had purchased the *Post*, then called the *Penny Paper*, in 1881. The sheet had a circulation of 13,000 in 1883, but, by 1892, the *Post* had a circulation of more than 85,000, the largest in the state. Scripps achieved this growth by undercutting the subscription price of his competitors, controlling costs, hiring talented executives and reporters, and paying close attention to local issues. These tactics and his understanding of vertical integration eventually allowed Scripps to pioneer the American newspaper chain.[26]

However, in 1892 Scripps was expanding the *Post's* production facilities and battling the Cincinnati *Times-Star* for the afternoon newspaper market. He was also trying to get out from under the thumb of his advertisers, the biggest group of which was out-of-state nostrum sellers. His strategy was to encourage local advertising and do whatever he could to increase subscription revenues.

Amick's plan met Scripps' needs and its outlines were visible two days before the suspicious consumption article appeared in the *Lancet-Clinic*. On March 5, 1892, *The Cincinnati Post* ran a three-column spread about William Amick and his discovery, headlined: "I've Found It!" Given the medical information the report contained, Amick probably authored the article, as later court records showed he often did, or he may have found a gullible reporter. The *Post* printed the story as its own. As far as Scripps was concerned Dr. Amick was a credible local physician and his announcement was something the paper's competitors did not have. The arrangement was mutually beneficial.[27]

The *Post* article proclaimed, "Koch Outdone by a Cincinnati Physician." It began, "Doctor, do you cure consumption? ' I have done so and am doing it today.'" The story reiterated the claims of Amick's forthcoming *Lancet-Clinic* piece, leading the unnamed reporter to gush: "These remarkable reports of the Cincinnati physician, confirmed as they are by eminent confreres, will cause a profound sensation in the medical circles of the Nation and of the world." On March 7, the day the *Lancet-Clinic* published Amick's article, the *Post* provided a front-page account, including a statement *Lancet-Clinic* editor Richardson never made: "My opinion has already been given as to Dr. Amick's wonderful and practical remedy."[28]

Amick used the new medium of wire service dispatch to his advantage. As many smaller papers did, the March 6, 1892, edition of the *St. Louis Republic*, in a section marked "Special to the Republic," summarized the *Post's* March 5 article, emphasizing, "Dr. A.B. Richardson, editor of *The Lancet and Clinic*, will testify to the cure." Subsequent court records and copies of telegrams confirmed that Amick wrote his own wire reports.[29]

Amick unveiled the cornerstone of his strategy on March 9. The *Post* announced on its front page that the paper would test his treatment in patients of its choosing. The *Post* again claimed the *Lancet-Clinic* had endorsed the cure and that its fame had spread to a thousand newspapers.[30]

The *Post* described how the testing would be scrupulously fair, seeking patients who were potentially curable, but not associated with Amick. Shortly thereafter it reported that Amick would begin treating Mrs. S.A. Madison, a woman who had suffered from asthma for eighty-seven years. Two weeks later it pronounced Mrs. Madison cured. Then it recorded consumption success stories, beginning with Mrs. John Hayes. The *Post* called Amick, "A Modern Joshua" who turned back life's setting sun.[31] This was all within the first month.

Cincinnati's elite physicians were apoplectic but powerless. Richardson published a second editorial demanding that Amick disclose his secret remedy. After Amick sent copies of the journal's disavowed article to Cincinnati's physicians, along with a circular on how to purchase his cure, many called him a quack and demanded his expulsion from the local medical society.[32]

Physician leaders made a fuss about Amick's secrecy, but that was not the real issue, even though the AMA's *Code of Ethics* prohibited proprietary nostrum use, secret or not. For example, almost all medical journals advertised Antikamnia for pain and, although the nostrum's owner never described the ingredients, physicians used it because it made modest claims and seemed to work.[33] Likewise, they readily accepted Listerine as an antiseptic. Amick's problem was that he publicly boasted he could do something that well-educated physicians were certain he could not do: cure consumption. Boastful pretending was the definition of quackery.

If William Amick had been operating in Illinois and Rauch had still been a member of the State Board of Health, Rauch might have arrested him for unethical behavior, but probably not gotten a conviction. With no licensing law Ohio was far less of a threat. The *Lancet-Clinic* editor noted a year earlier that a medical graduate was free to wander about the state advertising and disposing of his favorite remedies. He commented, "Although we sincerely despise a man who will resort to such dishonest practices, yet we are unable to deny him the right to do so."[34]

The Cincinnati College of Medicine and Surgery fired Amick two months after the *Lancet-Clinic* published his article and the regular physician community of Cincinnati shunned him. This was the most Cincinnati's doctors could do. Marion announced his retirement from the medical college to devote his time to William's business.[35]

The *Post* made Amick a local celebrity and encouraged physicians to use his product. On May 4, 1892, it announced that he had purchased a private residence, with plans to make it into a compounding laboratory, and that Marion would be joining him, followed by: "Reports from physicians who have been testing the Amick consumption and asthma cures are coming in thick and fast." Between April 1, 1892, and December 31, 1892, The *Post* printed eleven reports on Amick and his cure.[36]

Evidence suggests that the public testing idea originated with William Amick, not the newspaper, and that the *Post* did not regularly use this publicity stunt. There was only one similar example over the next two years and the *Post* compared it to Amick. Shortly after Amick appeared, Irvine Mott, a Cincinnati homeopathic physician, announced a cure for Bright's disease (renal failure). On April 23, 1892, the *Post's* headlines read: "Medical Science—The Queen City Blessed with It.—Dr. Irvine K. Mott Scores a Grand Success—In the Treatment of Deadly Bright's Disease—Wonderful Achievement of a Young Physician.—A Discovery as Interesting as That of Dr. Amick."[37]

The *Post* reported a test of Mott's claim in 1894, which, by then, also included a cure for diabetes. The paper reminded readers: "Some time ago when the Post printed the statement that Dr. Amick, one of the city's physicians claimed that he could cure consumption it was telegraphed far and wide, and was one of the biggest scenarios in the medical world. A test was made of his claim and every report was eagerly read all over the country."[38]

Mott agreed that the *Post* could select twelve patients for testing and he would choose five for treatment. He announced that Harvard Medical College would confirm the results. His treatment was based on three proprietary preparations he named lyco-carbon, kalin, and brucin. Two months after beginning the test, the *Post* declared that all five patients had been cured and that Harvard's professors were astonished. Mott had all he needed to turn his newspaper notoriety into public promotion. Over the next ten years his kidney disease advertisements reproduced the *Post's* coverage, emphasizing his Harvard connection, in newspapers and lay journals.[39]

Except there was no Harvard connection. After a three-year battle, Harvard forced Mott to cease using its name in 1904 and in 1905 *Collier's Weekly* described Mott as a typical quack. Undeterred, Mott continued to advertise his cure for Bright's disease and diabetes, dropping Harvard, but referring to the *Post's* 1894 tests, almost until his death in 1920.[40]

Mott pursued the usual course of physicians and faux physicians who pitched false cures. He made a pretense of scientific credibility and then advertised his services to an unsuspecting public. William Amick had bigger ambitions. Like Listerine's Lawrence and Lambert, he wanted America's physicians to use and promote his product. He convinced Thomas Spivey, president of the Victor Safe and Lock Company, to join Marion and him in founding the Amick Chemical Company. The company started producing its chemical treatment for consumption in August 1892 with an initial capitalization of $300,000. None of the organization's principals were chemists, nor did the company ever claim that it hired a chemist.[41]

The Chicago *Herald's* business manager, S.G. Sea, sent a letter to the *Post* on October 7, 1892, describing his miraculous recovery from consumption under Amick's treatment. Soon enough Sea joined the Amick Chemical Company, adding the final piece.[42]

Amick's plan was to pay newspapers, such as the *Post*, to report tests of his cure and then to send newspaper accounts across the country as if they were medical studies. However, he needed another layer of medical respectability to do this outside of Ohio, which was impossible with traditional journals such as the *Lancet-Clinic* and the *St. Louis Medical and Surgical Journal.* The latter publication had sided with the *Lancet-Clinic* in June, announcing that Amick had "gone bodily over to the quacks."[43] But Amick had a better option in St. Louis, a medical journal with broader circulation and fewer scruples, *The Medical Brief.*

Joseph Lawrence was a wealthy man by 1892, thanks to the hidden and synergistic relationship between Listerine and his journal. Lawrence had lowered the subscription price of *The Medical Brief* back to a dollar and claimed that, in its twentieth year, 50,000 physicians read the *Brief.* There were seven mentions of Listerine by different writers in the 1892 volume and twenty-three advertisements for the product.[44]

Lawrence obliged Amick with a short summary of his *Lancet-Clinic* piece in the July 1892 issue, emphasizing Amick's ideas on asthma and making no mention of the professional furor his discredited publication raised. *The Medical Brief* reprinted the entire *Lancet-Clinic* article in September, inserting an advertisement for the Amick Chemical Company, whose product was "Tested, indorsed, and adopted in practice by six thousand physicians." The *Brief* appended an additional five pages of physician testimonials and concluded with the Amick Company's boast: "We have enough reports like the foregoing to fill every page in this Journal were it necessary to publish them." Readers could not tell advertising hyperbole from medical journalism in the sixteen-page story. Over the next four months, the *Brief* published two more full-page advertisements for the Amick Chemical Company.[45]

All of the *Brief's* insertions about Amick's consumption cure were paid advertisements, even if readers did not always know it. The *Medical Summary* of Philadelphia, a competitor of *The Medical Brief,* published Amick's sixteen-page article-cum-promotion in December 1892, and clearly identified it as advertising.[46]

By now Amick had what he needed from the *Brief.* He put his pitch in front of Lawrence's readers, but, as he had done with his *Lancet-Clinic* article, he intended to combine the medical legitimacy the *Brief* afforded with the marketing reach of newspapers. On Sunday, December 25, 1892, an upstart New York City paper, the *Recorder,* announced a new contest to its Christmas Day readers. The paper would give a thousand dollar prize to anyone who could provide a meritorious treatment for the dread disease of consumption. In hindsight this had to be Amick's idea.[47]

The *Recorder* was a good fit for Amick. The paper was an entrepreneurial endeavor of tobacco magnate James B. Duke. It entered the crowded New York City newspaper market in 1891 and used ambitious, creative, and costly tactics to build circulation and revenues. The *Recorder* was the first to use color printing. It had the highest paid staff in New York, with many well-known names, and paid particular attention to women's issues. Within two years the paper claimed to have the second largest newspaper circulation in New York City. However, splashy journalism and Duke's money were not enough. The paper was up for sale by 1895 and the *Recorder* folded in 1896.[48]

The New York *Recorder's* 1892 consumption contest announcement occupied a full page, stressing the importance of the event and implying that the only reason scientists had not found a cure for mankind's greatest killer was because they lacked a modest financial incentive. It noted that physicians in Cincinnati were particularly interested in the challenge because of the successful work of one of their number.

The *Recorder* ran three more articles on the competition between Christmas and New Year's Eve, 1892, emphasizing a large portrait of Pasteur and increasing reports from Cincinnati: "Has Koch a Rival?" Could Dr. W.R. Amick, whose cure had been endorsed by the *Lancet-Clinic*, be induced to enter the *Recorder's* contest? The *Post* telegraphed the *Recorder*, "The Cincinnati *Post's* public tests of Dr. Amick's treatment for consumption in this city were in every respect successful, and confirm the doctor's claims."[49]

The *Recorder's* readers must have been elated on New Year's Eve to find that the modest Cincinnati doctor was willing to let the *Recorder* make any test of his discovery that it wished. The *Recorder* declared, "The St. Louis Medical Brief, the leading medical journal of the Southwest, in today's issue in a learned article discussing all the known treatments of consumption, indorses Dr. Amick's discovery." Amick had ties with the *Brief*, but there was no such discussion in the December issue.[50]

Just one week after opening the competition, on New Year's Day, 1893, the *Recorder* announced that that the challenge was closed to all entrants except Dr. W.R. Amick of Cincinnati. Among the numerous supporting interviews the *Recorder* claimed to have, including Koch and Virchow in Germany, it did not offer one from America's leading bacteriologist, Lieutenant Colonel George Sternberg, who would have been easy to find because he was in New York assisting with a cholera epidemic.[51]

The next four months were a repeat of the Cincinnati *Post* experience on a larger stage. The *Recorder* built suspense around its test of Amick's cure in twelve consumption patients. A January 1893 report headlined, "Koch Failed; Will Amick?" All patients had tragic stories and some signs of tuberculosis, but there were no sputum analyses. Each description included enough medical terminology to appeal to physicians and confuse laymen such as, "vocal fremitus increased over both lungs." The *Recorder* invariably reminded physicians to contact Amick for free samples of his treatment.[52]

There were at least twenty-six *Recorder* articles in 1893 describing patient recruitment and progress until the paper announced, on April 23, 1893, that all patients were cured or only a few weeks away from complete recovery. The *Recorder* devoted two full pages to congratulating itself and Amick, the winner of its competition. It also published more than one hundred testimonials from satisfied patients and physicians.[53]

As the *Recorder's* story progressed, telegraph wires planted Amick's name in hundreds of small newspapers. The Phillipsburg (Kansas) *Herald* printed a dispatch from New York on March 9, 1893, detailing the *Recorder's* sensational contest, its wonderful early results, and particulars on how Dr. Amick's cure could be obtained. The Buffalo (New York) *Sunday Morning News* proclaimed "Consumption Cured" on April 23, the same day the *Recorder* declared Amick's victory. On May 15, 1893, the *Recorder* announced that it had received notification of over two hundred newspapers mentioning the contest and Dr. Amick's cure in the past week alone.[54]

Amick's product gained momentum with every wire service report. According to the Amick Chemical Company, 1,256 physicians ordered medicines between February 1 and March 15, 1893. Physicians as far away as Los Angeles advertised that they cured consumption with Dr. Amick's chemical treatment.[55]

Papers that competed with Amick's chosen publications were silent on his miraculous results; as if they knew it was no more than another gilded age stunt. While the *Post* trumpeted Amick's wonders, the *Cincinnati Enquirer* and the Cincinnati *Times-Star* ignored the whole thing.[56] Likewise, New York's major papers, the *Times*, the *Herald*, the *World*, and the *Tribune*,[57] never covered Amick while his story filled the *Recorder*.

If the other papers knew that Amick's miraculous cure was not real news, they made no effort to expose his quackery. Competing newspapers turned a blind eye to Amick because they too profited from nostrum advertising and were in no position to unmask someone else's medical deception. The *Cincinnati Enquirer* ran an article on May 7, 1892, headlined, "A Medium for Cheats—How Frauds Are Worked through the Mails," which detailed how insurance companies, land swindlers, detective agencies, and other undesirables, without naming nostrum sellers, misused the postal service. At the same time, the paper offered numerous advertisements for mail-order consumption cures.[58]

Although there was a conspiracy of silence based on shared interests, the newspaper complicity had deeper roots. In "The Great American Fraud" Samuel Hopkins Adams described a common contractual "red clause" that voided an advertiser's agreement if the newspaper's state took legislative action restricting the sale of proprietary medicines. Adams wrote, "With a few honorable exceptions, the press of the United States is at the beck and call of the patent medicines. Not only do the newspapers modify news possibly affecting these interests, but they sometimes become their active agents."[59]

As the newspaper scenario played out in New York City and the other papers winked, it was almost as if the *Recorder* was in on the ruse. The *Recorder*, seeking a cure for world's deadliest human disease, never presented its contest or Amick's successes on the front page. The reports typically followed the business, sports, and society sections. Perhaps the paper's more serious journalists also knew what was up.

Amick's treatment was likely harmless, but his scheme's pernicious message did far more than promote another bogus nostrum. It threatened the professional infrastructure that guarded medicine's science and preserved its special status. The message was that newspaper editors and newspaper readers were as qualified to evaluate medical information as anyone else. This was a direct challenge to academic physicians, scientists, and medical journal editors. Cincinnati's medical establishment castigated Amick internally, but did nothing more. Despite the *Recorder's* repeated announcements of a sure cure for consumption, which included numerous physician testimonials, New York's physicians were silent.[60]

One impediment to physician action was professional ethics, which discouraged public criticism of fellow physicians. However, a more potent deterrent was the nostrum-seller's frequent use of legal tools, in this case anti-defamation laws, which favored the plaintiff.[61] When the *Ohio Medical Journal* accused Amick of marketing a false cure in 1893, he sued every faculty member of the Ohio Medical College, the journal's owner, for libel. Neither the College nor the Cincinnati newspapers reported the outcome of the suit, but the *Post* named all fourteen physician defendants in an article praising Amick, "the savant who spent 11 years of his life in the study of consumption."[62] Most physicians were reasonably fearful of this kind of publicity.

If Amick had any concerns with physician opposition to his cure, he had to be reassured by the verdict in the latest high-profile libel trial. Texas gardener William Radam began marketing his Microbe Killer as a cure-all in 1886, and in 1893 physician-pharmacist, R.G. Eccles, analyzed the product. Eccles reported that Radam's Microbe Killer was almost entirely water with a small amount of sulfuric acid and vigorously attacked Radam's claims in a pharmacy trade journal. Radam sued Eccles and the journal for libel and lost on the first round. But Radam won his appeal, based on a technical ruling.[63]

The narrow appellate decision, reported on June 24, 1893, reinforced the nostrum-seller's use of the courts to silence medical objections. Equally reassuring was the Chicago *Tribune's* announcement of the decision for Radam, one of its advertisers. The paper's three-column account headlined, "Radam's Microbe Killer in Court—Evidence of Its Phenomenal Curative Virtues Decided to Be Absolutely Conclusive." It was all good news. The phony Microbe Killer made Radam a wealthy man, even after Adams exposed it in 1905.[64]

Shortly after the New York triumph, Amick's company took its promotional machine to Chattanooga, where his agents planned to fill the pages of Adolph Ochs' Chattanooga *Times*. Ochs was feeling the same pressures as Scripps. He was going from bank to bank seeking loans and fending off the early effects of the Panic of 1893.[65] The *Times* was ready to board the Amick Express.

For his part Reeves was laboring over his microscope and enjoying his retirement. The Connecticut Medical Society had elected him an honorary member that spring and, in return, he sent the Society a note of appreciation and several slides. He was preparing a book on medical microscopy and planned to make a slide presentation in September at the Washington, D.C., meeting of the Pan-American Medical Congress. Chattanooga's avuncular pathologist was not looking for a fight.[66]

⽇ 19 ⽇

Professional Indifference
to Professional Enemies

The Chattanooga *Times* reported on July 8, 1893, that the weather was unusually warm throughout the South and that a black man accused of killing two girls had been lynched in Kentucky. The *Times* also mentioned that fifteen boxes of Amick's chemical cure for consumption had arrived at the city health department and that city physician Holland would give it a thorough trial. The brief article advised readers that this was the remedy for consumption which had received the New York Recorder's prize of $1,000 several months ago.[1]

The *Times*, along with dozens of other papers, printed a wire dispatch from Cincinnati the next day. This account, headlined, "Almost Miraculous," related that Mrs. Hayes, a consumptive from North Bend, Ohio, who had been given up for dead a year ago, was now recovering nicely under Dr. Amick's almost miraculous care. Thousands of consumptives regularly wrote to Dr. Amick, but his only aim was to make the cure available to his brother physicians.[2]

The paper announced on July 25 that eleven seriously ill consumptives who had been treated by the city's physician were now almost completely recovered. The report stated that the local medical consensus pronounced Amick's treatment "the most important discovery medical science has yet brought to light," while also noting that this information had been sent by wire to the country's press. The *Times* continued covering Amick's consumption remedy over the next several days, adding the names of Chattanooga doctors who were now firm believers in the Amick cure.[3]

Two Chattanoogans did not follow the script; one of whom was the paper's owner. Even before the New York *Times*, Adolph Ochs' famed journalistic objectivity hid a talent for exploiting a dispute.[4] The Cincinnati *Post* and New York *Recorder* faithfully praised Amick and avoided any negative coverage, but Ochs' Chattanooga *Times* promised readers an "open court" to evaluate Amick's treatment. The second person was Reeves. Reeves saw more than another quack cure and he was undeterred by ethical constraints against physician criticism or fears of litigation. He confronted Amick on his own grounds, the pages of the *Times*.

Reeves penned an angry letter to the *Times* on August 2, 1893, which the paper printed the next day. He quoted the *Times*' promise of an open court and attacked Ochs' complicity: "We have before us a medical question—an issue in which your indorsement is wholly worthless; for the reason that you are a newspaper, not a learned physician capable of striking the difference between the methods of medical quackery and the necessary painstaking labors in formulating medical truth."[5]

Reeves avoided calling Amick a quack. Instead he accused Amick of using the methods of quackery, such as forming a for-profit company, sending out slick brochures, undertaking his studies in the public press, and selling his cure. He seemed to be aware, unlike some of his colleagues, that labeling someone a quack was by itself (*per se*) defamatory and difficult to defend.

Reeves put his name and reputation in the line. He claimed that the city physician had no bacteriologic proof that any of the patients under his care had tuberculosis and, when Reeves had confronted him and offered to perform microscopic examinations, he (Holland) declined. Reeves told the *Times'* editor that he had ordered a sample of Amick's treatment and would give it a fair trial, under scrupulous supervision, as soon as possible. The *Times* appended a response, agreeing to the conditions set by Reeves, although its unnamed writer could not resist defending Amick as "a practitioner of standing and responsibility in Cincinnati."

The *Times* continued to report success stories over the next weeks, with minimal objections from Reeves' fellow physicians. Only one other *Times* letter raised doubts. Two Chattanooga physicians wrote on August 7 that one of the patients Amick claimed to have cured never had consumption. One of the doctors stated he had little interest in the open court, but he believed Amick had not discovered anything except "the efficacy of printer's ink." When medical editors paid Amick notice, they responded tepidly. The *North Carolina Medical Journal* observed that the daily press was being filled with reports of Amick's cure and wondered if this was merely advertising subterfuge. Deciding that it was, the *Journal* refused to accept Amick's advertisements.[6]

Reeves followed his published criticism and his willingness to publicly test Amick's cure with a third move that raised the stakes for everyone. He sent dozens of postal cards to the physicians Amick had named as satisfied users. He asked recipients to share their chemical treatment experience with him, observing that Amick had made Chattanooga a "head center for sending out in the secular press wonderful cures which are pure fabrication."[7]

Amick's friends in Cincinnati passed the card to Amick, who moved to silence Reeves. Amick ordered Milton Gosdorfer, a company agent who was secretly writing articles for the *Times*, to file a complaint with the postal service. A deputy U.S. marshal arrested Reeves on August 26, 1893, for violating federal postal laws. As Gosdorfer interrogated him, Reeves was first puzzled, then irate. If he had sent his inquiry in a letter, there would have been no issue, but communicating potentially defamatory statements via postal cards subjected Reeves to a five thousand dollar fine and five years' imprisonment per offense. The federal commissioner overseeing the arrest released Reeves on a thousand dollar bond and set a grand jury date for October. Gosdorfer publicly threatened Reeves with a civil suit if he continued defaming Amick.[8]

The Chattanooga papers reported the facts of the prominent doctor's arrest and the *Times* finally put its own reporter on the story, calling Amick's action his company's "Biggest Ad." Scripps' Cincinnati *Post* provided another spin. It boasted that Cincinnati physician Amick "Gets Back." Amick, it said, was tired of being abused by the medical profession.

He had Reeves arrested for violating postal laws and Reeves confessed to sending the offending card. In a backhanded compliment, the Cincinnati report referred to sixty-four-year-old Reeves as "a patriarch in the profession, being nearly three score and ten."[9]

Medical journals paid little attention to Reeves' arrest at first. James Baldwin in Ohio gave it a brief notice and, in language more typical of Baldwin than Reeves, promised that Reeves was "ready to wipe up the earth with the fraud." When the Philadelphia *Medical News* covered the event, it quoted Reeves as planning to keep after Amick, "though there be as many devils in the way as there are tiles on the houses of Chattanooga."[10]

For his part, Reeves returned to preparing slides for the September 5–8 Pan American Medical Congress in Washington, D.C. Several of Reeves' longtime associates attended the Congress and congratulated him on his opposition to Amick. The night before his microscopic presentation Reeves got word that Amick had made good on his threat and had filed a $25,000 civil suit against him. He seemed to welcome the news, smiling when he heard it.[11]

The editor of the *Medical News,* George Gould, also attended the Congress and afterwards Reeves and Gould became close friends. Reeves relished the meeting. He wrote to the conference chairman William Pepper a week after the Congress ended, complimenting his "guiding hand in winning the success of this incomparable venture." He signed the letter, "Your Old Friend, James E. Reeves."[12]

As Reeves awaited his October grand jury hearing on postal law violations, Amick flooded the country's newspapers with wire dispatches. He presented himself as a bold and maligned innovator, on a level with Pasteur. Like many other papers, the St. Joseph (Missouri) *Herald* reported on October 1, 1893, that Cleveland's physicians were successfully using Amick's cure. The article implied a medical conspiracy against Amick, concluding: "The majority of the profession interviewed evidently believe Amick, but many of them accuse him of violating the code."[13]

Reeves' day in court was short and definitive. The federal grand jury in Chattanooga returned a decision of no true bill on October 9, 1893, refusing to indict him for violating postal laws. Reeves told reporters that if the object was intimidation, "The wrong man was waked up." The Chattanooga *Times* presented the matter even-handedly and asked Reeves about his test cases. He responded that the most hopeful user of the Amick cure had died in thirty days, two had quit the treatment, and the remaining three had not improved. He assured the paper's readers that "a cure for consumption worthy of the name would need neither newspaper advertisements nor criminal arrest and damage suits to bring it before the public."[14]

Reeves' success in Amick's criminal suit now made the matter personal for a handful of other physicians. Gould praised his courage in *The Medical News*, criticizing his fellows for their fear of libel suits and medical editors for their nostrum advertising, and the *St. Louis Medical and Surgical Journal* reprinted Gould's words. The Philadelphia County Medical Society passed a resolution on October 18, 1893, commending Reeves for his bravery and reiterating that no one who advertised a secret nostrum could be considered a physician in good standing. At least four other journals published the Philadelphia County Medical Society's resolution, adding their own editorial endorsements.[15]

Cincinnati's James Culbertson provided the most spirited response, although Culbertson had his own agenda. When Culbertson edited the *Journal of the American Medical Association* from 1891 to 1893, he safeguarded regular physicians' interests by denigrating pharmacists and other practitioners who competed with regulars.[16] As owner of the *Lancet-Clinic*, Culbertson used Reeves' notoriety to pound regular medicine's competitors and increase his journal's visibility.

Culbertson posted a note in the *Lancet-Clinic* implying that Reeves had won a civil lawsuit when he had actually faced criminal charges. He followed this with a two-page diatribe against quackery and the public press, ending with: "The Amick Cure people are not the only quacks in this city and State, for the newspaper columns are full of the gush of a myriad of the ilk." Culbertson's condemnation of quackery and newspapers was standard regular physician invective, which nostrum-sellers and irregular practitioners often ignored or marketed as a badge of distinction. But Culbertson provided Amick with a point of attack and he took it. Amick sued Culbertson for $50,000 for calling him a quack.[17]

Amick soon filed another lawsuit against St. Louis College of Physicians and Surgeons for $150,000. The college's journal, *The St. Louis Clinique*, had repeated Culbertson's description of Reeves' legal encounter, included three other articles denouncing Amick as a quack, and added Gould's more accurate description of Reeves' victory in a criminal proceeding.[18]

Amick filed four civil libel suits in 1893 and Reeves had a role in three of them. The first was an April 1893 claim for $150,000 against the Ohio Medical College, before Reeves had heard of Amick. The next, in September, was for $25,000 against Reeves personally. The third was in November for $50,000 against Culbertson and the fourth was for $150,000 in December against the St. Louis College of Physicians and Surgeons, both of whom had cited Reeves in their attacks on Amick. Culbertson, who was a medical publisher and not a practitioner, relished the spectacle, writing: "Measured by the number of suits and the amount sued for, the Amick Company is the worst damaged firm or corporation in the world."[19]

An anonymous writer for the *British Medical Journal* saw Amick's unique threat to American medicine differently, more as Reeves did. It was not just a typical episode of quackery; it was a frontal assault on medical science. The *Journal's* Philadelphia correspondent singled out Amick: "he used the lay press to advertise his 'cure' by means of the reading notice—a great institution with us—and by means of 'doctored' press dispatches sent to the newspapers of the land, mixed up with real news and as if themselves real bits of news." The writer praised Reeves: "Finally, one physician in the whole country rose up and denounced the imposture. That brave man was Dr. J. C. Reeves [*sic*], of Chatanooga [*sic*], Tenn."[20]

The correspondent put his finger on the problem. The threat was Amick's misappropriation of "the reading notice," the news part of the newspaper and most Americans' source of scientific information. Amick did more than slip in the occasional endorsement and pay for outrageous advertising claims. His inflated medical credentials and his pseudo-scientific patient testing appeared in the same public arena as Koch and Pasteur, men of genuine accomplishment. If Amick could steal this space, no community was safe.

Amick's legal action against the Ohio Medical College never reappeared, but the Cincinnati *Post* reported Amick's success in his $150,000 claim against the St. Louis *Clinique* and the College of Physicians and Surgeons in February 1894. The notice did not mention the amount of damages, but its writer promoted Amick: "This medical journal questioned the merits of the Amick treatment for consumption, which many physicians here say is the only cure for this disease." The same report showed up in numerous other papers. A far less visible notice in the *St. Louis Post-Dispatch* reported that judge had awarded Amick a nominal twenty-five dollars in damages.[21]

The suit against Culbertson was changed to criminal libel, with a potential penalty of up to five hundred dollars and/or six months in jail. Preliminary testimony, published by Culbertson, showed how the Amick Company had a cozy relationship with the press and sent its own wire dispatches. William Amick did not testify, but, during the proceedings, brother Marion appeared as a bumbling co-conspirator who knew nothing about the company or its secret formula. Marion dealt with the question of quackery by stating that a quack was a rascally person with no diploma, whereas he and his brother were educated men. Culbertson's attorney presented evidence that a quack was someone who pretended to do what he could not. The following exchange transpired when Marion was asked the about his consumption cure: "Question: You still claim to have a cure for consumption? M.L. Amick: Yes, in the majority of cases. Question: How large a majority? M.L. Amick: Twenty-five percent." The grand jury refused to indict Culbertson and Culbertson announced his triumph in July 1894 and the impending demise of the Amick Chemical Company.[22]

Culbertson's legal and journalistic attacks may have heartened his physician readers, but they did not deter his target because Amick operated in a different arena. He continued to coax sympathetic commentary from other medical journals, doing so under Culbertson's nose in *The Cincinnati Medical Journal*. He advertised in the *Medical Brief* that while doctors disagreed on whether it was ethical to use his cure, thousands did. He boasted that the Amick Chemical Company sent seven thousand shipments to physicians in March 1894 compared to nineteen hundred in March 1893. When Reeves' attorney deposed Amick in October 1894, Amick claimed that his company had supplied treatments to forty thousand doctors. He sent that information via wire dispatch throughout the country as a "remarkable fact."[23]

Amick promoted his cure to doctors by pitching himself as an expert in consumption and defender of country physicians against America's medical elite. He railed against sanitarians who argued that consumption was a contagious disease caused by the tubercle bacillus. Consumptives did not want to deal with quarantine and separation and many practicing physicians did not want to stigmatize their patients. Amick was ever-ready to oppose the forced isolation of consumptives, while justifying the soundness of his product.[24]

Culbertson's assertion that Amick was done, mostly at Culbertson's hands, was self-serving and premature, but Culbertson correctly assessed Amick's worsening financial situation. Despite his grandiose numbers and opportunistic opposition to the germ theory, Amick was in trouble. His company's capital had plummeted from $300,000 in 1892, to $60,000 in 1895. He needed a convincing win, which he planned to get against Chattanooga naysayer, James Reeves.[25]

Amick was barely in Reeves' thoughts. While his lawyer was collecting evidence for the suit, Reeves was using his lucid and graceful pen to educate his fellow physicians.

Numerous medical authorities wanted physicians to add microscopy to their medical practice, as they had adopted the stethoscope, thermometer, and ophthalmoscope. In a prize-winning essay William Hays argued in 1893, as Reeves had done in 1882, that a working knowledge of microscopic technique was essential for the diagnosis and management of many common diseases. Good medical practice required microscopic information and the alternative to doing it yourself, relying on professional clinical laboratories, was not feasible for most physicians.[26]

Physicians needed a practical handbook to guide them. Microscopic societies held workshops for devotees of microscope technology and urban salons allowed interested amateurs to show their slides, but there was little guidance for busy doctors. Medical schools were just beginning to introduce students to bench science and the last American handbook on medical microscopy was written in 1871, before the germ theory, stains, microtomes, and oil immersion.[27]

The most recent handbook, London physician Frank Wethered's 1892 *Guide to the Use of the Microscope in Medical Practice*, was almost worthless. The *Journal of the American Medical Association* practically asked Reeves to take the baton in its review of Wethered: "It seems astonishing that at this time no better, simpler, or more practical recommendations can be made to the physician than those here set forth."[28]

Reeves published his 237-page *Hand-Book of Medical Microscopy for Students and General Practitioners* in September 1894. The book was small enough to fit in a physician's coat pocket, with a strong binding, high-quality paper, clearly-marked sections, and seventy-five illustrations, twenty-six in color. Reeves wrote that all progressive physicians should use the microscope in their practice. They must learn to do their own microscopic work or, if possible, find someone to do it for them. He quickly got to basics: how to buy the right equipment for the money, what lenses to get, how to use them, and how to prepare and stain specimens. The bulk of the book was devoted to interpreting common microscopic findings in infections, cancer, urine, blood, sputum, and feces. He dedicated the work to Frances Reeves and placed the copyright in her name: "My beloved wife and only companion in microscopy."[29]

Medical editors praised the effort. The *Journal of the American Medical Association*, which had panned Wethered's book two year earlier, wrote: "In the production of this little volume the author has turned his long practical experience to good account. He has succeeded in condensing in a minimum space a great deal of material of especial interest to the practitioner." Culbertson, in the Cincinnati *Lancet-Clinic*, was sympathetic to the kind words to Frances: "they speak to the heart of an affection and a sentiment that commands at once our esteem and admiration for the appreciative author and his beloved wife." To Culbertson, the book succeeded in placing within easy reach all the information a physician might need. Baldwin's *Columbus Medical Journal* opined, "Taken as a whole, the work is to be most heartily commended as one of our most valuable and practical treatises on Medical Microscopy." The *Virginia Medical Monthly* counseled, "Get it, is our advice to every practitioner."[30]

Reeves wrote to his daughter Annie in March 1895 that his book was selling well,

550 copies in the first five months. He told her that he had agreed to take charge of the bacteriology and microscopy laboratories at the next session of Vanderbilt University's medical college. He was seemingly in good health and good spirits as the Amick trial approached.[31]

Amick's suit went to trial in Chattanooga on April 11, 1895, and lasted a day and a half. The plaintiff charged Reeves with falsely and maliciously defaming him in his August 2, 1893, letter to the Chattanooga *Times*.[32]

Amick offered the story of his New York success, verified by the *Recorder*, as evidence of his legitimacy. He told jurors that he had been gracious enough to send samples of his cure to any physician who requested them, only charging doctors ten dollars for a month's supply of medicine after that. He claimed he had been persecuted by Reeves who called him a humbug and a bare-faced fraud, terms that did not appear in Reeves' August 2 letter to the *Times*. The plaintiff reminded the jury that all great medical discoveries had been accompanied by denunciations and his attorney took this sentiment to another level: "Every doctor who ventures a little in advance of his profession gets in front of an armed mob."

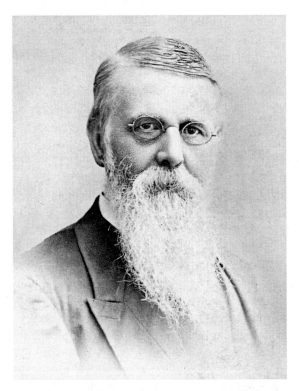

James Reeves in 1895. In April 1895 Cincinnati physician William Amick accused Reeves of libel in a dramatic courtroom trial. Reeves had charged Amick with promoting a false consumption cure by lying about its benefits, inducing local physicians to collaborate, and paying the Chattanooga *Times* to print his falsehoods as news (courtesy Barbara Boren).

The defense sought to show that Amick deserved Reeves' approbations. Reeves' attorney, W.B. Garvin, presented copies of Amick's marketing materials claiming that he had an absolute remedy for consumption and that he could cure the disease by treating patients through the mail. He called numerous Chattanooga doctors to the stand who testified that consumption could not be cured by mail order. The defense provided evidence that Amick's news articles printed by the *Times* during July and August 1893 were written by Milton Gosdorfer, the Amick Company's paid agent. Dr. Holland, the city physician, stated that he never tested the Amick cure as Gosdorfer's *Times'* articles reported he had. Garvin showed that many of the cases Amick claimed to have cured in Chattanooga were either dead from consumption or never had the disease.

Garvin challenged Amick's assertion that Reeves had libelously defamed Amick as a humbug by establishing that those words had been purloined from a *Times* interview that the paper never printed. The defense asserted that Reeves was an authority on the diagnosis of tuberculosis and the *Times* had offered him an open court of public opinion, to which Reeves had responded by writing truthfully and without malice. As he summed up the hours of testimony, Reeves' attorney reminded the jury of the stakes: "Why, a [favorable] verdict of this jury, even for one cent, would be worth a million dollars to them [Amick], because it would be a virtual endorsement of their claims, and be sent by wire all over the country within one hour from the delivery of such a verdict. They would send it out world-wide, 'Dr. Amick's cure vindicated.'"[33]

Amick's attorney countered that Reeves' actions were clearly malicious. He submitted a letter Reeves had written to Amick after Reeves' release from the criminal charges in 1893. The lengthy missive, reminiscent of Reeves' public attack on John Carlile in 1855 and his pamphlet denouncing Hupp in 1879, left few stones unthrown. Reeves called out Amick to his face with a list of his actions, included sending one of his manufactured newspaper articles about Reeves to the chairman of the arrangements committee of the 1893 Pan-American Congress. Why hadn't Amick tested his cure in the great Cincinnati hospital? "Indeed, why did you not go to the Pan-Congress and there convince the multitude of your grand discovery of a cure for consumption?" Reeves condemned Amick in his personal letter far more than he had in public. The document left no doubt that Reeves considered Amick a fraud and a sinner.

Following twelve hours of testimony and spirited summaries, the judge instructed the jury that despite Reeves' measured phrasing, his letter to the editor of the *Times* from August 1893 was *per se* libelous under Tennessee law. The pivotal matter was whether Reeves' statements were true. If they were, no matter how harshly written, there was no libel and the matter was settled. If there were questions of fact, then Reeves' motive was important. Did he act out of malice or in good faith and in the public interest?

After ten minutes deliberation, the jury returned a verdict in Reeves' favor. A few hours later the *Times* congratulated Reeves in its afternoon edition. The paper's story highlighted Reeves' noble motives and ignored the unpleasant journalistic and professional details the trial brought to light: "Dr. Reeves, having been tried by a jury of his peers, stands acquitted of any intention to malign a medicine compounder, and the inference was obvious, was working in what he considered the interest of the public." Among the facts not reported by the *Times* was that it had hired an Amick Company agent, Gosdorfer, with no oversight of his reporting, and that the Amick Company paid the *Times* double its usual advertising rates so that Gosdorfer's deceitful material would appear as reading matter.[34]

Except for Wheeling, where the dailies kept an eye on Reeves, newspapers outside Chattanooga ignored the trial. The Wheeling *Intelligencer* wrote, "Dr. Reeves vindicated," followed by a brief summary of the events. In the same notice the *Intelligencer* reported on "A very peculiar incident" associated with the case. S.G. Sea, the consumptive Chicago *Herald* business manager who had joined the Amick Chemical Company in 1892 after being cured by Amick's remedy, had died the previous week in New Mexico from consumption.[35]

The medical press was more engaged, but it preferred to report the courtroom disclosures that played into its anti-competitive narrative. Within a week of the trial's conclusion, the *Philadelphia Polyclinic* wrote, "Reeves Vindicated," emphasizing that

Reeves had forced the Chattanooga papers to admit that they were paid to present Amick's advertising as news. Gould reminded readers of the *Medical News* of Reeves' first victory in his criminal suit and started a campaign to raise two hundred dollars to pay for copies of the trial transcript as a "'stiffener of the moral backbone' of physicians in their fight with the nostrum vendors."[36]

To physicians who cared, such as Gould, this drama represented one physician's courageous battle against the forces of quackery. They overlooked what the trial said about regular physician complicity. Reeves had been approached by Amick's agent and told that it would be worth his while to endorse the product. He chose to publicly expose the fraud when others remained silent. Reeves' trial uncovered multiple improprieties committed by Chattanooga doctors, including assertions that patients were recovering when they weren't. Doctors paid Amick $10 for the medicines, but Amick encouraged them to charge patients as much as they could.

Physician leaders condemned this kind of self-serving physician behavior, but not in public. They preferred to deal with it internally, which generally meant ineffectively. Gould wrote in the *Medical News* about an unethical physician ring of self-referral and patient-stealing, asking: "Are we all proceeding, without protest and without solicitude, to ruin and individualism, and to utter neglect of the principles and practices whereby alone we can still keep a noble *esprit de corps* within the profession, and save it from the all-conquering crush of greed and commercialism?"[37] (author's italics). With the trial transcript in front of them, Gould and his fellow medical leaders had no comment on the exposure of physician shortcomings in Chattanooga. For them, it was better to keep such transgressions inside medicine's walls. Reeves normally took the same approach, but this case was different. Here the interests of his community took precedence.

Baldwin, who was a close friend of Gould as well as Reeves, chided Gould for stealing the Reeves Fund idea from him, but the drive to collect two hundred dollars to print copies of the trial transcript languished. Gould had donations from just fourteen physicians by June 1895 and he labeled the results: "Professional Indifference to Professional Enemies." He pointed out that English physicians had rallied around a physician cricket-player. Couldn't American physicians do the same for one who had so selfishly fought quackery on their behalf? In July the *Journal of the American Medical Association* picked up Gould's campaign and made it a national cause: "The Journal heartily indorses the sentiments of the Medical News, and urges every member of the American Medical Association to send his subscription of at least 50 cents to Dr. Reeves for a copy of this report."[38]

This step broke the ice. Over the next few months Gould printed subscribers' names in the *Medical News* as their donations arrived and, in September, he announced success. The James E. Reeves Fund contained $225, sent by sixty-five contributors in forty-one cities. The money was sent to Reeves to reprint copies of the trial transcript and cover legal expenses. The donors included Gould, Baldwin, and several of the country's better-known physicians: Baltimore's William Osler, AMA *Journal* editor, John B. Hamilton, and Battle Creek, Michigan's John Kellogg. Gould emphasized the danger that he saw: "The success of the suit of Amick vs. Reeves would have emboldened all forms of quackery and spread universal intimidation."[39]

James Culbertson, the *Lancet-Clinic's* owner and tenacious regular medicine advocate, never shared Gould's personal admiration of Reeves' battle; he tended to see Reeves' work as an extension of his own campaigns. Culbertson printed a brief notice following the verdict that J.R. (*sic*) Reeves in Chattanooga had exposed the fraudulent Amick Consumption Combine (*sic*). Two weeks later he reprinted the *Polyclinic* article, which focused on condemnation of the lay press. Culbertson did not contribute to the Reeves Fund and, in 1896, after Reeves died, he gave himself full credit for stopping Amick: "his [Amick's] plans were thwarted through a ventilation of the business in the *Lancet-Clinic* pages."[40]

The Amick consumption ruse succumbed to the weight of its false pretenses and its legal failures. William Amick left Cincinnati for his home town of Scipio, Indiana in September 1895 and Marion Amick returned to his practice. William developed consumption within a year and died in 1900. Marion avoided the stigma of William's business and at his death in 1904 was popularly recognized as one of Cincinnati's leading physicians. Family members told others that Marion had made $50,000 with William's consumption cure.[41]

From 1897 until 1903 Henry Roos ran the Amick Chemical Company and offered treatments for diseases of the lungs and air passages, but he did not advertise in medical journals, instead providing newspapers with occasional testimonials from grateful users. The company disappeared after 1903.[42]

Amick was the first and most ambitious physician to market a secret nostrum to physicians by organizing fake tests in the popular press. Historians of nineteenth-century quackery have not mentioned the episode, the strategy, or similar examples. Likewise, Reeves' pursuit was unique and his peers knew this. While medical editors, society officers, and licensing authorities often appointed themselves quack-chasers and protectors of the medical marketplace, they did not call each other out in postal cards and newspapers.

Once the Amick trial was done, Reeves returned to his routine. He had the energy to attend the May AMA meeting in Baltimore, where the delegates elected him a trustee of the organization, but his health began failing. His personal doctor, P.D. Sims, could find nothing wrong. In September, Reeves struggled to entertain his visiting son and two daughters and he and Sims became convinced there was a problem. Reeves worried it might be liver cancer.[43]

After his family returned home, Reeves took the train to Baltimore, where, in early October he met with Osler, who felt the liver nodules that confirmed Reeves' fatal diagnosis of cancer. To thank Osler for his time, Reeves sent him three collectible medical books as soon as he returned to Chattanooga. Gould heard of Reeves' meeting with Osler and planned a visit to Baltimore, but Reeves left for Chattanooga on October 15, before Gould could make the trip. Gould penned Reeves an affectionate note the same day, hoping to hear from him and Osler on the outlook.[44]

The word that Reeves was seriously ill spread quickly. Gould was distraught and wrote Reeves almost daily for the next several months. Gould and other physicians, including Louis Wilson from Wheeling, Baldwin from Columbus, and future AMA president Nicholas Senn from Chicago, travelled to Chattanooga to wish him and Frances well.[45]

Gould sent encouragement from Philadelphia's best-known doctors and several physicians corresponded with each other about Reeves. Gould wrote Reeves on November 24, 1895, "This Sunday morning I wonder how you are? I am rather blue from much work and worry and from solicitude about you. Senn wrote me a nice note, and Osler wrote that he would send you a line. Dear Osler!" Two days later Gould sent a letter to Baldwin that the Chattanooga *Times* later reprinted in Reeves' obituary: "It is very good of you to write to me so fully about dear old Reeves. We shall, then, have to give him up! It is very sad. We need such men as he in the profession…. He is one of the best and truest men in the profession, as you say, and has done noble work for us all and for humanity."[46]

Reeves viewed his fate with resignation. Chattanooga's mayor, Adolph Ochs' brother George Ochs, sent a note to Wheeling's mayor, George Caldwell, in December: "Dr. Reeves is now lying on his death-bed and may pass away any day … though his body has generally wasted, his mind still retains all its faculties, and he speaks with equanimity of his approaching end." Papers throughout the country carried a short dispatch a few days later announcing that "James Edmund Reeves, bacteriologist and physician of more than national eminence," was dying.[47]

Family and friends came to Reeves' bedside. Sims visited his patient once or twice a day during Reeves' last weeks and another physician, D.E. Nelson, slept in Reeves' house at night. Reeves told the family he wished to be buried next to his son in Wheeling and, knowing liver cancer was a rare disease, he wanted his abdominal organs sent to Osler.[48]

Within hours of his passing on January 4, 1896, Chattanooga's afternoon paper ran a lengthy obituary. The following morning, the *Times* devoted an entire page to Reeves and the Chattanooga Medical Society called a special meeting to honor him. The afternoon funeral service was filled with the city's leading citizens. Physicians performed the autopsy that Reeves requested and, following the Chattanooga memorial, Sims accompanied Reeves' body to Wheeling.[49]

The Wheeling papers reported Reeves' death and his body's journey to West Virginia. The *Intelligencer* described him as an eminent microscopist, but remembered his sanitary career, recognizing him as the author and advocate of the law creating the State Board of Health. On January 7, two days after the Chattanooga services, another large group of physicians and friends, augmented by many of Reeves' former patients, paid its respects. Wheeling's Mayor Caldwell was one of the pallbearers as Reeves was laid to rest in Greenwood Cemetery.[50]

Numerous newspapers printed a short notice of Reeves' death, but it was a minor event outside of Chattanooga and Wheeling. Irving Watson's *Physicians and Surgeons of America* presented a biography of Reeves in January 1896 based on Samuel Woods' 1885 sketch for the *New England Medical Monthly*. Reeves must have approved this publication because it contained a recent photograph and was clearly written before his death. The entry summarized his life, omitting Woods' testimonial to Reeves' character. Most medical journals that mentioned his passing referred to this information. Only the *Medical News*, edited by Gould's successor, J. R. Goffe, was more expansive: "Dr. Reeves was the type of man that the profession can ill afford to lose—broad-minded, progressive and aggressive, rigidly honest and ethical. The profession of medicine is nobler that he has lived." The president of the Association of American Physicians reminded Reeves' colleagues that "his undoubted courage and moral strength are a bright example that should not be forgotten."[51]

Epilogue
Medical Professionalism

Louis Wilson organized the twenty-ninth annual meeting of the Medical Society of West Virginia in June 1896. He asked Reeves' sister, Ann Jarvis, to send a letter about her recently deceased brother, which Wilson read to the group. Wilson added his own experiences to Ann's recollections, citing Reeves' accomplishments and virtues, but also remembering his faults: "His natural fondness for controversy sometimes led him to exhibit too much the ardor of combat." But, overall, Wilson worshipped Reeves and the work he achieved: "The State Medical Society and the State Board of Health of West Virginia must ever stand as testimonials to his farsighted wisdom. Truly, with Horace, he might have said, 'I have builded a monument more durable than brass,' for as long as these institutions endure so will his memory and influence live and bless.[1]"

The West Virginia State Medical Association remembered Reeves over the next forty years, establishing a monument to the organization's founding in 1936 and listing Reeves' name at the top. The monument was placed near where Reeves lived when the Association was founded in 1867 and the Monument Commission's chairman singled out Reeves' contributions to West Virginia at its dedication: "The climax of this great physician's life I believe was the formulation of the West Virginia health laws." The Chattanooga *Times* noticed the event: "Monument in West Virginia Dedicated to Dr. Reeves, Old-Time Chattanoogan." The stone monument still stands in a small city park near Fairmont and the state medical association displays a copy of the monument's plaque on its entrance.[2]

For the most part though, West Virginia and his profession forgot about Reeves during the century after his death. Callahan did not cover Reeves in his two-volumes of West Virginia biographies in 1923, nor did more contemporary West Virginia historians, such Williams (1976) or Rice (1985) mention him. To this day he is not listed in the West Virginia Public Health Hall of Fame or noted anywhere at the West Virginia University School of Public Health. The twentieth century's medical literature cited him just five times. Four of these were brief biographical notes early in the century and one was a derogatory swipe by an American Medical Association historian in 1984 who described his microscopy handbook as part of a "naïve" and "pathetic" physician self-education movement.[3]

Reeves deserves better. Medical historian James Mohr authored a book in 2013 on the West Virginia Board of Health Act and its legal consequences. Mohr described Reeves as "one of the most significant—if little known—figures in American medical history." For medical-legal scholar Mohr: "The West Virginia Board of Health Act should probably have been named the Reeves Act."[4]

For today's health care professionals the personal meaning of Reeves' story is not about his accomplishments, but his professional development and his ethics, features that define each of them. Reeves was a prototypical medical innovator, an early adopter of new concepts. As such, he frequently crossed paths with others whom the innovation diffusion literature would characterize as late majority adopters and laggards. He made it a personal mission to bring the emerging lessons of medical science, ones that he often taught to himself, to others. His life-long student-teacher identity exemplified a core value of todays' medical professionalism.[5]

But Reeves saw medical science differently from many of his fellows, not through the lens of medical fraternity, but through the teaching of his faith, what medical ethicists now call external ideals. Here he differed from today's vision of medical professionalism, one that often gives practitioners and educators the comfort to define their ethical standards and the right to own their science.[6]

Chapter Notes

Prologue

1. "Dr. James E. Reeves," *The Sunday Times*, Chattanooga, TN, January 5, 1896, 5; "Funeral of Dr. Reeves," *The Daily Times*, Chattanooga, TN, January 6, 1896.

2. "Dr. James E. Reeves"; "Funeral of Dr. J.E. Reeves," *The Wheeling Daily Intelligencer*, Wheeling, WV, January 8, 1896.

3. "Dr. Reeves Dead," *The Chattanooga News*, Chattanooga, TN, January 4, 1896; "Dr. Reeves Dying," *Wheeling Register*, Wheeling, WV, December 20, 1895, 8.

4. William Osler, Personal letter, November 27, 1895; George M Gould, Personal letter, November 26, 1895; "Dr. James E. Reeves."

Chapter 1

1. David M. Ludlum, *The Weather Factor* (Boston, MA: American Meteorological Society, 1989). Gaillard Hunt, ed. *The First Forty Years of Washington Society Portrayed by the Family Letters of Mrs. Samuel Harrison Smith* (New York, NY: Charles Scribner's Sons, 1906), 296; Arthur M. Schlesinger, *The Age of Jackson* (Old Saybrook, CT: Konecky & Konecky, 1971; repr., 1971).

2. Louis D. Wilson, "James Edmund Reeves, M.D.," *Transactions of the Medical Society of the State of West Virginia* (1896): 1319–27; W. C. Wile (editor), "Our Gallery—James Edmund Reeves, M.D. of Wheeling, W. Va.," *New England Medical Monthly* 4 (1884): 480–83. Josiah Reeves was 19 or 20 when James was born, but probably younger than his wife. Information on Josiah Reeves' birth is from: Baltimore Conference of the Methodist Episcopal Church, Index Card, Unknown. Although he was probably born in 1810, census records consistently show him as a year or two younger than Nancy: Bureau of the Census, "1850 Federal Census for Barbour County, Virginia," 1850. Nancy Kemper was 19 or 20 when James was born. The online Findagrave index gives her birth year as 1803: Jim Tipton, "Find a Grave Search Form," in *Find a Grave* .This date makes her eight years older than her husband and one that I erroneously used in an earlier paper: John M. Harris, "James Edmund Reeves (1829–1896) and the Contentious 19th Century Battle for Medical Professionalism in the United States," *Journal of Medical Biography* (2014). A published genealogy of the Kemper family also provides conflicting birthdates, 1803 and 1810: Willis Miller and Wright Kemper, Harry Linn, *Genealogy of the Kemper Family in the United States* (Chicago: Geo. K Hazlitt & Co., 1899)73, Appendix v. Data from the more reliable 1850 and 1860 U.S. census records place her birth year around 1810: "1850 Federal Census for Barbour County, Virginia"; Bureau of the Census, "1860 Federal Census for Barbour County, Virginia," 1860 This date also suggests that she and her husband were of similar ages. 1830 census records showed the "J.W. Revers" household, all the proper ages for the J.W. Reeves family, one name removed from the Elizabeth Kemper household, also the proper age to be Nancy's sister: U.S. Census, "Fifth Census of the United States, 1830," 1830; Kemper, *Genealogy of the Kemper Family in the United States* Ancestry members, "Ancestry Family Trees" (Provo, UT: Ancestry.com, 2016).

3. Eugene Scheel, *Culpeper—A Virginia County's History through 1920* (Orange, VA: Green Publishers, Inc., 1982).

4. Church; "City Matters," *The Wheeling Daily Intelligencer*, Wheeling, WV, December 20, 1882, 4. A newspaper reference showed Josiah Reeves working as a lay preacher in 1853: "The Execution at Phillippi," *Cooper's Clarksburg Register* Clarksburg, VA November 2, 1853. Josiah's daughter Ann described him as a stern father and "a highly respected and esteemed Methodist minister": Wilson, "James Edmund Reeves, M.D.," 1320.

5. Richard P. Heitzenrater, *Wesley and the People Called Methodists*, second ed. (Nashville, TN: Abingdon Press).

6. On American Methodism: William W. Sweet, *Religion on the American Frontier 1783–1840*, vol. IV—The Methodists (Chicago: University of Chicago Press, 1946); John H. Wigger, *Taking Heaven by Storm—Methodism and the Rise of Popular Christianity in America* (Urbana and Chicago: University of Illinois Press, 2001). The "true church" metaphor, an essential part of Reeves' professional identity, likely came from Immanuel Kant (1724–1804), who, reflecting on Christianity, described an "invisible church" of persons united under the laws of virtue: Helmut Holzhey and Vilem Mudroch, *Historical Dictionary of Kant and Kantianism*, vol. 60, Historical Dictionaries of Religions Philosophies, and Movements (Lanham, MD: Scarecrow Press, 2005). His fellow German, Christoph Wilhelm Hufeland (1762–1836), physician to the Prussian king, used Kant's imagery

to portray his profession's dedication to science: "There has ever been an invisible church of genuine physicians, who, always faithful to nature, animated by her spirit, acted according to her intimation, and preserved her holy word": Christoph Wilhelm Hufeland, *Enchiridion Medicum; Oder, Anleitung Zur Medizinischen Praxis VermäChtniss Einer FüNfzigjäRigen Erfahrung* (Berlin: Jonas, 1836), 68. In English: *Enchiridion Medicum or Manual of the Practice of Medicine*, trans. Caspar Bruchhausen, sixth German edition (New York: William Radde, 1842), 75.

7. For information on Wesley's preaching see, among others: Heitzenrater, *Wesley and the People Called Methodists*; Stephen W. Rankin, "Wesley and War: Guidance for Modern Day Heirs?," *Methodist Review* 3 (2011): 101–39; John Wesley, "Sermon 88—on Dress," *Global Ministries of the United Methodist Church*, http://www.umcmission.org/; "Sermon 98—on Visiting the Sick," *Global Ministries of the United Methodist Church*, http://www.umcmission.org/; "Sermon 30—Upon Our Lord's Sermon on the Mount, 10," *Global Ministries of the United Methodist Church*, http://www.umcmission.org/; "Sermon 32—Upon Our Lord's Sermon on the Mount, 12," *Global Ministries of the United Methodist Church*, http://www.umcmission.org/; "Sermon 65—the Duty of Reproving Our Neighbour," *Global Ministries of the United Methodist Church*, http://www.umcmission.org/; "Sermon 86—A Call to Backsliders," *Global Ministries of the United Methodist Church*, http://www.umcmission.org/; Charles V. Chapin, "History of State and Municipal Control of Disease," in *A Half Century of Public Health*, ed. Mazÿck Ravenel (New York, NY: American Public Health Association, 1921), 133–60; David A. Loving, "The Development of American Public Health, 1850–1925" (University of Oklahoma, 2008).

8. A Mechanic, "For the United States Telegraph," *United States Telegraph*, Washington, D.C. March 6, 1829, 7. Knight's patent was contested by Ross Winan and the invention, while fanning interest in rail commerce, proved to be impractical. John H. White, *The American Railroad Passenger Car*, 2 vols., vol. 2 (Baltimore, MD: Johns Hopkins University Press, 1985).

9. E. R. Wicker, "Railroad Investment before the Civil War," in *Trends in the American Economy in the Nineteenth Century*, ed. The Conference on Research in Income and Wealth (Princeton, NJ: Princeton University Press, 1960), 503–46; "Railroad Investment before the Civil War"; John F. Stover, *History of the Baltimore and Ohio Railroad* (West Lafayette, IN: Purdue University Press, 1987); L.T.C. Rolt, *George & Robert Stephenson—The Railway Revolution* (Westport, CT: Greenwood Press, 1977), 146–175.

10. The Tom Thumb was the first practical locomotive built in the U.S. In 1829, however, the Stourbridge Lion, which was manufactured in England before Stephenson's *Rocket*, was purchased by the Delaware and Hudson Canal Company and made a trial run in Pennsylvania on August 8, 1829. It was too heavy for the company's wooden rails and was never used. P.H. Dudley, "The Inception and Progress of Railways," *Transactions of the New York Academy of Science* 5 (1886): 137–51.

11. Thomas Condit Miller and Hu Maxwell, West Virginia, *and Its People*, 3 vols., vol. 1 (New York, NY: Lewis Historical Publishing Company, 1913), 229; Ronald L. Lewis, *Transforming the Appalachian*

Countryside (Chapel Hill, NC: University of North Carolina Press, 1998).

12. William G. Thomas, *The Iron Way—Railroads, the Civil War, and the Making of Modern America* (New Haven, CT: Yale University Press, 2011); "Improved Rail-Road Cars," *Scientific American* 1, no. 1 (1845): 1.

13. Ritchie & Cook, Richmond, VA, "Proceedings and Debates of the Virginia State Convention of 1829–30," 1830. 144.

14. James Morton Callahan, *History of West Virginia—Old and New*, 3 vols., vol. 1 (Chicago and New York: The American Historical Society, Inc., 1923).

15. International Mother's Day Shrine, Photograph from Births page, December 16, 2015; 1830 census records showed the "J.W. Revers" household, with all of the proper ages for the J.W. Reeves family: "Fifth Census of the United States, 1830"; According to Rappahannock County records (formed from Culpeper County in 1833) Josiah. W. "Reavers" lived there in 1834, as did Josiah W. "Rivers" in 1835. There are no records of this or a similar family after 1835: Rappahannock County Clerk, Washington, VA, "County Tax Records," 1834, 1835; Tax records from 1839 place Josiah Reeves in Jacob Noel's district of Shenandoah County, which included New Market: "Personal Property Tax Records," Shenandoah County, Virginia, Shenandoah County, 1839; there is no record of Josiah's purchase of property, but he sold his house and land on lot #49 in New Market in 1842: Virginia Shenandoah County, Shenandoah County, Virginia, "Deed Book," 1842; John W. Wayland, *A History of Shenandoah County, Virginia* (Baltimore. MD: Regional Publishing Company, 1980), 141.

16. *A History of Shenandoah County, Virginia*. 489.

17. *A History of Shenandoah County, Virginia*; U.S. Census, "Sixth Census of the United States, 1840," 1840; Harry M. Strickler, *Forerunners—A History or Genealogy of the Strickler Families, Their Kith and Kin* (Harrisonburg, VA: Harry M. Strickler, 1925).

18. Wayland, *A History of Shenandoah County, Virginia*; "Sixth Census of the United States, 1840."

19. Shenandoah County, Virginia, "Personal Property Tax Records"; "Personal Property Tax Records," Shenandoah County, Virginia, Shenandoah County, 1840; "Personal Property Tax Records," Shenandoah County, Virginia, Shenandoah County, 1841; "Personal Property Tax Records," Shenandoah County, Virginia, Shenandoah County, 1842; "Personal Property Tax Records," Shenandoah County, Virginia, Shenandoah County, 1843.

20. The 1840 U.S. census showed Josiah W. Rives: "Sixth Census of the United States, 1840" and the list of slaveholders showed Joseph W. Rives: Nancy B. Stewart, "Lists of African Americans in Shenandoah County " (Edinburg VA: Shenandoah County Historical Society, 2016). The data in these files correlate with the county tax records, where Josiah Reeves' name is spelled correctly.

21. Wilson, "James Edmund Reeves, M.D.," 1320.

22. Shenandoah County, Virginia, "Deed Book"; Deed Book #1," Barbour County Recorder's Office, 1843.

23. Hu Maxwell, *The History of Barbour County, West Virginia* (Parsons, WV: McClain Printing Company, 1968; repr., 1968); Jane K. Mattaliano and Lois G. Omonde, *Milestones: A Pictorial History of Philippi,*

West Virginia, 1844–1994 (Virginia Beach, VA: The Donning Company, 1994).

24. Wolfe states that the family had five children in 1850 and that Ann was born in 1832 in Culpeper County: Howard H. Wolfe, *Mothers Day and the Mothers Day Church* (Kingsport, TN: Privately Printed, 1962). Sheets states that the family had three children in 1845, and that it moved to Philippi that year when Ann was twelve: L. Wayne Sheets, *Mother's Day—The Legacy of Anna Jarvis* (Parsons, WV: McClain Printing Company, 2013). Kendall, who knew Ann personally, said she was born in 1833: Norman F. Kendall, *Mothers Day—A History of Its Founding and Its Founder* (Grafton, WV: D. Grant Smith, 1937). Ann Jarvis' tombstone in Bala Cynwyd, Pennsylvania, shows her birth year as 1834: Tipton, "Find a Grave Search Form."

25. Personal communication Shrine.

26. "Sixth Census of the United States, 1840": Note: Reeves was misspelled as "Rievs" or "Riers" in this census.

27. "1850 Federal Census for Barbour County, Virginia."

28. Anna Jarvis, Anna Jarvis Papers (1864–1948), various years.

29. "Death of Rev. Reeves," *Wheeling Register*, Wheeling, WV, Dec. 21, 1882; Shenandoah County tax records, which are fairly complete, do not show Josiah Reeves after 1843. There are no comparable tax records for Barbour County, which might confirm Reeves' residence in Barbour County in 1843 or 1844: Eva Grimsley, 2016.; Deed records show that Josiah purchased lot #7 in Philippi in 1849 from Compton and note, "…now occupied by Reeves and Compton as a tailor and boot and shoemaking establishment." "Deed Book #2," Barbour County Recorder's Office, Multiple Years. 484.

30. This information appeared in a Connecticut journal that wanted to honor Reeves: Samuel Woods, "Our Gallery—James Edmund Reeves, M.D. Of Wheeling W. Va.," *New England Medical Monthly* 4 (1885): 480–83 481. It contained a number of personal details and was signed "UET." In 1885, Samuel Woods wrote to Reeves that he had prepared a biography of Reeves from 1848 to the present. He stipulated that Reeves could, "…use the narrative in any way you wish, but upon this condition, that, if published, the signature must be 'U.E.T.' signifying simply 'unus ex tribus,' 'one from three.' It was a signature selected for our common use by C.W. Callinder, James Neeson and myself when we left College in 1842 and went out in the world, as did Abraham, 'not knowing whither he went.': Personal letter, April 7, 1885, 1885; Wilson, "James Edmund Reeves, M.D."; Irving A. Watson, *Physicians and Surgeons of America: A Collection of Biographical Sketches of the Regular Medical Profession* (Concord, NH: Republican Press Association, 1896), 9–10.

31. Maxwell, *The History of Barbour County, West Virginia.*

32. Wilson, "James Edmund Reeves, M.D.," 1320; County real estate records don't clearly show where Josiah located his family dwelling or even when he bought the property, but the most likely transaction occurred in 1846, when he purchased five quarter-acre lots and three hillside acres from William Wilson for $100. He later sold this property to John Carlile, but that deed was not recorded. What was recorded

was that, in 1868 Samuel Woods, who had purchased this property from Carlile, sold one and a quarter acres, consisting of a "House and lot formerly owned and occupied by Josiah W. Reeves," for $980: "Deed Book #1," 582; "Deed Book #11," Barbour County Recorder's Office, 1868. 249.

33. Maxwell, *The History of Barbour County, West Virginia*; Mattaliano and Omonde, *Milestones: A Pictorial History of Philippi, West Virginia, 1844–1994.*

34. A.H. Redford, *History of the Organization of the Methodist Episcopal Church South* (Nashville, TN: Methodist Episcopal Church South, 1871), 444–445.

35. John Wesley, *Thoughts Upon Slavery*, second ed. (London: R. Hawes, 1774), 16.

36. Quotations in: C.C. Goen, *Broken Churches, Broken Nation—Denominational Schisms and the Coming of the American Civil War* (Macon, GA: Mercer University Press, 1985), 99.

37. Kendall, *Mothers Day—A History of Its Founding and Its Founder.* 9.

Chapter 2

1. Sir Gilbert Blane, *Elements of Medical Logick*, second ed. (London, UK: Thomas and George Underwood, 1821). William Osler, living at the epicenter of the dramatic nineteenth century changes in medicine and fully appreciative of them, artfully acknowledged their foundation in work by 17th and 18th century writers in 1913 William Osler, *The Evolution of Modern Medicine—A Series of Lectures Delivered at Yale University on the Silliman Foundation in April 1913* (New Haven, CT: Yale University Press, 1921).

2. N.S. Davis, *History of Medical Education and Institutions in the United States* (Chicago, IL: S.C. Griggs & Company, 1851); Richard Harrison Shryock, *Medical Licensing in America, 1650–1965* (Baltimore, MD: Johns Hopkins University Press, 1967).

3. Golden age: Chapman American Medical Association, "The Transactions of the American Medical Association" (Philadelphia, PA: The American Medical Association, 1848), 7; Davis, *History of Medical Education and Institutions in the United States.*

4. Henry E. Sigerist, *American Medicine*, trans. Hildegard Nagel (New York: W.W. Norton & Company, Inc., 1934), 132; Davis, *History of Medical Education and Institutions in the United States.*

5. The first formal study of medical college entrance requirements occurred in 1846–47: American Medical Association, "Proceedings of the National Medical Conventions Held in New York, May 1846 and Philadelphia, May 1847" (Philadelphia, PA: The American Medical Association, 1847), 79–82.; Davis, *History of Medical Education and Institutions in the United States.*

6. J. A. C. Grant, "The Gild Returns to America 1 & 2," *The Journal of Politics* 4, no. 3 & 4 (1942): 303–36, 458–77; Roy C. Smith, *Adam Smith and the Origins of American Enterprise: How the Founding Fathers Turned to a Great Economist's Writings and Created the American Economy* (New York, NY: Truman Talley Books, 2002). Most historians have followed Shyrock's lead that the forces of Jacksonian egalitarianism challenged the medical profession's organizational urges during the period: Shyrock, *Medical Licensing in America, 1650–1965.* See Paul Starr, *The Social Transformation of American Medicine—The*

Rise of a Sovereign Profession and the Making of a Vast Industry (New York: Basic Books, 1982). Berlant, however, argues that Jacksonian anti-monopoly movements were not directed at efforts to organize (i.e., corporations), but efforts by organizers to obtain unique market advantages. This response would not have opposed medical organization *per se.* Berlant does not address the broader Jacksonian cultural bias that arose against elitism in general: Jeffry Berlant, *Profession and Monopoly: A Study of Medicine in the United States and Great Britain* (Berkeley: University of California Press, 1975).

7. Davis, *History of Medical Education and Institutions in the United States*; For a detailed discussion of state licensure requirements see also American Medical Association, *The Transactions of the American Medical Association*, vol. 2 (Philadelphia, PA: American Medical Association, 1849), 326–332; and William G. Rothstein, *American Physicians in the 19th Century—From Sects to Science* (Baltimore, MD: Johns Hopkins University Press, 1992), Appendix II: 332–339; Steven M. Stowe, *Doctoring the South—Southern Physicians and Everyday Medicine in the Mid-Nineteenth Century* (Chapel Hill, NC: University of North Carolina Press, 2004); Abraham Jobe, *A Mountaineer in Motion—The Memoir of Dr. Abraham Jobe 1817–1906*, ed. David C. Hsuing (Knoxville, TN: University of Tennessee Press, 2009).

8. J. Boss, "The Medical Philosophy of Francis Bacon (1561–1626)," *Med Hypotheses* 4, no. 3 (1978): 208–20; "Medicine is a science which hath been (as we have said) more professed than laboured, and yet more laboured than advanced; the labour having been, in my judgment, rather in circle than in progression. For I find much iteration, but small addition." Francis Bacon, *The Advancement of Learning*, ed. Henry Morley, Project Gutenburg, ed. (London, UK: Cassell & Company, Limited, 1893). The Second Book: X.(3).

9. Robert B. Sullivan, "Sanguine Practices: A Historical and Historiographic Reconsideration of Heroic Therapy in the Age of Rush," *Bulletin of the History of Medicine* 68, no. Summer (1994): 211–34.

10. J. D. Rolleston, "F. J. V. Broussais (1772–1838): His Life and Doctrines: (Section of the History of Medicine)," *Proc R Soc Med* 32, no. 5 (1939): 405–13.

11. Blane, *Elements of Medical Logick*. 163.

12. Courtney R. Hall, "Jefferson on the Medical Theory and Practice of His Day," *Bulletin of the History of Medicine* 37, no. January 1, 1957 (1957): 235–45. 239.

13. See, in particular, Edward H. Clarke, Henry J. Bigelow, Samuel D. Gross et al., *A Century of American Medicine: 1776–1876* (Philadelphia: Henry C. Lea, 1876).

14. John S. Haller, Jr., *American Medicine in Transition, 1840–1910* (Urbana, IL: University of Illinois Press, 1981); Rothstein, *American Physicians in the 19th Century—From Sects to Science*; Charles E Rosenberg, "The Therapeutic Revolution: Medicine, Meaning and Social Change in Nineteenth Century America.," *Perspectives in Biology and Medicine* 20, no. 4 (1977): 485–506. 487.

15. See, for example, Erwin Ackerknecht, "Aspects of the History of Therapeutics," *Bulletin of the History of Medicine* 36, no. 5 (1962): 389–419.

16. C. H. Beecher, "The Management of Congestive Heart Failure," *New England Journal of Medicine* 209, no. 24 (1933): 1226–28.

17. For nineteenth-century applications: George Bacon Wood and Franklin Bache, *Dispensatory of the United States of America* (Philadelphia, PA: Grigg and Elliot, 1833); Robely Dunglison, *Medical Lexicon : A New Dictionary of Medical Science, Containing a Concise Account of the Various Subjects and Terms*, second ed. (Philadelphia, PA: Lea and Blanchard, 1839); for twentieth-century applications: Louis S. Goodman and Alfred Gilman, *The Pharmacological Basis of Therapeutics* (New York, NY: The Macmillan Company, 1955), 970–1001; The United States Pharmacopœial Convention Inc., *The Pharmacopeia of the United States of America* (Easton, PA: Mack Publishing Company, 1950); Jacalyn Duffin and Pierre Rene, "'Anti-Moine; Anti-Biotique': The Public Fortunes of the Secret Properties of Antimony Potassium Tartrate (Tartar Emetic)," *Journal of the History of Medicine and Allied Sciences* 46, no. 4 (1991): 440–56.

18. Everard Home, ed. *A Treatise on the Blood, Inflammation, and Gun-Shot Wounds by the Late John Hunter* (London, UK: John Richardson, 1794); Wendy Moore, *The Knife Man: Blood, Body Snatching, and the Birth of Modern Surgery* (New York, NY: Broadway Books, 2005); James Lind, *A Treatise on the Scurvy*, second ed. (London, UK: A Millar, 1757). He described his famous controlled trial on pp. 149–153; Edward Jenner, *An Inquiry Into the Causes and Effects of the Variola Vaccine* (London, UK: Sampson Low, 1798); The Parisian capability to systematically study large groups of hospital patients was the impetus for mid–19th century medical progress: W. F. Bynum, *Science and the Practice of Medicine in the Nineteenth Century* (Cambridge, UK: Cambridge University Press, 1994).

19. Benjamin Rush, *Medical Inquiries and Observations*, vol. 4 (Philadelphia: Thomas Dobson, 1796), 238, 193.

20. The 1819 edition of Blane's work was cited in 1820 by the American author Robely Dunglison, who presented similar views on medical knowledge of the time: Robely Dunglison, *On the Use of the Moxa : As a Therapeutical Agent / by Baron D.J. Larrey ; Translated from the French, with Notes, and an Introduction Containing a History of the Substance* (London, UK: Thomas and George Underwood, 1822); for a 20th century interpretation of Blane: "We realize further that all the errors prevalent at that time are still with us today, although in different ratio and different intensities." See: Lester S. King, "Medical Logic," *Journal of the History of Medicine and Allied Sciences* 33, no. 3 (1978): 377–85.; J. P. Ioannidis, "Why Most Published Research Findings Are False," *PLoS Med* 2, no. 8 (2005): e124.

21. Depending on the context, "empiric" meant either quackery or science to an early nineteenth-century regular physician. Regulars favored "empirical" evidence if it produced a medical theory: John Harley Warner, *The Therapeutic Perspective: Medical Practice, Knowledge, and Identity in America, 1820–1885* (Princeton, NJ: Princeton University Press, 1997). Regulars sometimes had to tell whether they meant "bad" empiricism, implying non–Baconian quackery or "good" empiricism meaning observational-based Baconian thinking. For example, Blane referred to both types of empiricists in his 1821 essay: Blane, *Elements of Medical Logick*, and Bartlett used the term empiric with both positive and negative connotations in 1844: Elisha Bartlett, *Essay on the Philosophy of*

Medical Science (Philadelphia, PA: Lea & Blanchard, 1844). In the 1847 *Code of Medical Ethics,* the physician writers clearly used empiricism solely as a derogatory concept, equivalent to quackery: AMA Committee on Medical Ethics, *Code of Medical Ethics of the American Medical Association* (Chicago: American Medical Association Press, 1847).

22. The United States Pharmacopœial Convention Inc., "The Pharmacopoeia of the United States of America," in *The General Convention for the Formation of the American Pharmacopoeia* (New York, NY: S. Converse, 1830).

23. S. J. Rogal, "Pills for the Poor: John Wesley's Primitive Physick," *Yale J Biol Med* 51, no. 1 (1978): 81–90; John B. Blake, "From Buchan to Fishbein: The Literature of Domestic Medicine," in *Medicine Without Doctors—Home Health Care in American History,* ed. Gunter B; Numbers Risse, Ronald L; Leavitt, Judith Walker (New York, NY: Science History Publications, 1977), 11–30; Charles E. Rosenburg, "'The Fielding H. Garrison Lecture': Medical Text and Social Context: Explaining William Buchan's *Domestic Medicine,*" *Bulletin of the History of Medicine* 57, no. Spring (1983): 22–42.

24. Thomson presented a powerful account of his life and the development of his system in the introduction to his *New Guide* Samuel Thomson, *New Guide to Health; or Botanic Family Physician,* second ed. (Boston, MA: E. G. House, 1825); Ronald L. Numbers, "Do-It-Yourself the Sectarian Way," in *Medicine Without Doctors,* ed. Gunter B.; Numbers Risse, Ronald L.; Leavitt, Judith Walker (New York, NY: Science History Publications, 1977), 49–72.

25. Haller describes several editions of Thomson's book. Like Haller, I have referenced the 1825 edition: John S. Haller, Jr., *The People's Doctors—Samuel Thomson and the American Botanical Movement, 1790–1860* (Carbondale, IL: Southern Illinois University Press, 2000); Thomson, *New Guide to Health; or Botanic Family Physician.* 7.

26. *New Guide to Health; or Botanic Family Physician.* 88; Thomson's botanicals were: the Emetic Herb (*Lobelia inflata*), cayenne (*Capsicum annuum*), powdered bayberry root (*Myrica cerifera*), poplar bark (*Populus tremudoides*), ginger root (*Zingiber officinale*), and rheumatic drops (a mixture of brandy, myrrh, and cayenne). Specifically, regulars did not use bayberry root for therapeutic purposes. Wood and Bache, *Dispensatory of the United States of America.*

27. Thomson, *New Guide to Health; or Botanic Family Physician.* 9.

28. Haller, *The People's Doctors—Samuel Thomson and the American Botanical Movement, 1790–1860.* Appendix H.

29. F. C. Waite, "American Sectarian Medical Colleges before the Civil War," *Bull Hist Med* 19 (1946): 148–66.

30. Williams, "The Thomsonian National Infirmary—Extracts from Dr. Williams's Speech in the Maryland House of Delegates," *The Boston Medical and Surgical Journal* 12, no. May 6 (1835): 200–6. 203, 206.

31. For general background on Hahnemann and homeopathy see: Thomas Lindsley Bradford, *The Life and Letters of Dr. Samuel Hahnemann* (Philadelphia: Boerickle & Tafel, 1895); Haller, *American Medicine in Transition, 1840–1910;* Harris L. Coulter, *Divided Legacy; The Conflict Between Homoeopathy and the*

American Medical Association, second ed. (Berkeley, CA: North Atlantic Books, 1982); John S. Haller, Jr., *The History of American Homeopathy: The Academic Years, 1820–1935* (New York, NY: Pharmaceutical Products Press, 2005); John C. Burnham, *Health Care in America: A History* (Baltimore, MD: Johns Hopkins University Press, 2015); Edzard Ernst, *Homeopathy: The Undiluted Facts* (Basel, Switzerland: Springer, 2016).

32. Samuel Hahnemann, *Organon Der Rationellen Heilkunde* (Dresden: Arnoldischen Buchandlung, 1810); *Organon of the Rational Art of Healing—Translated from the First Edition,* ed. Ernest Rhys, trans. C.E. Wheeler, Everyman's Library—Science (London, UK: J.M. Dent & Sons, Ltd., 1913); (*Organon der rationellen Heilkunde*). There is confusion about the English meaning of the *Organon's* title. In later editions the word "Heilkunde" or knowledge of healing, i.e., "medicine" or "therapeutics," was changed to "Heilkunst," or art of healing. In his 1913 English translation of the 1810 *Organon,* Wheeler translated the title as "Art of Healing," which is not consistent with Hahnemann's original efforts to present his approach as empirically-based science. As Schmidt noted, the *Organon* began within the medical scientific mainstream, but gradually moved into what regular physicians regarded as mysticism: J. M. Schmidt, "200 Years Organon of Medicine—A Comparative Review of Its Six Editions (1810–1842)," *Homeopathy* 99, no. 4 (2010): 271–7.

33. Hahnemann, *Organon of the Rational Art of Healing—Translated from the First Edition.*11–12.

34. *Organon of the Rational Art of Healing—Translated from the First Edition.* 3, 8.

35. *Organon of the Rational Art of Healing—Translated from the First Edition.* 102.

36. Andrew Duncan, Jr., *The Edinburgh New Dispensatory,* seventh ed. (Edinburgh, UK: Bell & Bradfute, 1813), 61–63; Belladonna is a toxic product of the leaves or root of the deadly nightshade plant. The ancient Greeks knew the properties of this drug and it was used over the centuries by physicians, wizards, and murderers. A liquid extract of deadly nightshade dilates the eyes, which, as a symbol of beauty and a window to the soul, inspired the Italian physician, Pietro Andrea Mattioli (1501–1577) to name it "belladonna," or beautiful lady. A German chemist isolated the active chemical, atropine, from nightshade roots in 1831. Atropine and similar agents are widely used today to inhibit neurotransmission in the brain and autonomic nervous system in diseases such as Parkinson's disease and asthma.

37. Samuel Hahnemann, *Materia Medica Pura,* trans. Charles Julius Hempel, first ed. (New York, NY: William Radde, 1846).

38. *Organon of the Rational Art of Healing—Translated from the First Edition.* 9.

39. Schmidt, "200 Years Organon of Medicine—A Comparative Review of Its Six Editions (1810–1842)";

40. Editor, "Homoeopathy," *The Boston Medical and Surgical Journal* 4, no. 3 (1831): 51–54.

41. See: Clarke, Bigelow, Gross et al., *A Century of American Medicine: 1776–1876.*

42. William E. Stempsey, ed. *Elisha Bartlett's Philosophy of Medicine,* vol. 83, Philosophy and Medicine (Dordrecht, The Netherlands: Springer, 2005); William Osler, "Elisha Bartlett—A Rhode Island Philosopher," in *An Alabama Student and Other Biographical Es-*

says (London: Oxford University Press, 1929; reprint, 1929), 108–58; Elisha Huntington, *An Address on the Life, Character, and Writings of Elisha Bartlett, M.D., M.M.S.S.* (Lowell, MA: Middlesex North Distric Medical Society, 1856).

43. Elisha Bartlett, "Account of the Hôtel-Dieu at Paris," *The American Journal of the Medical Sciences* 4 (1828): 376–83; "Account of La Charité at Paris," *The American Journal of the Medical Sciences* 6 (1829): 369–76. 369; "Account of the Hopital De La Pitie, Hopital De St. Antoine, Hopital Necker, Hopital Cochin, and Hopital Beaujon at Paris," *The American Journal of the Medical Sciences* 7 (1829): 117–22.

44. Russell M. Jones, "American Doctors and the Parisian Medical World, 1830–1840: Part 1," *Bulletin of the History of Medicine* 47, no. 1 (1973): 40–65; "American Doctors and the Parisian Medical World, 1830–1840: Part 2," *American Doctors and the Parisian Medical World, 1830–1840: Part 1* 47, no. 2 (1973): 177–204.

45. A. Morabia, "P. C. A. Louis and the Birth of Clinical Epidemiology," *J Clin Epidemiol* 49, no. 12 (1996): 1327–33.

Chapter 3

1. Huntington, *An Address on the Life, Character, and Writings of Elisha Bartlett, M.D., M.M.S.S.*; Osler, "Elisha Bartlett—A Rhode Island Philosopher"; David McCullough, *The Greater Journey—Americans in Paris* (New York, NY: Simon & Schuster, 2011); "The Steam-Ship Great Britain," *Scientific American* 1, no. 1 (1845): 2.

2. Pierre-Charles-Alexandre Louis, *Researches on the Effects of Bloodletting in Some Inflammatory Diseases*, trans. C.G. Putnam (Boston, MA: Hilliard, Gray, & Company, 1836); René-Théophile-Hyacinthe Laennec, *A Treatise on the Diseases of the Chest*, trans. John Forbes (London: T. and G. Underwood, 1821); J. H. Felts, "Henry Ingersoll Bowditch and Oliver Wendell Holmes: Stethoscopists and Reformers," *Perspect Biol Med* 45, no. 4 (2002): 539–48; Jacalyn Duffin, *To See with a Better Eye: A Life of R. T. H. Laennec* (Princeton, NJ: Princeton University Press, 1998).

3. Pierre-Charles-Alexandre Louis, *Anatomical, Pathological and Therapeutic Researches Upon the Disease Known Under the Name of Gastro-Enterite, Putrid, Adynamic, Ataxic, or Typhoid Fever, Etc., Compared with the Most Common Acute Diseases*, trans. Henry I. Bowditch, 2 vols. (Boston, MA: Isaac R. Butts, Hilliard Gray & Co., 1836); Lloyd G. Stevenson, "Exemplary Disease: The Typhoid Pattern," *Journal of the History of Medicine* 37, no. 2 (1982): 159–81.

4. B.E. Cotting, "Nature in Disease," *The Boston Medical and Surgical Journal* 47, no. 11 (1852): 223–31.

5. Elisha Bartlett, *The History Diagnosis and Treatment of Typhoid and of Typhus Fever; with an Essay on the Diagnosis of Bilious Remittent and of Yellow Fever* (Philadelphia, PA: Lea and Blanchard, 1842), 137–138.

6. See, for example, the British review of Bartlett's book, which expressed many of the current confusions: "Dr. Bartlett on Typhoid and Typhus Fever," *The British and Foreign Medical Review*, no. 33

(1844): 357–70; For a rough comparison of 18th and 19th century fevers to current terms for the diseases they likely represented, see Phyllis A. Richmond, "Glossary of Historical Fever Terminology," *Journal of the History of Medicine:* 16, no. 1 (1961): 76–77.

7. Bartlett, *The History Diagnosis and Treatment of Typhoid and of Typhus Fever; with an Essay on the Diagnosis of Bilious Remittent and of Yellow Fever.* 176–177.

8. W.W. Gerhard, "On the Typhus Fever, Which Occurred at Philadelphia in the Spring and Summer of 1836; Illustrated by Clinical Observations at the Philadelphia Hospital; Showing the Distinction between This Form of Disease and Dothinenteritis or the Typhoid Fever with Alteration of the Follicles of the Small Intestine. Part 1.," *The American Journal of the Medical Sciences* 38, no. February 1837 (1837): 289–322; Editor, "W.W. Gerhard: Typhoid Vs Typhus Fever," *JAMA* 181, no. 2 (1962): 154–55.

9. "Typhoid and Typhus Fever," *The Boston Medical and Surgical Journal* 27, no. 10 (1842): 171–72. 172.

10. Osler, "Elisha Bartlett—A Rhode Island Philosopher," 133.

11. Jobe, *A Mountaineer in Motion—The Memoir of Dr. Abraham Jobe 1817–1906.* 55.

12. Bartlett, *Essay on the Philosophy of Medical Science*; Erwin Ackerknecht, "Elisha Bartlett and the Philosophy of the Paris Clinical School," *Bulletin of the History of Medicine* 24, no. Jan (1950): 43–60.

13. The quotation from Bacon is at the beginning of Bartlett's 1844 book. It is from Book II of Bacon's *Novum Organon*, Aphorism X. The full aphorism, in English, is: "Therefore, a just and adequate natural and experimental history is to be procured, as the foundation of the whole thing; for we are not to fancy, or imagine, but to discover what are the works and laws of nature." Francis Bacon, *The Works of Francis Bacon—Containing Novum Organon Scientiarium*, ed. Baron Verulam, trans. Baron Verulam, vol. 4 (London, UK: M. Jones, 1815), 168. In Latin: *The Works of Lord Bacon*, 2 vols., vol. II (London, UK: Henry G. Bohn, 1854), 460.

14. Bartlett, *Essay on the Philosophy of Medical Science.* 184.

15. *Essay on the Philosophy of Medical Science.* FN1, 179.

16. *Essay on the Philosophy of Medical Science.* 292–293.

17. "Review—An Essay on the Philosophy of Medical Science," *The American Journal of the Medical Sciences* 19, no. July (1845): 141–44.

18. Charles Lee, "An Essay on the Philosophy of Medical Sciences by Elisha Bartlett, M.D.," *The New York Journal of Medicine and the Collateral Sciences* 4 (1845): 65–82. 74.

19. John Harley Warner, *Against the Spirit of System—The French Impulse in Nineteenth-Century American Medicine* (Princeton, NJ: Princeton University Press, 1998), 175; Owen Whooley, *Knowledge in the Time of Cholera—The Struggle Over American Medicine in the Nineteenth Century* (Chicago, IL: University of Chicago Press, 2013); Lester S. King, *Transformations in American Medicine* (Baltimore, MD: Johns Hopkins University Press, 1991).

20. "Review of the Philosophy of Medical Science," *The Boston Medical and Surgical Journal* 33, no. 13 (1845): 262–63. 263.

21. Osler, "Elisha Bartlett—A Rhode Island Philosopher."

22. I.N. Danforth, *The Life of Nathan Smith Davis* (Chicago, IL: Cleveland Press, 1907).

23. *The Life of Nathan Smith Davis*; Nathan S. Davis, *History of the American Medical Association from Its Organization Up to January 1855* (Philadelphia: Lippincott, Grambo and Company, 1855).

24. Association, "Proceedings of the National Medical Conventions Held in New York, May 1846 and Philadelphia, May 1847," 1847; Davis, *History of the American Medical Association from Its Organization Up to January 1855*; Robert B. Baker, "A National Code of Medical Ethics," *Before Bioethics: A History of American Medical Ethics from the Colonial Period to the Bioethics Revolution* (Oxford: Oxford University Press, 2014), www.oxfordscholarship.com.

25. Davis, *History of the American Medical Association from Its Organization Up to January 1855*, 37, 38.

26. Isaac Hays (editor), "National Medical Convention," *The American Journal of the Medical Sciences* 12, no. 23 (1846): 266–73. 266.

27. Association, "Proceedings of the National Medical Conventions Held in New York, May 1846 and Philadelphia, May 1847," 1847; Jones, "American Doctors and the Parisian Medical World, 1830–1840: Part 1."

28. Association, "Proceedings of the National Medical Conventions Held in New York, May 1846 and Philadelphia, May 1847," 1847. 36, 37.

29. "Proceedings of the National Medical Conventions Held in New York, May 1846 and Philadelphia, May 1847," 1847. 67.

30. "Proceedings of the National Medical Conventions Held in New York, May 1846 and Philadelphia, May 1847," 1847. 71.

31. Thomas Percival, *Medical Ethics or a Code of Institutes and Precepts, Adapted to the Professional Conduct of Physicians and Surgeons* (London: S. Johnson, St. Paul's Church Yard and R. Bickerstaff, 1803); Benjamin Rush, *Sixteen Introductory Lectures* (Philadelphia, PA: Bradford and Innskeep, 1811), 319–339; Ethics, *Code of Medical Ethics of the American Medical Association*.

32. Jonsen called the 1847 *Code*, "that very American political fiction," because of its unilateral nature. See Albert R. Jonsen, *A Short History of Medical Ethics* (New York, NY: Oxford University Press, 2000), 70.

33. Ethics, *Code of Medical Ethics of the American Medical Association*. 96, 97, 106.

34. Robert B. Baker, "The American Medical Ethics Revolution," in *The American Medical Ethics Revolution*, ed. Robert B. Baker, Arthur L. Caplan, Linda L. Emanuel, et al. (Baltimore, MD: Johns Hopkins University Press, 1999), 17–51. xxviii; C. D. Leake, "Theories of Ethics and Medical Practice," *JAMA* 208, no. 5 (1969): 842–7; Starr, *The Social Transformation of American Medicine- the Rise of a Sovereign Profession and the Making of a Vast Industry*; Berlant, *Profession and Monopoly: A Study of Medicine in the United States and Great Britain*.

35. Charles T. Ambrose, "The Secret Kappa Lamda Society of Hippocrates (and the Origin of the American Medical Association's Principles of Medical Ethics)," *Yale J Biol Med* 78, no. 1 (2005): 45–56; Baker, "A National Code of Medical Ethics."

36. Association, "The Transactions of the American Medical Association," 1848. 7.

37. "The Transactions of the American Medical Association," 1848. 9.

Chapter 4

1. Josiah's real estate transactions were recorded in Barbour County deed records, e.g.: "Deed Book #2."

2. Wilson, "James Edmund Reeves, M.D.," 1320.

3. "Deed Book #2," 101.

4. Loren C. Talbot, *History of the Talbots and Their Kinsmen* (Des Moines, IA: The Law Brief Company, 1951). Note the two spellings of the name, Talbot and Talbott. Maxwell acknowledged that the family used both versions: Maxwell, *The History of Barbour County, West Virginia*. For physician data see: Association, "The Transactions of the American Medical Association," 1848. 359–364.

5. Store location in "Deed Book #2," 484; Wilson, "James Edmund Reeves, M.D.," 1320; James E. Reeves, "Typhoid Fever in North Western Virginia," *Buffalo Medical Journal and Monthly Review* 12, no. 5 (1856): 257–78. 272.

6. Strickler, *Forerunners—A History or Genealogy of the Strickler Families, Their Kith and Kin.* 48. Also: U.S. Census, "Seventh Census of the United States, 1850," 1850; James E. Reeves, *A Practical Treatise on Enteric Fever; Its Diagnosis and Treatment: Being an Analysis of One Hundred and Thirty Consecutive Cases Derived from Private Practice and Embracing a Partial History of the Disease in Virginia* (Philadelphia, PA: J. B. Lippincott & Co., 1859); Woods, "Our Gallery—James Edmund Reeves, M.D., of Wheeling W. Va.," 481.

7. The AMA reported five regular physicians in Braxton County in 1848, only one of whom possessed a diploma: Association, "The Transactions of the American Medical Association," 1848; "Seventh Census of the United States, 1850."

8. The 1850 census information showing the living arrangement is contained on two pages and the ages listed are not entirely accurate. James is shown as 24 and Johnson N. as 23: "Seventh Census of the United States, 1850"; Festus P. Summers, *Johnson Newlon Camden—A Study in Individualism* (New York, NY: G.P. Putnam's Sons, 1937); William B. Atkinson, *A Biographical Dictionary of Contemporary American Physicians and Surgeons* (Philadelphia: D.G. Brinton, 1880); Otis K. Rice, *West Virginia: A History* (Lexington, KY: University Press of Kentucky, 1985); John Alexander. Williams, West Virginia, *and the Captains of Industry* (Morgantown, WV: West Virginia University Press, 2003).

9. Association, *The Transactions of the American Medical Association*. 281–299; Details on Hampden-Sidney from Wyndham B. Blanton, *Medicine in Virginia in the Nineteenth Century* (Richmond: Garrett & Massie Inc., 1933).

10. Association, "Proceedings of the National Medical Conventions Held in New York, May 1846 and Philadelphia, May 1847," 1847; *The Transactions of the American Medical Association*. 307.

11. Most information about Lydia is from a privately printed book that James Reeves wrote for his children in 1862, on Lydia's death. The copy he gave

to his daughter, Nancy is owned by Nancy's great granddaughter, Joan Webb: James E. Reeves, *Mrs Lydia Reeves: A Letter to Her Children—By Father* (Baltimore, MD: W.R. and D.S. Miller, 1862), Personal Publication; Additional information on the Martz family: John W. Wayland, *A History of Rockingham County, Virginia* (Dayton, VA: Ruebush-Elkins Company, 1912); Ralph Fraley Martz, *The Martzes of Maryland* (Frederick, MD: Ralph Fraley Martz, 1973); "Rockingham County Real Estate Assessments," Harrisonburg VA, 1850; Jacob Martz, Rockingham County, VA, "Last Will and Testament," 1850; In the 1850 census Jacob Martz estimated his property at $20,000: "Seventh Census of the United States, 1850."

12. The property Reeves purchased for his home was lots #35 and #36, later the location of the historic Peck-Crim-Chesser house at 14 Walnut Street: "Deed Book #3," Barbour County Recorder's Office, Multiple Years. The small parcel he sold was recorded in: "Deed Book #4," Barbour County Recorder's Office, Multiple Years.

13. Reeves, *Mrs Lydia Reeves: A Letter to Her Children—By Father.* 7.

14. These estimates of proximity are based on the lot locations as shown for Reeves: "Deed Book #3"; S. Woods in 1848: Samuel Woods, "Samuel Woods Papers," in *Woods, Samuel Family. Papers,* ed. University of West Virginia (Various: West Virginia and Regional History Center, Various) and 1856: "Samuel Woods Papers," Various; "Deed Book #22," Barbour County Recorder's Office, Multiple Years, 122; Undated MEC records at Crim UMC show that before 1861 Josiah, Nancy, and Emily Reeves were in a class led by Samuel Woods and that the Reeves family (was?) removed in 1861, probably after Samuel joined the Confederacy. Given that Josiah was ordained as a deacon in 1859, it seems likely that this class record predates 1859: Philippi Methodist Church, Record book of church membership, 1861+, 1861; Samuel Woods was 6 years older than James Reeves and Isabella Woods was 4 years older. In the 1860 census, the Reeves family had four children and the Woods family seven, all between ages 1 and 10: U.S. Census, "Eighth Census of the United States, 1860," 1860.

15. Description of Lydia from Reeves, *Mrs Lydia Reeves: A Letter to Her Children—By Father,* 14; Photograph courtesy of Joan Webb.

16. Talbot, *History of the Talbots and Their Kinsmen*; Bo Zaunders, *The Great Bridge Building Contest* (New York, NY: Harry N. Abrams, 2004).

17. Maxwell, *The History of Barbour County, West Virginia,* 278.

18. Barbour County (Reeves added to total) and Richmond city physician estimates from: Association, "The Transactions of the American Medical Association," 1848, 359–364. Virginia physician estimates based on: "Seventh Census of the United States, 1850," lxxiv and 272. A manual count of Barbour County from the 1850 census: "1850 Federal Census for Barbour County, Virginia" found eight physicians, including E.D. Talbott, vs. nine reported in the AMA's 1847 survey, thus these estimates are consistent. For an overview of the *ante-bellum* medical environment: Richard Harrison Shyrock,' *Medicine and Society in America: 1660–1860* (New York, NY: New York University Press, 1960; repr., 1963); also "The American Physician in 1846 and 1946—A Study in Professional Contrasts," *JAMA* 134, no. 5 (1947): 417–24.

Chapter 5

1. Stevenson, "Exemplary Disease: The Typhoid Pattern"; William Osler, *The Problem of Typhoid Fever in the United States* (Baltimore, MD: John Murphy Company, 1899), 3.

2. Reeves, *A Practical Treatise on Enteric Fever; Its Diagnosis and Treatment: Being an Analysis of One Hundred and Thirty Consecutive Cases Derived from Private Practice and Embracing a Partial History of the Disease in Virginia*; George Bacon Wood, *A Treatise on the Practice of Medicine,* 1 ed., 2 vols. (Philadelphia, PA: Grigg, Elliot, and Co., 1847).

3. P. Claiborne Gooch (editor), "Review: A Treatise on the Practice of Medicine by George B. Wood," *The Stethoscope and Virginia Medical Gazette* 2, no. 7 (1852): 399. Quotation p. 399.

4. Warner, *The Therapeutic Perspective: Medical Practice, Knowledge, and Identity in America, 1820–1885.*

5. Reeves, "Typhoid Fever in North Western Virginia," 257.

6. Today's physicians usually define enteric (typhoid) fever bacteriologically, not clinically. It is the febrile illness caused by one of several species of the bacterium *Salmonella enterica,* mainly *S. enterica* (typhi). With sanitation and antibiotic treatment, the diagnosis is far less common and far less ominous than it was for Reeves. Currently, in the U.S., there are fewer than 400 cases and one or two deaths annually from enteric fever. Most twenty-first-century American doctors will never see a case: Centers for Disease Control and Prevention, "National Typhoid and Paratyphoid Fever Surveillance," http://www.cdc.gov/nationalsurveillance/typhoid-surveillance.html; C. M. Parry, T. T. Hien, G. Dougan et al., "Typhoid Fever," *N Engl J Med* 347, no. 22 (2002): 1770–82; David A. Pegues and Samuel I. Miller, "Salmonella Species," in *Mandell, Douglas, and Bennett's Principles and Practice of Infectious Diseases, Updated Edition,* ed. John E. Bennett, Raphael Dolin, and Martin J. Blaser (Philadelphia, PA: Saunders, 2015), 2559–68.

7. C. Kuvandik, I. Karaoglan, M. Namiduru et al., "Predictive Value of Clinical and Laboratory Findings in the Diagnosis of the Enteric Fever," *New Microbiol* 32, no. 1 (2009): 25–30.

8. Reeves, "Typhoid Fever in North Western Virginia," 273.

9. "Typhoid Fever in North Western Virginia," 257.

10. Louis, *Anatomical, Pathological and Therapeutic Researches Upon the Disease Known under the Name of Gastro-Enterite, Putrid, Adynamic, Ataxic, or Typhoid Fever, Etc.: Compared with the Most Common Acute Diseases*; Elisha Bartlett, *The History, Diagnosis, and Treatment of the Fevers of the United States* (Philadelphia, PA: Lea and Blanchard, 1847); Austin Flint, *Clinical Reports on Continued Fever Based on Analyses of One Hundred and Sixty-Four Cases* (Philadelphia, PA: Lindsay & Blakiston, 1855).

11. AMA Committee on Medical Literature American Medical Association, *The Transactions of the American Medical Association,* vol. 3 (Philadelphia, PA: American Medical Association, 1850), 153–187.

12. Blanton, *Medicine in Virginia in the Nineteenth Century,* 135.

13. Reeves, "Typhoid Fever in North Western Virginia," 273.

14. *A Practical Treatise on Enteric Fever; Its Diagnosis and Treatment: Being an Analysis of One Hundred and Thirty Consecutive Cases Derived from Private Practice and Embracing a Partial History of the Disease in Virginia.* 14.

15. "Local Affairs—Virginia Medical Society," *Richmond Dispatch*, Richmond, VA April 28, 1859, 1; *A Practical Treatise on Enteric Fever; Its Diagnosis and Treatment: Being an Analysis of One Hundred and Thirty Consecutive Cases Derived from Private Practice and Embracing a Partial History of the Disease in Virginia.*

16. Wilson, "James Edmund Reeves, M.D."; Jarvis, "Anna Jarvis Papers (1864–1948)," various years.; George Bacon Wood, "George Bacon Woods Papers," in *Wood, George Bacon. Papers*, ed. The College of Physicians of Philadelphia (Various: Historical Medical Library, various years).

17. Reeves, *A Practical Treatise on Enteric Fever; Its Diagnosis and Treatment: Being an Analysis of One Hundred and Thirty Consecutive Cases Derived from Private Practice and Embracing a Partial History of the Disease in Virginia.* IX.

18. *A Practical Treatise on Enteric Fever; Its Diagnosis and Treatment: Being an Analysis of One Hundred and Thirty Consecutive Cases Derived from Private Practice and Embracing a Partial History of the Disease in Virginia.* 188.

19. Editor, "Book Review: A Practical Treatise on Enteric Fever; Its Diagnosis and Treatment; Being an Analysis of One Hundred and Thirty Consecutive Cases, Derived from Private Practice, and Embracing a Partial History of the Disease in Virginia," *The Boston Medical and Surgical Journal* 61, no. 4 (1859): 84.

20. "A Practical Treatise on Enteric Fever (Review)," *The Peninsular and Independent Medical Journal* II, no. 7 (1859): 409–10.

21. "Book Review: A Practical Treatise on Enteric Fever; Its Diagnosis and Treatment: Being an Analysis of One Hundred and Thirty Consecutive Cases, Derived from Private Practice, and Embracing a Partial History of the Disease in Virginia," *The American Journal of the Medical Sciences* 76, no. October (1859): 519–20, 520.

22. "Book Review: A Practical Treatise on Enteric Fever; Its Diagnosis and Treatment; Being an Analysis of One Hundred and Thirty Consecutive Cases, Derived from Private Practice, and Embracing a Partial History of the Disease in Virginia," 520.

23. American Medical Association, *The Transactions of the American Medical Association*, vol. 13 (Philadelphia, PA: American Medical Association, 1860), 779.

24. Pennsylvania's Medical School Catalogues do not mention Reeves' book for 1860–61 or 1860–62; George Bacon Wood, *A Treatise on the Practice of Medicine*, 6 ed., 2 vols. (Philadelphia, PA: J.B. Lippincott and Co, 1866).

25. John Ashhurst, Jr., ed. *Transactions of the International Medical Congress* (Philadelphia, PA: The International Medical Congress, 1877), FN2, 254; Charles Smart, *The Medical and Surgical History of the War of Rebellion—Medical History Part 3*, 2 vols., vol. 1 (Washington, D.C.: Government Printing Office, 1888); Blanton, *Medicine in Virginia in the Nineteenth Century*, FN126, 254.

26. Flint apologized for the errors of his ways in his review of the third edition of Bartlett's *Fevers*: Austin Flint (editor), "Review of the History, Diagnosis, and Treatment of the Fevers of the United States, by Elisha Bartlett, M.D., Third Edition," *Buffalo Medical Journal and Monthly Review* 8 (1853): 186; The total page count for all thirty-six issues in Volumes 6–8 (1850–53) was 2,496. Flint's reports were: Austin Flint, "Report of Clinical Observations on Continued (Typhus and Typhoid) Fever. Based on Analysis of Fifty-Two Cases," *ibid.* 6 (1850–51): 129–48, 93–214, 57–82, 321–46, 85–401, 49–66; "Second Clinical Report on Continued Fever—Based on an Analysis of Forty-Eight Cases," *Buffalo Medical Journal and Monthly Review* 7 (1851–52): 65–80, 172–83, 216–37, 80–98, 321–38, 85–401; Austin Flint (editor), "Supplement to Reports on Continued Fever—Symptoms Distinctive of Typhoid and Typhus Fever. Identity of These Two Types. Diagnosis, Etc.," *ibid.*, no. 8 (1852): 249–75; "The Management of Continued Fever," *Buffalo Medical Journal and Monthly Review* 7 (1852): 513–41, 76–93; and Austin Flint, "Third Clinical Report on Continued Fever—Based on an Analysis of Sixty-Four Cases," *ibid.* 8 (1852–53): 6–31, 76–104, 45–58; Warren Winkelstein, Jr., "Austin Flint, Clinician Turned Epidemiologist," *Epidemiology* 18, no. 2 (2007): 279.

27. In his third report, Flint also acknowledged the recent work of English physician William Jenner in helping him understand the autopsy findings in typhoid and typhus fevers: Flint, "Third Clinical Report on Continued Fever—Based on an Analysis of Sixty-Four Cases," 89.

28. *Clinical Reports on Continued Fever Based on Analyses of One Hundred and Sixty-Four Cases.*

29. Flint (editor), "The Management of Continued Fever," 529, 530.

30. "The Management of Continued Fever," 530, 527.

31. "The Management of Continued Fever," 529.

32. Editor, "Book Review: Clinical Reports on Continued Fever by Austin Flint, M.D.," *The Southern Journal of the Medical and Physical Sciences* 2, no. 3 (1854–1855): 202–5.

33. American Medical Association, *The Transactions of the American Medical Association*, vol. 6 (Philadelphia, PA: American Medical Association, 1853), 115.

34. Warner, *The Therapeutic Perspective: Medical Practice, Knowledge, and Identity in America, 1820–1885*, 60.

Chapter 6

1. Reeves, *Mrs Lydia Reeves: A Letter to Her Children—By Father*. The two Presiding Elders (similar to District Superintendents today) who baptized James' children, Moses Ticknell (1853) and Gordon Battelle (1858), were from the Clarksburg District, Western Virginia Conference, of the MEC: Henry J. Fox and W. B. Hoyt, *Fox and Hoyt's Quadrennial Register of the Methodist Episcopal Church and Universal Church Gazetteer: 1852–1856* (Hartford, CT: Case, Tiffany, & Co., 1852); Brett T. Miller, Personal Communication, May 16, 2016. For a discussion of how Josiah Reeves named his children after famous men, see: Wolfe, *Mothers Day and the Mothers Day Church*, 252.

2. James E. Reeves, "Case of Puerperal Convul-

sions, in Which Neuralgic Symptoms Were Singularly Exhibited," *Buffalo Medical Journal and Monthly Review* 12, no. 3 (1856): 129–33; in 1911 the New York City Health Commissioner estimated that more than 50 percent of the births in the U.S. were attended by midwives: Thomas Darlington, "The Present Status of the Midwife," *American Journal of Obstetrics and Diseases of Women and Children* 63, no. 5 (1911): 870–76; Rothstein asserted that in 1847, "physicians performed most obstetrical cases in America"; however, this was probably not correct: Rothstein, *American Physicians in the 19th Century—From Sects to Science*, 109.

3. L. C. Chesley, "History and Epidemiology of Preeclampsia-Eclampsia," *Clin Obstet Gynecol* 27, no. 4 (1984): 801–20; S. Ong, "Pre-Eclampsia: A Historical Perspective," in *Pre-Eclampsia: Current Perspectives on Management*, ed. Philip Baker and John Kingdom (Boca Raton, FL: CRC Press, 2004); For an earlier American description of puerperal convulsions and their treatment, see: Norman Lyman, "Remarks on the Nature and Treatment of Peurpural Convulsions," *The New England Journal of Medicine and Surgery* 13, no. 4 (1824): 337–56 and Robely Dunglison, ed. *The Cyclopaedia of Practical Medicine*, 4 vols., vol. 1 (Philadelphia, PA: Lea & Blanchard, 1845); Fleetwood Churchill, *On the Theory and Practice of Midwifery*, second ed. (London, UK: Henry Renshaw, 1850), data on pp. 415–416. Churchill was acknowledged as an authority in 1845 by American author Robely Dunglison: Dunglison, *The Cyclopaedia of Practical Medicine*, and his book as a standard American text again in 1852: Editor, "On the Theory and Practice of Midwifery. By Fleetwood Churchill," *Buffalo Medical Journal and Monthly Review* 12, no. 6 (1852): 755.

4. Francis H. Ramsbotham, *The Principles and Practice of Obstetric Medicine and Surgery* (London, UK: John Churchill, 1856); for information on standard obstetrical texts of the period see: University of Pennsylvania, "Catalogue of the Trustees Officers and Students of the University of Pennsylvania," ed. University of Pennsylvania (Philadelphia, PA: University of Pennsylvania, 1858–59); William P. Dewees, *A Compendious System of Midwifery*, 12th ed. (Philadelphia, PA: Blanchard and Lea, 1853).

5. Charles D. Meigs, *Obstetrics—The Science and the Art*, second ed. (Philadelphia, PA: Blanchard and Lea, 1852); James E. Reeves, "On All Sides a Learned Doctor," *New Orleans Medical and Surgical Journal* 18, no. 8 (1891): 581–96. 584.

6. Meigs, *Obstetrics—The Science and the Art*. 455.

7. Meigs translated the first, second, and fourth editions of Velpeau's *Treatise* in 1831, 1838, and 1852: Alfred-Armand-Louis-Marie Velpeau, *Elementary Treatise on Midwifery: Or Principles of Tokology and Embryology.*, trans. Charles D. Meigs, first American ed. (Philadelphia: J. Grigg, 1831); *Elementary Treatise on Midwifery: Or Principles of Tokology and Embryology.*, trans. Charles D. Meigs, second American ed. (Philadelphia: Grigg & Elliot, 1838); *Complete Treatise on Midwifery: Or Principles of Tokology and Embryology.*, trans. Charles D. Meigs, fourth American ed. (Philadelphia: Lindsay and Blakiston, 1852). For the history of eclampsia: Ong, "Pre-Eclampsia: A Historical Perspective."

8. Meigs, *Obstetrics—The Science and the Art*. 457.

9. Chesley, "History and Epidemiology of Preeclampsia-Eclampsia."

10. Bynum, *Science and the Practice of Medicine in the Nineteenth Century*; Gordon Jones, "Obstetrical Practice in Civil War Times," *JAMA* 184, no. 5 (1963): 254–61; Committee on Obstetrics: Association, "The Transactions of the American Medical Association," 1848. 225–234; Committee on Educational Reform: "Proceedings of the National Medical Conventions Held in New York, May 1846 and Philadelphia, May 1847," 1847, 63–78; for English practice see Churchill's 1866, textbook: Fleetwood Churchill, *On the Theory and Practice of Midwifery*, fifth ed. (London, UK: Henry Renshaw, 1866) and A. B. Steele, "The Treatment of Puerperal Eclampsia," *Br Med J* 2, no. 609 (1872): 240–1; for German practice, which showed similar reluctance to induce labor, see Karl Schroeder, *Manual of Midwifery—Including the Pathology of Pregnancy and the Puerperal State*, trans. Charles H. Carter, third ed. (New York, NY: D. Appleton and Company, 1878); Meigs remained a visible advocate of induction to treat eclampsia, although some other American obstetricians were more cautious: Wm H. Byford, *A Treatise on the Theory and Practice of Obstetrics* (New York, NY: William Wood & Co, 1870).

11. *Proceedings of the Pathological Society of Philadelphia*, (Philadelphia, PA: J.B. Lippincott & Co., 1860), 239–240.

12. Milton Bettmann, "Report of a Case of Fibrinous Bronchitis, with a Review of All Cases in the Literature," *The American Journal of the Medical Sciences* 123, no. 2 (1902): 304–29.

13. *James E. Reeves V. Thomas Skidmore* (1859).

14. Price comparisons based on general price index 1856–1938 from: Bureau of the Census, Washington, D.C., Department of Commerce, "Historical Statistics of the United States: 1789–1945," 1949. 231–232; and GDP deflator 1938–2017 from: U.S. Bureau of Economic Analysis, Washington, D.C., "Gross Domestic Product (Implicit Price Deflator) " 2018. See also Robert Sahr, "Inflation Conversion Factors for Years 1774 to Estimated 2027 " (Corvallis, OR: Oregon State University, 2018).

15. George Rosen, *Fees and Fee Bills: Some Economic Aspects of Medical Practice in Nineteenth Century America* ed. Henry E. Sigerist, Supplement 6 to the Bulletin of the History of Medicine (Baltimore, MD: Johns Hopkins University Press, 1946).

16. Shyrock, "The American Physician in 1846 and 1946—A Study in Professional Contrasts"; Stowe, *Doctoring the South—Southern Physicians and Everyday Medicine in the Mid-Nineteenth Century*; Rothstein, *American Physicians in the 19th Century—From Sects to Science*.

17. For examples of billing advice, see "Letters from Boston" B., "Letters from Boston," *The Cincinnati Medical Observer* 2, no. 2 (1857): 79–80 and "Medical Fees (editorial)," *Cincinnati Medical Observer* 2, no. 3 (1857): 134–35.

18. "Protest of the Majority," *Cooper's Clarksburg Register* Clarksburg, VA May 18, 1853; "Political Meeting," *Cooper's Clarksburg Register*, July 12, 1854.

19. Michael F. Holt, *The Rise and Fall of the American Whig Party: Jacksonian Politics and the Onset of the Civil War* (Oxford, UK: Oxford University Press, 1999).

20. Tyler G. Anbinder, *Nativism and Slavery: The Northern Know Nothings and the Politics of the 1850s*

(Oxford, UK: Oxford University Press, 1992); Thomas J. Curran, *Xenophobia and Immigration, 1820–1930* (Woodbridge CT: Twayne Publishers, 1975).

21. John David Bladek, "'Virginia Is Middle Ground': The Know Nothing Party and the Virginia Gubernatorial Election of 1855," *The Virginia Magazine of History and Biography* 106, no. 1 (1998): 35–70. FN1, 35.

22. Until this meeting, there was no mention of James Reeves in the local Democratic press, although his father appeared on several occasions: James E. Reeves, "Another Huzzah for Wise, M'comack and Bocock!—Ratification Meeting in Barbour," *Cooper's Clarksburg Register*, Clarksburg, VA February 21, 1855, 1.

23. "Eighth Census of the United States, 1860," 516–521; Kevin H Williams, "Barbour (W)Va 1860 Slave Schedule Federal Census," in *USGenWeb Census Project* http://www.us-census.org/ (Idaho: USGen-Net, 2003).

24. "For the Register," *Cooper's Clarksburg Register* Clarksburg, VA April 4, 1855.

25. A local newspaper showed Carlile announcing his Clarksburg practice in December 1851 "John S. Carlile—Attorney at Law," *Cooper's Clarksburg Register* Clarksburg, VA December 3, 1851, 4; Charles Holden (Secretary), "Democratic Meeting," *ibid.*, March 10, 1852.

26. "From the Parkersburg News: John S. Carlile," *ibid.*, May 2, 1855, 2.

27. "Mr. Carlile in Barbour County," *Cooper's Clarksburg Register* Clarksburg, VA May 16, 1855, 2.

28. Bladek, "'Virginia Is Middle Ground': The Know Nothing Party and the Virginia Gubernatorial Election of 1855." Barbour County vote p. 56.

29. "The Result in This Congressional District," *Cooper's Clarksburg Register* Clarksburg, VA June 13, 1855, 2.

30. Philip Morrison Rice, "The Know-Nothing Party in Virginia, 1854–1856 (Concluded)," *The Virginia Magazine of History and Biography* 55, no. 2 (1947): 159–67.

31. George H. Douglas, *The Golden Age of the Newspaper* (Westport, CT: Greenwood Press, 1999); Patrick Novotny, *The Press in American Politics, 1787–201* (Santa Barbara, CA: Praeger, 2014); "Seventh Census of the United States, 1850" Table XLVIII, p: lxiv; table XLIX, p: lxv; "1860 Federal Census for Barbour County, Virginia." Table: "The Public Press," 321; Richard L. Forstall, U.S. Department of Commerce, "Population of States and Counties of the United States: 1790–1990," 1996; Lorman A. Ratner, Paula T. Kaufman, and Dwight L. Teeter, Jr., *Paradoxes of Prosperity: Wealth-Seeking Versus Christian Values in Pre-Civil War America* (Urbana, IL: University of Illinois Press, 2009).

32. Dan King, "Quackery—Its Causes and Effects, with Reflections and Suggestions," *The Boston Medical and Surgical Journal* 48, no. 11 (1853): 209–15.

33. The actual amount of space on this day was 13 percent, based on fraction of column-inches devoted to medical cures and nostrums. "Announcements," *Cooper's Clarksburg Register* Clarksburg, VA August 8, 1856, 3.

34. Miller and Maxwell, West Virginia, *and Its People*; Balthasar Henry Meyer, ed. *History of Transportation in the United States Before 1860* (Washington, D.C.: Carnegie Institution of Washington, 1917); Stover, *History of the Baltimore and Ohio Railroad*.

35. George A Dunnington, *History and Progress of the County of Marion, West Virginia: From Its Earliest Settlement by the Whites Down to the Present, Together with Biographical Sketches of Its Most Prominent Citizens* (Fairmont, WV: George A. Dunnington, 1880); Callahan gives January 1852 as the date the B&O arrived at Fairmont Callahan, *History of West Virginia—Old and New*, but this seems to be an error. The date was June 1852 according to multiple sources.

36. Campbell Gibson, Washington, D.C., U.S. Bureau of the Census, "Population of the 100 Largest Cities and Other Urban Places in the United States: 1790 to 1990," 1998.

37. For an overview of Southern medical sectionalism during the pre-war period see John Harley Warner, "A Southern Medical Reform: The Meaning of the Antebellum Argument for Southern Medical Education," in *Science and Medicine in the Old South*, ed. Ronald L. Numbers and Todd L. Savitt (Baton Rouge, LA: Louisiana State University Press, 1989), 206–25.

38. University of Pennsylvania, "Catalogue of the Trustees Officers and Students of the University of Pennsylvania," ed. University of Pennsylvania (Philadelphia, PA: University of Pennsylvania, 1859–60); Joseph Carson, *A History of the Medical Department of the University of Pennsylvania* (Philadelphia, PA: Lindsay and Blakiston, 1869); Frederick P. Henry (editor), *Standard History of the Medical Profession of Philadelphia* (Chicago, IL: Goodspeed Brothers, 1897); Howard A. Kelly and Walter L. Burrage, *Dictionary of American Medical Biography* (New York, NY: D. Appleton and Company, 1928); James H. Cassedy, "The Microscope in American Medical Science, 1840–1860," *Isis* 67, no. March (1976): 76–97.

39. Stover, *History of the Baltimore and Ohio Railroad*, 99.

40. For general histories of Brown's raid and the events leading to the outbreak of the Civil War see: David M. Potter, *The Impending Crisis: 1848–1861* (New York, NY: Harper & Row, 1976) and James M. McPherson, *Battle Cry of Freedom—The Civil War Era*, ed. C. Vann Woodward, 11+ vols., vol. 6, The Oxford History of the United States (Oxford, UK: Oxford University Press, 1988). For western Virginia specifics: Mark A. Snell, West Virginia, *And the Civil War*, ed. Doug Bostick, Civil War Sesquicentennial Series (Charleston, SC: The History Press, 2011); Virginius Dabney, *Virginia—The New Dominion: A History from 1607 to the Present* (Charlottesville, VA: University Press of Virginia, 1971).

41. Pennsylvania, "Catalogue of the Trustees Officers and Students of the University of Pennsylvania," 1859–60, "Catalogue of the Trustees Officers and Students of the University of Pennsylvania," ed. University of Pennsylvania (Philadelphia, PA: University of Pennsylvania, 1860–61).

42. "Catalogue of the Trustees Officers and Students of the University of Pennsylvania," 1860–61.

Chapter 7

1. Maxwell, *The History of Barbour County, West Virginia*; Atkinson, *A Biographical Dictionary of Contemporary American Physicians and Surgeons*. 493; Howard A. Kelly, *A Cyclopedia of American Medical Biography*, 2 vols., vol. II (Philadelphia, PA: W. B. Saunders Co, 1912), 194–195.

2. Dunnington, *History and Progress of the County of Marion, West Virginia: From Its Earliest Settlement by the Whites Down to the Present, Together with Biographical Sketches of Its Most Prominent Citizens.*

3. Kazuko Uchimura, "Coal Operators and Market Competition: The Case of West Virginia's Smokeless Coalfields and the Fairmont Field, 1853–1933," *West Virginia History* 4, no. 2 (2010): 59–86; "Eighth Census of the United States, 1860," 516–521.

4. Sale price recorded in "Deed Book #7," Barbour County Recorder's Office, Multiple Years; Reeves, *Mrs Lydia Reeves: A Letter to Her Children—By Father;* The purchase deed was not recorded until 1865, but it notes that Reeves' house was bounded by properties owned by Stone and Pierpont. The 1860 census also shows Stone and Pierpont families located near Reeves. It is likely that he purchased his house when he moved in 1860 and did not record the purchase until after the end of the Civil War: "Deed Book #14," Marion County Recorder's Office, Multiple Years.

5. Richard Orr Curry, *A House Divided—A Study of Statehood Politics and the Copperhead Movement in West Virginia* (Pittsburgh, PA: University of Pittsburgh Press, 1964); W. Hunter Lesser, *Rebels at the Gate—Lee and McClellan on the Front Line of a Nation Divided* (Naperville, IL: Sourcebooks, Inc., 2004).

6. Curry, *A House Divided—A Study of Statehood Politics and the Copperhead Movement in West Virginia.* Quotation FN #31, 34.

7. "Eighth Census of the United States, 1860," 516–521; Diane Davis Darnley, "Camp Carlile," ed. Mike Keller, *e-WV: The West Virginia Encyclopedia* (Charleston, WV: West Virginia Humanities Council 2011), http://www.wvencyclopedia.org/articles/822.

8. Whitelaw Reid, Ohio, *In the War—Her Statesmen, Soldiers, and Generals*, 2 vols., vol. 1 (Columbus, OH: Eclectic Publishing Company, 1893), 48.

9. Lesser, *Rebels at the Gate—Lee and McClellan on the Front Line of a Nation Divided*. 55; John W. Shaffer, *Clash of Loyalties—A Border County in the Civil War* (Morgantown, WV: West Virginia University Press, 2003).

10. For Porterfield's account of the battle at Philippi see Maxwell, *The History of Barbour County, West Virginia*. 250–251.

11. Number from: George A. Otis, *The Medical and Surgical History of the War of Rebellion—Surgical History*, ed. Joseph K. Barnes, 2 vols., vol. 2—Part 2, The Medical and Surgical History of the War of Rebellion (Washington, D.C.: Government Printing Office, 1877) and George A. Otis and D.L. Huntington, *ibid.*, vol. 2—Part 3 (1883). It includes non-war-related amputations. The number was verified by Alfred Jay Bollet, *Civil War Medicine—Challenges and Triumphs* (Tucson, AZ: Galen Press, 2002).

12. "The J.E. Hanger Story," Hanger, Inc., http://www.hanger.com/history/Pages/The-J.E.-Hanger-Story.aspx; For an informal, unsourced, but presumably accurate account of James Hanger, see Bob O'Connor, *The Amazing Legacy of James E. Hanger, Civil War Soldier* (West Conshocken, PA: Infinity Publishing, 2014).

13. Maxwell, *The History of Barbour County, West Virginia*, 267.

14. Lesser, *Rebels at the Gate—Lee and McClellan on the Front Line of a Nation Divided*, 150.

15. Curry, *A House Divided—A Study of Statehood Politics and the Copperhead Movement in West Virginia.*

16. David R. Zimring, "'Secession in Favor of the Constitution': How West Virginia Justified Separate Statehood During the Civil War," *West Virginia History (New Series)* 3, no. 2 (2009): 23–51; For biographical information on Pierpont, see Dunnington, *History and Progress of the County of Marion, West Virginia: From Its Earliest Settlement by the Whites Down to the Present, Together with Biographical Sketches of Its Most Prominent Citizens.*

17. Shaffer, *Clash of Loyalties—A Border County in the Civil War;* Ruth Woods Dayton, *Samuel Woods and His Family* (Charleston, WV: Hood-Heserman-Brodhag Company, 1939), 23.

18. John Alexander Williams, "The New Dominion and the Old: Ante-Bellum and Statehood Politics as the Background of West Virginia's Bourbon Democracy," *West Virginia History* 33, no. 4 (1972): 317–407; James Morton Callahan, *Semi-Centennial History of West Virginia* (Charleston, WV: Semi-Centennial Commission of West Virginia, 1913).

19. Granville Parker, *The Formation of the State of West Virginia and Other Incidents of the Late Civil War* (Wellsburg, WV: Glass & Son, Book and Job Printers, 1875), 78.

20. "Death of Rev. Gordon Battelle," *Daily Intelligencer*, Wheeling, WV, August 8, 1862, 2; There were multiple "camp fevers" during the war. Although historically typhus was known as "camp fever," it was relatively rare, based on physician diagnosis. Typhoid was thirty times more common than typhus. See Smart, *The Medical and Surgical History of the War of Rebellion—Medical History Part 3*. 191"; Obsequies to Mr. Battelle," *Daily Intelligencer*, Wheeling, WV, August 11, 1862, 2.

21. Reeves, *Mrs Lydia Reeves: A Letter to Her Children—By Father*, p. 8.

22. In the book for the children Reeves wrote, "... during the last two or three years of her life she had abandoned all thought of seeing you become men and women." *Mrs Lydia Reeves: A Letter to Her Children—By Father*, pp. 10–11.

23. Lydia's brother was Dorilas Jackson Martz, who served in Virginia's 97th Militia Infantry Regiment. Her cousin was the better known Dorilas Henry Lee Martz who served in the 10th Virginia Volunteer Infantry: Historical Data Systems, "U.S. Civil War Soldier Records and Profiles, 1861–1865," (Duxbury, MA Historical Data Systems, 2009), Wayland, *A History of Rockingham County, Virginia*, and Martz, *The Martzes of Maryland.*

24. For descriptions of 19th century medical terms, particularly "cholera morbus" see Dunglison, *Medical Lexicon : A New Dictionary of Medical Science, Containing a Concise Account of the Various Subjects and Terms*, Wood, *A Treatise on the Practice of Medicine*, and G. S. Rousseau and D. B. Haycock, "Coleridge's Choleras: Cholera Morbus, Asiatic Cholera, and Dysentery in Early Nineteenth-Century England," *Bull Hist Med* 77, no. 2 (2003): 298–331.

25. Reeves, *Mrs Lydia Reeves: A Letter to Her Children—By Father.*

26. Wood, *A Treatise on the Practice of Medicine.* Quotation Vol. 2, 765. One can speculate what present-day diagnoses might explain Lydia's early death. Given the history Reeves left, doctors today might attribute her chronic despair and episodic arm and leg numb-

ness to depression complicated by a functional neurological disorder, only a slightly better understood version of the nervous temperament and hysteria that Reeves and Wood may have diagnosed. E Broussolle, F Gobert, T Danaila et al., "History of Physical and 'Moral' Treatment of Hysteria," *Frontiers of Neurology and Neuroscience* 35 (2014): 181–97. But they would probably consider other possibilities as well, including a chronic infectious disease superimposed on an anatomic abnormality, such as rheumatic heart disease complicated by infective endocarditis. J. Ezell, "A 34-Year-Old Woman with Fever, Tachycardia, Vomiting, and Hemiparesis," *J Emerg Nurs* 30, no. 3 (2004): 275–7, L. L. Pelletier, Jr., and R. G. Petersdorf, "Infective Endocarditis: A Review of 125 Cases from the University of Washington Hospitals, 1963–72," *Medicine (Baltimore)* 56, no. 4 (1977): 287–313. The final scene did not describe a mental illness. Her fever, vomiting, and neurologic symptoms pointed to an underlying infection. However, in 1862, even if doctors had examined her blood microscopically and noticed the evidence of many white corpuscles, as they could have, they would not have considered the possibility that invisible organisms were growing inside her. They would have sought another explanation, such as a miasmatic poison. A full understanding of the germ theory was more than a generation away.

27. For Irwin see "Tribute of Respect," *Daily Intelligencer*, Wheeling, WV, November 24, 1863, 2; for Mather see F.P. Pierpoint, *Annual Report of the Adjutant General of the State of West Virginia for the Year Ending December 31, 1864*, Annual Report of the Adjutant General of the State of West Virginia (Wheeling, WV: State of West Virginia, John F.M. McDermot, Printer, 1864), 138 and "Eighth Census of the United States, 1860"; Charles Henry Ambler, *Sectionalism in Virginia from 1776 to 1861* (Chicago: University of Chicago Press, 1910).

28. For William Arnett see: George W. Atkinson, *Bench and Bar of West Virginia* (Charleston, WV: Virginian Law Book Company, 1919), 34–36; for Jonathan Arnett see: James Morton Callahan, *Genealogical and Personal History of the Upper Monongahela Valley—West Virginia*, ed. Bernard L. Butcher, 3 vols. (New York, NY: Lewis Historical Publishing Company, 1912), volume 2.; Dayton, *Samuel Woods and His Family*.

29. Reeves' younger brother, Joseph Henry Clay, moved to Baltimore and publicly announced his Union sympathies in January 1861: "Mass Meeting," *Sun*, Baltimore, MD, January 7, 1861, 2 but he devoted his energies to business: Ron V. Jackson, "Maryland, Compiled Census and Census Substitutes Index, 1772–1890" (Provo, UT: Ancestry.com, 1999); Jarvis, "Anna Jarvis Papers (1864–1948)," various years. His parents were recognized as Union sympathizers in Philippi: John W. Shaffer, *Union and Confederate Soldiers and Sympathizers of Barbour County, West Virginia* (Baltimore, MD: Genealogical Publishing Company, 2005); however they joined Joseph in Baltimore in 1861, where Josiah continued his tailoring: "Death of Rev. Reeves." At some point during the War Reeves' sister Emily married James T. Simms and they, along with Reeves' other brother, Thomas Asbury, moved to Brazil to work on the railroad. The facts surrounding this event are hazy at best; see: Wolfe, *Mothers Day and the Mothers Day Church* and Jarvis, "Anna Jarvis Papers (1864–1948)," various years. In Webster, where his sister Ann and her husband had offered her

home to the invading General McClellan in 1861, his brother-in-law Granville Jarvis continued with his mercantile business: Wolfe, *Mother's Day and the Mother's Day Church*, Sheets, *Mother's Day—The Legacy of Anna Jarvis.*

30. Rankin, "Wesley and War: Guidance for Modern Day Heirs?"

31. Kendall, *Mother's Day—A History of Its Founding and Its Founder.* 10.

32. Sheets, *Mother's Day—The Legacy of Anna Jarvis.* 19; Wolfe, *Mother's Day and the Mother's Day Church.*

33. Dayton, *Samuel Woods and His Family.*

34. Wilson, "James Edmund Reeves, M.D."; S.T. Wiley, *History of Preston County (West Virginia)* (Kingwood, WV: Journal Printing House, 1882); "Death of Mrs. Dr. J.E. Reeves," *The Wheeling Daily Intelligencer*, Wheeling, WV, January 12, 1872, 4; "Seventh Census of the United States, 1850."

35. Snell, West Virginia, *and the Civil War.*

36. Dennis M. Zembala, Washington, D.C., Department of the Interior, "Baltimore and Ohio Railroad Fairmont Bridge," Unknown.

37. Thomas Bland Camden, *My Recollections and Experiences of the Civil War or a Citizen of Weston During the Late Unpleasantness* (Parsons, WV: The Friends of the Louis Bennett Public Library, 2000); Atkinson, *A Biographical Dictionary of Contemporary American Physicians and Surgeons*; Summers, *Johnson Newlon Camden—A Study in Individualism.*

Chapter 8

1. John Duffy, *The Sanitarians—A History of American Public Health* (Urbana, IL: University of Illinois Press, 1992); Editor, "Lemuel Shattuck (1793–1859): Prophet of American Public Health," *American Journal of Public Health* 49, no. 5 (1959): 676–77; William J. Novak, *The People's Welfare: Law and Regulation in Nineteenth-Century America* (Chapel Hill, NC: University of North Carolina Press, 1996); Wilson G. Smillie, *Public Health: Its Promise for the Future* (New York, NY: The Macmillan Company, 1955); George Rosen, *A History of Public Health—Expanded Edition*, second ed. (Baltimore, MD: Johns Hopkins University Press, 1993); Loving, "The Development of American Public Health, 1850–1925"; Henry I. Bowditch, *Public Hygiene in America* (Boston, MA: Little, Brown and Company, 1877); W.G. Lumley and E. Lumley, *The New Sanitary Laws: Namely the Public Health Acts, 1848 & 1858 and the Local Government Act, 1858* (London, UK: Shaw and Sons, Fetter Lane, 1871).

2. Howard D. Kramer, "Effect of the Civil War on the Public Health Movement," *The Mississippi Valley Historical Review* 35, no. 3 (1948): 449–62; Many histories of Civil War medicine recount the story of the USSC, but the firsthand account written in 1866 by Charles Stillé remains the most detailed and, in many ways, most interesting Charles Stillé, *History of the United States Sanitary Commission—Being the General Report of Its Work During the War of the Rebellion* (Philadelphia, PA: J.B. Lippincott & Co, 1866).

3. Bollet, *Civil War Medicine—Challenges and Triumphs*; Bynum, *Science and the Practice of Medicine in the Nineteenth Century*; Stillé, *History of the United States Sanitary Commission—Being the Gen-*

eral Report of Its Work During the War of the Rebellion.

4. J.J. Woodward, *The Medical and Surgical History of the War of the Rebellion—Medical History Part 1*, ed. Joseph K. Barnes, 2 vols., vol. 1 (Washington, D.C.: Government Printing Office, 1870); Horace Herndon Cunningham, *Doctors in Gray—The Confederate Medical Service* (Gloucester, MA: Peter Smith, 1970); George Worthington Adams, *Doctors in Blue* (Dayton, OH: Morningside House, Inc., 1985).

5. Stillé, *History of the United States Sanitary Commission—Being the General Report of Its Work During the War of the Rebellion*, 91.

6. Bonnie Ellen Blustein, "'To Increase the Efficiency of the Medical Department: A New Approach to U.S. Civil War Medicine," *Civil War History* 33, no. 1 (1987): 22–41.

7. The Congress of the United States, Washington, D.C., "Public Acts of the Thirty-Seventh Congress of the United States," 1862, 378–379.

8. Frank R. Freemon, "Lincoln Finds a Surgeon General: William A. Hammond and the Transformation of the Union Army Medical Bureau," *Civil War History* 33, no. 1 (1987): 5–21; American Medical Association, *The Transactions of the American Medical Association*, vol. 10 (Philadelphia, PA: American Medical Association, 1857), 513–587; John T. Greenwood, "Hammond and Letterman: A Tale of Two Men Who Changed Army Medicine," *Institute of Land Warfare Publications* (2003), https://www.ausa.org/publications/hammond-and-letterman-tale-two-men-who-changed-army-medicine; Bonnie Ellen Blustein, *Preserve Your Love for Science—Life of William A. Hammond, American Neurologist*, ed. Charles Webster and Charles Rosenberg, Cambridge History of Medicine (Cambridge, UK: Cambridge University Press, 2002).

9. William A. Hammond and Jonathan Letterman, "Two Reports on the Condition of Military Hospitals: Grafton, Va, and Cumberland, Md.," (New York, NY: United States Sanitary Commission, 1862).

10. "Two Reports on the Condition of Military Hospitals: Grafton, Va, and Cumberland, Md.," 1862. 21.

11. Editor, "Surgeon-General of the U.S. Army," *The Cincinnati Lancet and Observer* 5, no. 6 (1862): 364–65.

12. "Surgeon-General of the U.S. Army," *The Boston Medical and Surgical Journal* 66, no. 13 (1862): 283.

13. "The Week," *The American Medical Times* 4 (1862): 239.

14. Greenwood, "Hammond and Letterman: A Tale of Two Men Who Changed Army Medicine," 3.

15. Woodward, *The Medical and Surgical History of the War of the Rebellion—Medical History Part 1*. Appendix 45.

16. The Congress of the United States, *The Congressional Globe—37th Congress 3rd Session*, ed. John C. Rives, The Congressional Globe (Washington, D.C.: John C. Rives, 1862), 1271, 720.

17. *The Congressional Globe—37th Congress 3rd Session*. 1270, 720.

18. Margaret Humphreys, *Marrow of Tragedy—The Health Crisis of the American Civil War* (Baltimore, MD: Johns Hopkins University Press, 2013); Shauna Devine, *Learning from the Wounded—The Civil War and the Rise of American Medical Science* ed. Gary W. Gallagher, Peter S. Carmichael, Caroline E. Janney, et al., Civil War America (Chapel Hill, NC: University of North Carolina Press, 2014).

19. Editor, "Article XII—a Treatise on Hygiene with Special Reference to the Military Service," *The American Journal of the Medical Sciences* 92, no. Oct. 1863 (1863): 411–32; William A. Hammond, *A Treatise on Hygiene: With Special Reference to the Military Service* (Philadelphia, PA: J.B. Lippincott & Co., 1863).

20. J.J. Woodward, *The Medical and Surgical History of the War of the Rebellion—Medical History Part 2*, ed. Joseph K. Barnes, 2 vols., vol. 1 (Washington, D.C.: Government Printing Office, 1879) 688, FN 718; George Bacon Wood, *A Treatise on the Practice of Medicine*, 5 ed., 2 vols. (Philadelphia, PA: J.B. Lippincott and Co., 1858); for information on blue mass: Norbert Hirschhorn, Robert G. Feldman, and Ian Greaves, "Abraham Lincoln's Blue Pills: Did Our 16th President Suffer from Mercury Poisoning?," *Perspectives in Biology and Medicine* 44, no. 3 (2001): 315–32; T. H. Walker, "Treatment of Camp Diarrhea (Reprinted from Chicago Medical Journal)," *The New England Journal of Medicine* 67, no. September 4 (1862): 103–4.

21. Woodward, *The Medical and Surgical History of the War of the Rebellion—Medical History Part 2*, 719.

22. The History of the War records 12,344 physicians serving in the Union Army between 1861 and 1865, of whom 189 were regular officers: Smart, *The Medical and Surgical History of the War of Rebellion—Medical History Part 3*, p. 901. I have assumed, along with other historians, that this number represented 12,344 unique individuals. For information on the three women physicians who participated in the Union Army see: Humphreys, *Marrow of Tragedy—The Health Crisis of the American Civil War*, 53–62. According to 1860 census data, there were 36,616 persons who identified as physicians in the Union states and territories. I estimate that 85 percent of these persons were regulars in some degree of active practice: "Eighth Census of the United States, 1860."

23. "Calomel in the Army," *The New York Times*, New York, NY, June 7, 1863.

24. Along with many books on the subject, cited previously, also: Gert Brieger, "Therapeutic Conflicts and the American Medical Profession in the 1860's," *Bulletin of the History of Medicine* 41, no. 3 (1967): 215–22.

25. For a list of journals, see: Woodward, *The Medical and Surgical History of the War of the Rebellion—Medical History Part 2*. FN 719.

26. Editor, "Calomel and Tartar Emetic in the Army," *The American Medical Times* 6, no. June 20, 1863 (1863): 297.

27. Woodward, *The Medical and Surgical History of the War of the Rebellion—Medical History, Part 2*. FN 719.

28. Editor, "Editor's Table," *The Cincinnati Lancet and Observer* 6, no. 6 (1863): 369–77.

29. American Medical Association, *The Transactions of the American Medical Association*, vol. 14 (Philadelphia, PA: American Medical Association, 1864).

30. *The Transactions of the American Medical Association*, 32.

31. Editor, "Medical Intelligence," *The Boston Medical and Surgical Journal* 72, no. 22 (1865): 455–56;

"William Alexander Hammond, M.D.," in *American Biography—A New Cyclopedia*, ed. Unknown (New York, NY: The American Historical Society, 1918), 343–52.

32. "The Case of Surgeon-General Hammond," *The Boston Medical and Surgical Journal* 71, no. 6 (1864): 125–27.

33. "The Case of Surg. Gen. Hammond," *The Cincinnati Lancet and Observer* 7, no. 11 (1864): 689–90.

34. Stephen Smith (editor), "Our Sanitary Defences," *The American Medical Times* 1, no. July 21, 1860 (1860): 46–47.

35. "Sanitary Interests of New York," *The American Medical Times* 6, no. January 10, 1863 (1863): 21–22.

36. Gert H. Brieger, "Sanitary Reform in New York City: Stephen Smith and the Passage of the Metropolitan Health Bill," *Bulletin of the History of Medicine* 40, no. 5 (1966): 407–29; for details on the legislative process: James C. Mohr, *The Radical Republicans and Reform in New York During Reconstruction* (Ithaca, NY: Cornell University Press, 1973).

37. Council of Hygiene and Public Health of the Citizens' Association of New York, *Report Upon the Sanitary Condition of the City* (New York, NY: D. Appleton and Company, 1865).

38. *Report Upon the Sanitary Condition of the City.* xliii.

39. *Report Upon the Sanitary Condition of the City.* xii, xiii.

40. Stephen Smith, *The City That Was* (New York, NY: Frank Allaben, 1911), 145–146. See also Brieger, "Sanitary Reform in New York City: Stephen Smith and the Passage of the Metropolitan Health Bill."

41. Bowditch, *Public Hygiene in America*. For a description of the 1886 New York law: 397–400.

42. Jane Boswell Moore, "Grafton Hospital," *Daily Intelligencer*, Wheeling, WV, March 12, 1863, 2; Committee of Maryland, "Third Report," ed. G. S. (Chairman) Griffith (Baltimore, MD: United States Christian Commission, 1864); M. Hamlin Cannon, "The United States Christian Commission," *The Mississippi Valley Historical Review* 38, no. 1 (1951): 61–80; Smart, *The Medical and Surgical History of the War of Rebellion—Medical History Part 3*. 963; "Sherman, Socrates Norton (1801–1873)," *Biographical Directory of the United States Congress* (Washington, D.C.), http://bioguide.congress.gov/scripts/biodisplay.pl?index=S000350.

43. A Sufferer, "Statement Concerning the Accident on the Baltimore Road on the 24th Ult.," *Daily Intelligencer*, Wheeling, WV, November 5, 1864, 2.

44. James E. Reeves, "Case of Ovariotomy," *The American Journal of the Medical Sciences* 51, no. April (1866): 397–403.

45. "Case of Ovariotomy," 398.

46. "Case of Ovariotomy," 398.

47. H. R. Spencer, "The History of Ovariotomy: (Section of the History of Medicine)," *Proc R Soc Med* 27, no. 11 (1934): 1437–44; Edwin M. Jameson, *Clio Medica—Gynecology and Obstetrics* (New York, NY: Hafner Publishing Company, 1962; repr., 1962).

48. Editor, "Ovariotomy in London Hospitals," *BMJ* 1(205), no. December 1, 1860 (1860): 933; Jameson, *Clio Medica—Gynecology and Obstetrics*. For an overview of the development of ovariotomy in the nineteenth century see: Sally Frampton, "Defining Difference: Competing Forms of Ovarian Surgery in

the Nineteenth Century," in *Technological Change in Modern Surgery: Historical Perspectives on Innovation*, ed. Thomas Schlich and Christopher Crenner (Rochester, NY: University of Rochester Press, 2017), 51–70. Note that by the late nineteenth century the operation was more routine and increasingly used for what would now be considered medically inappropriate reasons: John Studd, "Ovariotomy for Menstrual Madness and the Pre-Menstrual Syndrome—19th Century History and Lessons for Current Practice.," *Gynecology and Endocrinology* 22 (2006): 411–15.

49. T. Spencer Wells, "On the Treatment of Large Ovarian Cysts and Tumours," *BMJ* 2(51), no. December 21, 1861 (1861): 656–58, "On the Treatment of Large Ovarian Cysts and Tumours," *BMJ* 2(52), no. December 28, 1861 (1861): 679–81; Editor, "Progress of the Medical Sciences—Treatment of Large Ovarian Cysts and Tumors," *The American Journal of the Medical Sciences* 43, no. April 1862 (1862): 550–54.

50. The ovarian mass weighed six pounds and contained multiple cystic areas. "The smaller cavities, sometimes communicating with each other, contained a cream or pus-like fluid; the larger, for the most part, a glutinous, viscid matter." James E. Reeves, "Case of Ovariotomy," *ibid.* 51, no. April (1866): 397–403, 400. Using today's terminology, the mass was likely a benign ovarian mucinous cystadenoma or a malignant ovarian mucinous cystadenocarcinoma: Schorge JO, Hoffman BL, Schaffer JI, Halvorson LM, Bradshaw KD, Cunningham F, Calver LE., "Pelvic Mass," in *Williams Gynecology*, ed. Schorge JO Hoffman BL, Schaffer JI, Halvorson LM, Bradshaw KD, Cunningham F, Calver LE (New York, NY: McGraw-Hill, 2012).

51. Reeves, "Case of Ovariotomy," 402; Wilson, "James Edmund Reeves, M.D."

52. Otis and Huntington, *The Medical and Surgical History of the War of Rebellion—Surgical History*. 169, 427, 572, 573.

53. Smart, *The Medical and Surgical History of the War of Rebellion—Medical History Part 3*; George A. Otis, *The Medical and Surgical History of the War of Rebellion—Surgical History*, ed. Joseph K. Barnes, 2 vols., vol. 2—Part 1, The Medical and Surgical History of the War of Rebellion (Washington, D.C.: Government Printing Office, 1870); *The Medical and Surgical History of the War of Rebellion—Surgical History*, George A. Otis and D.L. Huntington, *ibid.*, vol. 2—Part 3 (1883).

54. Quoted in: George H. Torney, "Surgery of the Battlefield," *New York State Journal of Medicine* 12, no. 9 (1912): 483–88.

55. DeWitt Clinton Peters, *The Life and Adventures of Kit Carson—The Nestor of the Rocky Mountains from Facts Narrated by Himself* (New York, NY: W. R. C. Clark & Co., 1858); Woodward, *The Medical and Surgical History of the War of the Rebellion—Medical History Part 1*. Appendix 235.

56. *The Medical and Surgical History of the War of the Rebellion—Medical History Part 1*. Appendix 230–233; Warner, "The Idea of Southern Medical Distinctiveness: Medical Knowledge and Practice in the Old South."

57. Smart, *The Medical and Surgical History of the War of Rebellion—Medical History Part 3*. 896–964.

Chapter 9

1. John H. Traylor, "Relative Strength of the Two Armies," *Confederate Veteran* 12, no. 11 (1904): 534–36; Frederick H. Dyer, *A Compendium of the War of the Rebellion* (Des Moines, IA: Dyer Publishing Company, 1908); Charles H. Ambler and Festus P. Summers, *West Virginia—The Mountain State*, second ed. (Englewood Cliffs, NJ: Prentice Hall, Inc., 1958) estimated 9,000 Confederates from West Virginia; Shaffer, *Clash of Loyalties—A Border County in the Civil War* estimated 10,000–15,000 Confederates; much of the Confederacy's data were destroyed, making existing estimates of Southern state contributions and mortality a subject of ongoing debate: William L. Fox, *Regimental Losses in the American Civil War: 1861–1865* (Albany, NY: Albany Publishing Company, 1889); Civil War Trust, "Civil War Casualties," Civil War Trust, http://www.civilwar.org/education/civil-war-casualties.html.

2. Dayton, *Samuel Woods and His Family*. 16.

3. Cognoscious, "Barbour County," *The Wheeling Daily Intelligencer*, Wheeling, WV, January 11, 1868, 1.

4. Williams, *West Virginia and the Captains of Industry*.

5. Williams, "The New Dominion and the Old: Ante-Bellum and Statehood Politics as the Background of West Virginia's Bourbon Democracy"; Robert M Bastress, "The Constitution of West Virginia," West Virginia Humanities Council, http://www.wvencyclopedia.org/articles/1558

6. Woods, "Samuel Woods Papers," Various. Letter of February 25, 1872, cited by Randall Scott Gooden, "The Completion of a Revolution: West Virginia from Statehood through Reconstruction" (University of West Virginia, 1995) 336.

7. Barry Mowell, "Bourbon Democracy," in *Encyclopedia of Populism in America: A Historical Encyclopedia*, ed. Alexandra Kindell and Elizabeth S. Demers (Santa Barbara, CA: ABC-CLIO, LLC, 2014), 86–88; For an example of the pejorative term "Bourbon Democracy" see: "The Allegiance Question—A Prominent Southern Journal," *The Daily Evening Telegraph*, Philadelphia, PA, October 10, 1868, 4; For an example of Southern acceptance of "Bourbon Democracy" see: "Charleston Convention," *Wheeling Register*, Wheeling, WV, March 11, 1876, 1; Richard Orr Curry, "Crisis Politics in West Virginia, 1861–1870," in *Radicalism, Racism, and Party Alignment: The Border States During Reconstruction*, ed. Richard Orr Curry (Baltimore, MD: Johns Hopkins Press, 1969), 80–104. 104; Mark Wahlgren Summers, *The Ordeal of the Reunion—A New History of Reconstruction* (Chapel Hill, NC: University of North Carolina Press, 2014).

8. American Medical Association, *The Transactions of the American Medical Association*, vol. 17 (Philadelphia, PA: American Medical Association, 1866); Based on reported members, AMA membership was 3,000 of the 40,000 total regulars. AMA membership numbers are those of living permanent members from *The Transactions of the American Medical Association*. Physician population estimates are for 1871 from *The Transactions of the American Medical Association*, vol. 22 (Philadelphia, PA: American Medical Association, 1871), 155. Note that U.S. census data, based on self-report, including irregu-lars, estimated 62,383 U.S. physicians in 1870. There is little question that AMA membership in 1866 was less than 10 percent of regular physicians.

9. "West Virginia State Teachers Association," *The Wheeling Daily Intelligencer*, Wheeling, WV, August 4, 1866, 3; Burton J. Bledstein, *The Culture of Professionalism—The Middle Class and the Development of Higher Education in America* (New York, NY: W.W. Norton & Company, 1978).

10. "Accidents," *The Wheeling Daily Intelligencer*, Wheeling, WV, January 11, 1866, 4; "Sunstruck," *The Wheeling Daily Intelligencer*, Wheeling, WV, July 17, 1866, 4.

11. In 1855 the AMA decided that local societies must not change the *Code* to remain eligible for AMA membership. See: American Medical Association, *The Transactions of the American Medical Association*, vol. 8 (Philadelphia: American Medical Association, 1855), 56.

12. C. Snyder, "Our Ophthalmic Heritage. Julius Homberger, M.D," *Arch Ophthalmol* 68 (1962): 875–8; Rosemary Stevens, *American Medicine and the Public Interest* (New Haven, CT: Yale University Press, 1971); George Weisz, *Divide and Conquer : A Comparative History of Medical Specialization* (Oxford, UK: Oxford University Press, 2006).

13. Association, *The Transactions of the American Medical Association*. See pp. 55–65.

14. *The Transactions of the American Medical Association*. Quotation p. 64.

15. *The Transactions of the American Medical Association*, 504

16. *The Transactions of the American Medical Association*, 508–509.

17. *The Transactions of the American Medical Association*, 512.

18. The AMA and its journal repeatedly stated the AMA's doctrine on physician advertising: Nathan S. Davis, "Ethical Advertising (editorial)," *JAMA* 1, no. 18 (1883): 540–42. The issue was put to rest in 1982 when the U.S. Supreme Court upheld a Federal Trade Commission order prohibiting the AMA from restricting truthful, non-deceptive physician advertising: *American Medical Association Et Al. V Federal Trade Commission*, 638 Federal Reporter, 2nd Series (1982).

19. For a list of 1866 AMA attendees, members, and a summary of AMA rules see Association, *The Transactions of the American Medical Association*; For a list of medical organizations and hospitals in West Virginia and dates of founding, see *The Transactions of the American Medical Association*, vol. 24 (Philadelphia, PA: American Medical Association, 1873), pp. 312, 332.

20. "Medical," *The Wheeling Daily Intelligencer*, Wheeling, WV, March 1, 1867, 4.

21. Medical Society of West Virginia, *Transactions of the Medical Society of West Virginia—Including Proceedings of the Medical Convention Held at Fairmont April 10, 1867* (Wheeling: Medical Society of West Virginia, 1868), 3.

22. Example of Todd's marketing: "Dr. A.S. Todd—Dear Sir," *Daily Intelligencer*, Wheeling, WV, October 25, 1858, 3; J.H. Newton, G.G. Nichols, and A.G. Sprankle, *History of the Pan-Handle; Being Historical Collections of the Counties of Ohio, Brooke, Marshall and Hancock, West Virginia* (Wheeling: J.A. Caldwell, 1879), 260. The AMA frequently threatened to expel

medical societies that did not accept and enforce the *Code*: Association, *The Transactions of the American Medical Association.* 56. In 1866 the AMA expelled Iowa physician Asa Horr, a former president of the Dubuque County Medical Society, for violating the *Code: The Transactions of the American Medical Association.* 32; William B. Atkinson, *Physicians and Surgeons of the United States* (Philadelphia: Charles Robson, 1878), 237.

23. Virginia, *Transactions of the Medical Society of West Virginia—Including Proceedings of the Medical Convention Held at Fairmont April 10, 1867*; AMA data reported 395 regular physicians in WV in 1871: Association, *The Transactions of the American Medical Association.* 155; List of WV counties and dates of formation. "West Virginia Counties," State of West Virginia, http://www.wv.gov/local/Pages/default.aspx.

24. Virginia, *Transactions of the Medical Society of West Virginia—Including Proceedings of the Medical Convention Held at Fairmont April 10, 1867*, 8.

25. *Transactions of the Medical Society of West Virginia—Including Proceedings of the Medical Convention Held at Fairmont April 10, 1867*, 9, 11.

26. *Transactions of the Medical Society of West Virginia—Including Proceedings of the Medical Convention Held at Fairmont April 10, 1867*, 12; "The Baltimore and Ohio Railroad Company—Indignation Meeting at Fairmont," *The Wheeling Daily Intelligencer*, Wheeling, WV, November 24, 1866, 2; Gooden, "The Completion of a Revolution: West Virginia from Statehood through Reconstruction."

27. Atkinson, *A Biographical Dictionary of Contemporary American Physicians and Surgeons.* 392; Medical Society of West Virginia, *Transactions of the Medical Society of the State of West Virginia* (Wheeling, WV: Medical Society of West Virginia, 1870); *Transactions of the Medical Society of the State of West Virginia* (Wheeling, WV: Medical Society of West Virginia, 1874).

28. American Medical Association, *The Transactions of the American Medical Association*, vol. 18 (Philadelphia, PA: American Medical Association, 1867); "The National Medical Association," *The Wheeling Daily Intelligencer*, Wheeling, WV, May 14, 1867, 4

29. Virginia, *Transactions of the Medical Society of West Virginia—Including Proceedings of the Medical Convention Held at Fairmont April 10, 1867*, 18.

30. *Transactions of the Medical Society of West Virginia—Including Proceedings of the Medical Convention Held at Fairmont April 10, 1867*, 23.

31. "The Union Meeting Last Night," *The Wheeling Daily Intelligencer*, Wheeling, WV, February 23, 1866, 2.

32. Association, *The Transactions of the American Medical Association.* 288–313. The five states that predated the Civil War, but did not have a state medical society in 1867 (plus date of admittance to the U.S.) Louisiana (1812), Alabama (1819), Arkansas (1836), Florida (1845), and Minnesota (1858).

33. "Deed Book #14," "Deed Book #17," Marion County Recorder's Office, 1867.

Chapter 10

1. "Personal," *The Wheeling Daily Intelligencer*, Wheeling, WV, November 9, 1867, 4.

2. Records from Wheeling's Fourth Street (now Chapline Street) Methodist Church go back to 1870. These show Dr. James E. and Mary V. Reeves as members that year, noting Mary's death in 1872 and James' resignation in 1881: Fourth Street Record: Full Membership Approximately 1870–1920 Hand-written Ledger, 1920; "A Fireman," *The Wheeling Daily Intelligencer*, Wheeling, WV, November 28, 1867, 4; Advertisement, "Home—Life Insurance Company," *ibid.*, May 8, 1868, 2.

3. Charles V. Chapin, "The Evolution of Preventive Medicine," *JAMA* 76, no. January 22, 1921 (1921): 215–22.

4. "At a Meeting of the New Board of Health," *The Wheeling Daily Intelligencer*, Wheeling, WV, March 27, 1865, 2; Meeting of the City Council," *The Wheeling Daily Intelligencer*, Wheeling, WV, March 3, 1866, 4; "Notice to Carters," *The Wheeling Daily Intelligencer*, Wheeling, WV, March 12, 1866, 2";To the Citizens of Wheeling," *The Wheeling Daily Intelligencer*, April 19, 1866, 2; "The City Health Office," *The Wheeling Daily Intelligencer*, Wheeling, WV, May 21, 1867, 4.

5. "Our Readers May Be Aware," *The Wheeling Daily Intelligencer*, Wheeling, WV, June 18, 1866, 4; "The City Health Office"; "The Duties of the Health Officer," *The Wheeling Daily Intelligencer*, Wheeling, WV, November 2, 1866, 4.

6. "Mayor Sweeney's Message," *The Wheeling Daily Intelligencer*, Wheeling, WV, February 15, 1867, 1.

7. "Traitors in Wheeling: Below Will Be Found a Complete List of the Traitors and Rebels of Wheeling, Va., Who Voted May 23, 1861, for the Infamous Ordinance of Secession, Adopted by the Usurpers in the Richmond, Va., Convention," ed. University of Virginia Library (Unknown: Unknown, 1861); "The Wrong Man," *Daily Intelligencer*, Wheeling, WV, August 22, 1862, 3; "City Council," *The Wheeling Daily Intelligencer*, Wheeling, WV, June 19, 1867, 4; "The Sanitary Conditions of the City," *The Wheeling Daily Intelligencer*, Wheeling, WV, June 20, 1867, 4.

8. "Information Wanted," *The Wheeling Daily Intelligencer*, Wheeling, WV, May 20, 1867, 4; Where Shall Dead Horses Be Buried?," *The Wheeling Daily Intelligencer*, Wheelign, WV, September 25, 1867, 4; "Meeting of the City Council," *The Wheeling Daily Intelligencer*, Wheeling, WV, November 14, 1867, 4.

9. Medical Society of West Virginia, *Transactions of the Medical Society of West Virginia—Annual Address of John Frissell M.D.—President of the Society* (Wheeling, WV: Medical Society of West Virginia, 1869), 83–101.

10. John Frissell, Frissell Scrapbook: John Frissell Papers University of West Virginia Library WV and Regional History Collection, 1879; The document is in private hands today and has been described by: Kate Quinn, "A Heinous Offence," *Upper Ohio Valley Historical Review* 30, no. 1 (2007): 3–8. One could argue that Reeves did not write it, as it is unsigned and written in the third person. But it contains a number of details that would be best known by Reeves. Moreover, the third person narrative was typical for Reeves.

11. Reeves' original constitution was removed from the printed *Transactions* during publication. The document is missing pages 59–62: Virginia, *Transactions of the Medical Society of West Virginia—Including Proceedings of the Medical Convention Held at Fairmont April 10, 1867.* The membership lan-

guage, however, was printed in the Wheeling *Intelligencer:* "The Fairmont *Vedette*," *The Wheeling Daily Intelligencer*, Wheeling, WV, April 13, 1867, 2.

12. *Transactions of the Medical Society of West Virginia—Minutes of the First Annual Meeting* (Wheeling, WV: Medical Society of West Virginia, 1868).

13. "Election of Health Officer," *The Wheeling Daily Intelligencer*, Wheeling, WV, July 16, 1868, 4; Biographical information on Weisel in: Newton, Nichols, and Sprankle, *History of the Pan-Handle; Being Historical Collections of the Counties of Ohio, Brooke, Marshall and Hancock, West Virginia*, p. 254.

14. Samuel Jepson, "The Healing Arts in the Pan-Handle," in *History of the Upper Ohio Valley*, ed. Gibson L Cranmer (Madison, WI: Brant & Fuller, 1890), 563–93; "Medical Association," *The Wheeling Daily Intelligencer*, Wheeling, WV, October 21, 1868, 4; James E. Reeves, "Remarks on the Contagiousness of Enteric Fever—Made Before the Wheeling and Ohio County Medical Society," *The Medical Record* 4, no. March 1, 1869 (1869): 49–51. 50.

15. American Public Health Association, *Public Health Papers and Reports—Volume VIII Presented at the Tenth Annual Meeting of the American Public Health Association—Indianapolis, Ind. Oct 17–20, 1882* (Boston: American Public Health Association, 1883), 231; Wilson, "James Edmund Reeves, M.D." 1323; "City Council," *The Wheeling Daily Intelligencer*, Wheeling, WV, March 17, 1869, 4.

16. For information on McGinnis see Jepson, "The Healing Arts in the Pan-Handle," 584; "City Council"; "An Ordinance," *The Wheeling Daily Intelligencer*, Wheeling, WV, March 23, 1869, 2.

17. "City Council"; "Health Officer's Notice," *The Wheeling Daily Intelligencer*, Wheeling, WV, March 23, 1869, 2.

18. Report of Committee on Disinfectants Association, *The Transactions of the American Medical Association*. 129; In addition to previously cited references on the Civil War, see also: Howard D. Kramer, "Effect of the Civil War on the Public Health Movement," *The Mississippi Valley Historical Review* 35, no. 3 (1948): 449–62; The Civil War, Efficiency, and the Sanitary Impulse, 1845–1870" in John Harley Warner and Janet A. Tighe, eds., *Major Problems in the History of American Medicine and Public Health*, Major Problems in American History (Boston, MA: Houghton Mifflin Company, 2001).

19. Medical Society of West Virginia, *Transactions of the Medical Society of West Virginia—Minutes of the Second Annual Meeting* (Wheeling, WV: Medical Society of West Virginia, 1869), 102–118. 104.

20. Anonymous, Pamphlet, 1879. 2.

21. Newton, Nichols, and Sprankle, *History of the Pan-Handle; Being Historical Collections of the Counties of Ohio, Brooke, Marshall and Hancock, West Virginia*; Atkinson, *A Biographical Dictionary of Contemporary American Physicians and Surgeons*; Jepson, "The Healing Arts in the Pan-Handle"; George W. Atkinson and Alvaro Franklin Gibbens, *Prominent Men of West Virginia* (Wheeling, WV: W. L. Callin, 1890).

22. Sydney E. Ahlstrom, *A Religious History of the American People*, second ed. (New Haven, CT: Yale University Press, 2004); for self-prepared biographies on Hupp, see: Atkinson, *Physicians and Surgeons of the United States*, 292–293 and Atkinson, *A Biographical Dictionary of Contemporary American Physi-*

cians and Surgeons, 292–293; Newspaper account: John C. Hupp, "Local Traditional Reminiscences of Pioneer Life," *The Daily Intelligencer*, Wheeling, WV, May 31, 1864, 1.

23. American Medical Association, *The Transactions of the American Medical Association*, vol. 11 (Philadelphia, PA: American Medical Association, 1858); Atkinson and Gibbens, *Prominent Men of West Virginia*; Gibson L Cranmer, *History of Wheeling City and Ohio County, West Virginia, and Representative Citizens* (Chicago, IL: Biographical Pub. Co., 1902); John C. Hupp, *Vaccination and Its Protective Power in the State of West Virginia: A Report to the Governor, November 8, 1870* (Wheeling, WV: John Frew, Public Printer, 1871).

24. Jepson, "The Healing Arts in the Pan-Handle," 573.

25. "A Number of the Medical Profession...," *The Wheeling Daily Intelligencer*, Wheeling, WV, November 22, 1869, 3.

26. "Proceedings of the Medical Convention," *The Weekly Register*, Point Pleasant, WV, December 2, 1869, 3.

27. "To the Medical Profession," *Spirit of Jefferson*, Charlestown, WV, May 10, 1870, 2; Virginia, *Transactions of the Medical Society of the State of West Virginia*.

28. AMA data reported 395 regular physicians in WV in 1871: Association, *The Transactions of the American Medical Association*. 155. There were approximately 5,600 physician members of state medical societies in 1873: *The Transactions of the American Medical Association* and, assuming 80 percent of physicians in the U.S. census were practicing regulars, roughly 50,000 practicing physicians: U.S. Census, "Ninth Census of the United States, 1870," 1870. Physicians could belong to a local medical society and not a state society, but they could have also belonged to both. Even assuming no overlap, the available data show that most physicians did not participate in any form of organized medicine. The MSWV had 306 members in 1901 and 75 meeting attendees: Medical Society of West Virginia, *Transactions of the Medical Society of the State of West Virginia* (Wheeling, WV: Medical Society of West Virginia, 1901). The 1900 U.S. Census reported 1,885 physicians in West Virginia: U.S. Census, "Twelfth Census of the United States, 1900," 1900, and I have conservatively assumed that 80 percent of these were practicing regulars: Starr, *The Social Transformation of American Medicine- the Rise of a Sovereign Profession and the Making of a Vast Industry* 99); Oliver Garceau, *The Political Life of the American Medical Association* (Hamden, CT: Archon Books, 1961).

29. "Hand Hurt," *The Wheeling Daily Intelligencer*, Wheeling, WV, April 6, 1870, 4; "Head Cut," *The Wheeling Daily Intelligencer*, Wheeling, WV, June 16, 1870, 4; "Seriously Injured," *The Wheeling Daily Intelligencer*, Wheeling, WV, September 5, 1870, 4; "Frightful Fall," *The Wheeling Daily Intelligencer*, Wheeling, WV, September 23, 1870, 1; "Board of Supervisors," *The Wheeling Daily Intelligencer*, Wheeling, WV, January 31, 1870, 4; "City Council," *The Wheeling Daily Intelligencer*, Wheeling, WV, February 16, 1870, 4. The one local organization Reeves did join was the West Virginia Historical Society, which was heavily dominated by physicians and counted Boston's Dr. Oliver Wendell Holmes as a correspon-

ding member: "West Virginia Historical Society," *The Wheeling Daily Intelligencer,* Wheeling, WV, February 10, 1870, 4.

30. Wilson, "James Edmund Reeves, M.D.," 1325; James E. Reeves, *The Physical and Medical Topography, Including Vital, Manufacturing and Other Statistics of the City of Wheeling* (Wheeling: Daily Register Book and Job Office, 1870).

31. Number of copies from: James Edmund Reeves (editor), "The Health of Wheeling," *The West Virginia Medical Student* 1, no. 1 (1875): 25–28. Favorable notices cited in: James E. Reeves, *The Health and Wealth of the City of Wheeling—Including Its Physical and Medical Topography; Also General Remarks on the Natural Resources of West Virginia.* (Baltimore: The Sun Book and Job Office, 1871). Review in: Edward S. Dunster (editor), "The Physical and Medical Topography, Including Vital, Manufacturing, and Other Statistics, of the City of Wheeling (Review)." *The New York Medical Journal* 11, no. 3 (1870): 315.

32. John D. Wilsey, *American Exceptionalism and Civil Religion: Reassessing the History of an Idea* (Downers Grove, IL: InterVarsity Press, 2015); John Wesley, *Notes on the Bible* (Grand Rapids, MI: Christian Classics Ethereal Library, 1754). 1529; Reeves, *The Physical and Medical Topography, Including Vital, Manufacturing and Other Statistics of the City of Wheeling.*

33. Stephen Smith (editor), "Rational Medicine," *The American Medical Times* 1, no. August 25, 1860 (1860): 136–37. 137.

34. Reeves, *The Physical and Medical Topography, Including Vital, Manufacturing and Other Statistics of the City of Wheeling.* 8.

35. Rudolph Virchow, *Collected Essays on Public Health and Epidemiology,* ed. L.J. Rather, trans. Anne Gismann, 2 vols., vol. 2, Resources in Medical History (Canton, MA: Science History Publications/U.S.A., 1985), 193–266. 236.

36. J. David Hacker, "Decennial Life Tables for the White Population of the United States, 1790–1900," *Historical Methods* 43, no. 2 (2010): 45–79; James C. Riley, *Rising Life Expectancy: A Global History* (Cambridge, UK: Cambridge University Press, 2001).

37. Editor, "Salutatory," *The Medical Times* 1, no. October 1, 1870 (1870): 9–10.; James E. Reeves, "Letter from Wheeling," *ibid.,* no. November 15, 1870: 62–63, 62.

38. "Letter from Wheeling W. Va.," *The Medical Times* 1, no. February 1, 1871 (1871): 160–61; "Medical Notes I. Dysentery," *The Medical Times* 1, no. June 1, 1871 (1871): 315–16; "Medical Notes Ii. Diphtheria," *The Medical Times* 1, no. July 15, 1871 (1871): 371–72; "Medical Notes Iii. Scarlet Fever," *The Medical Times* 1, no. August 1, 1871 (1871): 394–95; "Medical Notes IV. Enteric or Typhoid Fever," *The Medical Times* 1, no. August 15, 1871 (1871): 415–17; Reeves contributed six articles to Volume 1, as did William Pepper and journal editor James Tyson. See James H. Hutchinson (editor) and James Tyson (editor), *The Medical Times,* 41 vols., vol. 1 (Philadelphia, PA: J.B. Lippincott & Co., 1870–71), 469–475.

39. Reeves, "Medical Notes Iii. Scarlet Fever," 395.

40. Medical Society of West Virginia, *Transactions of the Medical Society of the State of West Virginia* (Wheeling, WV: Medical Society of West Virginia, 1872).

41. For biographical information on Bland, see

Atkinson, *A Biographical Dictionary of Contemporary American Physicians and Surgeons.* 310; Adolescentulus, "West Virginia Medical Society," *The Wheeling Daily Intelligencer,* Wheeling, WV, June 4, 1870, 2; Virginia, *Transactions of the Medical Society of the State of West Virginia.*

42. American Medical Association, *The Transactions of the American Medical Association,* vol. 21 (Philadelphia, PA: American Medical Association, 1870) 29.

43. Latin: "very young man."

44. "West Virginia Medical Society."

45. "Medical Society of West Virginia," *ibid.,* November 15.

Chapter 11

1. Reeves, *The Health and Wealth of the City of Wheeling—Including Its Physical and Medical Topography; Also General Remarks on the Natural Resources of West Virginia.*; The local paper wrote that the book was "prepared and published by himself": "Health and Wealth of Wheeling," *The Wheeling Daily Intelligencer,* Wheeling, WV, February 22, 1871, 3.

2. *The Health and Wealth of the City of Wheeling—Including Its Physical and Medical Topography; Also General Remarks on the Natural Resources of West Virginia.* iv.

3. *The Health and Wealth of the City of Wheeling—Including Its Physical and Medical Topography; Also General Remarks on the Natural Resources of West Virginia..* Quotations pp. 1, 10, 11, 12.

4. Bowditch, *Public Hygiene in America.*

5. Reeves, *The Health and Wealth of the City of Wheeling—Including Its Physical and Medical Topography; Also General Remarks on the Natural Resources of West Virginia,* 12, 20.

6. Virchow, *Collected Essays on Public Health and Epidemiology.* Quotations pp. 215, 216.

7. E. D. Mapother, *Lectures on Public Health—Delivered at the Royal College of Surgeons,* second ed. (Dublin, Ireland: Fannin & Co., 1867). Quotation pp. 555–556.

8. A.N. Bell, ed. *The Sanitarian,* vol. 4 (New York, NY: The Sanitarian, 1876)

9. For example Willemijn Dicke and Martin Albrow, "Reconstituting the Public-Private Divide under Global Conditions.," *Global Social Policy* 5, no. 2 (2011): 227–48.

10. Benjamin Franklin, "The Papers of Benjamin Franklin," (New Haven, CT: Yale University, 2006); Carla J. Mulford, email, 3/29/2017, 2017.

11. Reeves, *The Health and Wealth of the City of Wheeling—Including Its Physical and Medical Topography; Also General Remarks on the Natural Resources of West Virginia.* 91, 96.

12. *The Health and Wealth of the City of Wheeling—Including Its Physical and Medical Topography; Also General Remarks on the Natural Resources of West Virginia.*

13. "We Notice in Our Exchanges...," *The Wheeling Daily Intelligencer,* Wheeling, WV, March 17, 1871, 2.

14. Editor, "The Health and Wealth of the City of Wheeling, West Virginia," *The Boston Medical and Surgical Journal* 7 (1871): 199; "The Health and Wealth of the City of Wheeling," *The Medical Times*

1, no. April 15, 1871 (1871): 265; "From Lippincott's Medical Times," *The Wheeling Daily Intelligencer,* Wheeling, WV, April 18, 1871, 4.

15. Reeves, *The Health and Wealth of the City of Wheeling—Including Its Physical and Medical Topography; Also General Remarks on the Natural Resources of West Virginia,* 121.

16. "Death of Mrs. Dr. J.E. Reeves"; *Mamma's Last Gift* (Wheeling, WV1871), Personal Publication.

17. "Health Officer's Notice," *The Wheeling Daily Intelligencer,* Wheeling, WV, April 13, 1872, 3; "Hand Crushed," *The Wheeling Daily Intelligencer,* Wheeling, WV, April 19, 1872, 4; "That Small-Pox Case," *The Wheeling Daily Intelligencer,* Wheeling, WV, April 20, 1872, 4.

18. Virginia, *Transactions of the Medical Society of the State of West Virginia;* Anonymous.

19. In 1878, Robert Cochran, a respected judge, blasted Hupp in the local press: "Come down from your exalted chronic vanity, and incomprehensible, *ponderous,* pomposity, unless, indeed, you expect to add a new chapter to your Pickwickian autobiography..." (italics in original): "The Board of Education—Reply of Judge Cochran to Dr. J.C. Hupp," *Wheeling Register,* July 31, 1878, 4.

20. "State Medical Society," *The Wheeling Daily Intelligencer,* Wheeling, WV, June 8, 1872, 3.

21. Greenleaf Cilley and Jonathan P. Cilley, *The Mount Desert Widow: Genealogy of the Gamble Family of Maine from the First Landing on the Coast of Mount Desert Down to the Present Day* (Rockland, ME: Knox County Historical and Genealogical Magazine, 1895), 104; Wilson, "James Edmund Reeves, M.D."; "Deed Book #60," Ohio County Recorder's Office, 1873; For Reeves' residences see J. Wiggins, *J. Wiggins & Co.'S Wheeling Directory 1874–5* (Cleveland, OH: J. Wiggins & Co., 1874), Advertisement, "For Rent," *The Wheeling Daily Intelligencer,* Wheeling, WV, November 5, 1879, 4, W.L. Callin, *Callin's Wheeling City Directory* (Wheeling, WV: W.L. Callin, 1880).

22. For Baird's term as Wheeling mayor see: "Meeting of the New Council," *The Daily Intelligencer,* Wheeling, WV, January 30, 1863, 3, "Butternut Meeting at Triadelphia," *The Daily Intelligencer,* Wheeling, WV, March 9, 1863, 3, "City Council," *The Daily Intelligencer,* Wheeling, WV, January 29, 1864, 3; Atkinson, *A Biographical Dictionary of Contemporary American Physicians and Surgeons.* 444.

23. "Assault," *The Wheeling Daily Intelligencer,* Wheeling, WV, December 20, 1872, 4; "Police Court," *The Wheeling Daily Intelligencer,* Wheeling, WV, December 21, 1872, 4.

24. Stephen Smith, "Historical Sketch of the American Public Health Association," *Public Health Papers and Reports* 5 (1880): xvii–liv. xi.

25. Further information on APHA founders: Kelly and Burrage, *Dictionary of American Medical Biography.* 919–920; James C. Mohr, *Doctors & the Law: Medical Jurisprudence in Nineteenth-Century America* (New York, NY: Oxford University Press, 1993)"; Obituary—Edward Houghton Janes," *The Brooklyn Medical Journal* 7, no. 4 (1893): 289; York, *Report Upon the Sanitary Condition of the City;* T.A. Thacher, *Biographical and Historical Record of the Class of 1835 in Yale College* (New Haven, CT: Tuttle, Morehouse, and Taylor, 1881); Kelly and Burrage, *Dictionary of American Medical Biography;* "Death of

Carl Pfeiffer, Architect," *The American Architect and Building News* 23, no. 648 (1888): 241; Arthur R. Reynolds, "Three Chicago and Illinois Public Health Officers: John H. Rauch, Oscar C. De Wolf, and Frank W. Reilly," *Bulletin of the Society of Medical History of Chicago* 1, no. 2 (1911): 89–108; F. Garvin Davenport, "John Henry Rauch and Public Health in Illinois 1877–1891," *Journal of the Illinois State Historical Society* 50, no. 3 (1957): 277–94; James H. Cassedy, "Edwin Miller Snow: An Important American Public Health Pioneer," *Bulletin of the History of Medicine* 35, no. 1 (1961): 156–62.

26. Only Harris and Janes attended the 1872 AMA meeting: American Medical Association, *The Transactions of the American Medical Association,* vol. 23 (Philadelphia, PA: American Medical Association, 1872); For biographical information on Logan see Howard A. Kelly and Walter L. Burrage, *American Medical Biographies* (Baltimore, MD: The Norman, Remington Company, 1920), pp. 173–714.

27. Association, *The Transactions of the American Medical Association,* 47.

28. Smith, "Historical Sketch of the American Public Health Association."

29. "City Council," *The Wheeling Daily Intelligencer,* Wheeling, WV, February 13, 1873, 4; Editor, "Regulating the Sale of Kerosene," *ibid.,* March 11, 3; A search of online newspaper sources for information on the kerosene issue (http://genealogybank.com,, http://chroniclingamerica.loc.gov/, and a relatively contemporary index of West Virginia law showed no references to a kerosene, coal oil, or illuminating oil safety or purity law: Charles E. Hogg, ed. *Hogg's West Virginia Code,* 3 vols. (St Paul, MN: West Publishing Company, 1914); West Virginia stood in contrast to Michigan, where an 1875 physician-led effort resulted in a law regulating illuminating oils: American Medical Association, *The Transactions of the American Medical Association,* vol. 27 (Philadelphia, PA: American Medical Association, 1876), 354.

30. Elisha Harris, "Record of Proceedings," *Public Health Reports and Papers* 2 (1876): 532–52. 537.

31. Among Woodward's many accomplishments were the first two volumes of *The Medical and Surgical History of the War of the Rebellion.* In the second, 1879, volume he cited data that Reeves had presented in several publications, referring to him as, "my friend," Dr. James E. Reeves, of Wheeling, West Virginia": Woodward, *The Medical and Surgical History of the War of the Rebellion—Medical History Part 2.* 425, 794; For information on Woodward see Humphreys, *Marrow of Tragedy—The Health Crisis of the American Civil War,* Devine, *Learning from the Wounded—The Civil War and the Rise of American Medical Science ,* Kelly and Burrage, *American Medical Biographies.*

32. Those APHA members who did travel to the two 1873 meetings were Snow (RI), Bell (NY), Dean (NY), Toner (DC), Woodworth (DC), and Woodward (DC): Harris, "Record of Proceedings," 536–539; Association, *The Transactions of the American Medical Association.*

33. *The Transactions of the American Medical Association.* 94; Further discussion of the anti-laboratory, anti-experimental bias of American medicine during this period: Warner, *The Therapeutic Perspective: Medical Practice, Knowledge, and Identity in America, 1820–1885.*

34. Association, *The Transactions of the American Medical Association.* 80. 83.
35. *The Transactions of the American Medical Association.* 90. 93.
36. *The Transactions of the American Medical Association.* 205, 211, 225, 257–258, 270; Thomas P. Gariepy, "The Introduction and Acceptance of Listerian Antisepsis in the United States," *Journal of the History of Medicine and Allied Sciences,* 49, no. 2 (1994): 167–206.
37. Joseph Lister, "Illustrations of the Antiseptic System of Treatment in Surgery," *The Lancet* 90, no. 2309 (1867): 668–69; "On a New Method of Treating Compound Fracture, Abscesses, Etc.—With Observations on the Conditions of Suppuration," *The Lancet* 89, no. 2273 (1867): 326–29; David W. Yandell, "Thirty Surgical Cases Treated with Carbolic Acid as a Dressing," *Richmond and Louisville Medical Journal* 7, no. 6 (1869): 651–65; Gert H. Brieger, "American Surgery and the Germ Theory of Disease," *Bulletin of the History of Medicine* 40, no. 2 (1966): 135–45; Gariepy, "The Introduction and Acceptance of Listerian Antisepsis in the United States."

Chapter 12

1. "Cholera and How to Disarm It," *The Wheeling Daily Intelligencer,* Wheeling, WV, June 24, 1873, 3; "A Necessary Action," *The Wheeling Daily Intelligencer,* Wheeling, WV, June 26, 1873, 2.
2. APHA records show the names of 29 persons, counting the speakers, at the opening presentations, plus "many other physicians and citizens." In light of subsequent statements that a quorum of twenty-five members had never been present, it is hard to believe that more than fifty people attended the opening meeting: Harris, "Record of Proceedings," 539.
3. A.N. Bell (editor), "The American Public Health Association," *The Sanitarian* 1, no. 9 (1873). 407–28; Elisha Harris (editor), "Contents," *Public Health Reports and Papers* 1 (1875): i–vii; Jarvis had already published several commentaries on good living: Rosalba Davico, ed. *The Autobiography of Edward Jarvis (1803–1884),* Medical History Supplement Number 12 (London, UK: Wellcome Institute for the History of Medicine, 1992) and Reeves later reprinted his essay at his own expense: Advertisement, "The Physical and Moral Causes of Bad Health in American Women," *The West Virginia Medical Student* 1, no. 1 (1875): 40.
4. Carroll Smith-Rosenberg, "The Female Animal: Medical and Biological Views of Women," in *No Other Gods: On Science and American Social Thought,* ed. Charles E. Rosenberg (Baltimore, MD: Johns Hopkins University Press, 1997), 54–70, 61; Carroll Smith-Rosenberg and Charles Rosenberg, "The Female Animal: Medical and Biological Views of Woman and Her Role in Nineteenth-Century America," in *Women and Health in America—Historical Readings,* ed. Judith Walzer Leavitt (Madison, WI: University of Wisconsin Press, 1984), 12–27.
5. There is no extant version of the complete paper, but it was extensively abstracted by the New York *Times:* "The Causes of Bad Health in American Women," *The New York Times,* November 12, 1873.
6. Harris, "Record of Proceedings," 539–540.
7. Billings: American Medical Association, *The Transactions of the American Medical Association,* vol. 30 (Philadelphia, PA: American Medical Association, 1879), 275–291; APHA member list: "List of Members of the Association," *Public Health Papers and Reports* 5 (1880): 244–56.
8. Charles B. Davenport, "Biographical Memoir of Frederick Augustus Porter Barnard: 1809–1889," ed. Unknown, *Biographical Memoirs of the National Academy of Sciences* (Washington, D.C.: National Academy of Sciences, 1938), http://www.nasonline.org/publications/biographical-memoirs/.; F.A.P. Barnard, "The Germ Theory of Disease and Its Relations to Hygiene," *Public Health Reports and Papers* 1 (1875): 70–87; For contemporary overviews of the evolution of the germ theory see: Bynum, *Science and the Practice of Medicine in the Nineteenth Century* and Roy Porter, *The Greatest Benefit to Mankind—A Medical History of Humanity* (New York, NY: W.W. Norton and Company, 1997); Mazÿck Ravenel, "The American Public Health Association: Past, Present, and Future," in *A Half Century of Public Health,* ed. Mazÿck Ravenel (New York, NY: American Public Health Association, 1921), 13–55. 21.
9. Barnard, "The Germ Theory of Disease and Its Relations to Hygiene," 80.
10. "The Germ Theory of Disease and Its Relations to Hygiene," 82.
11. "The Germ Theory of Disease and Its Relations to Hygiene," 87.
12. Candice Millard, *Destiny of the Republic* (New York: Doubleday, 2011).
13. Numerous authors have argued that there was delayed uptake of the germ theory in the United States, generally attributing it to a lack of American laboratory science and/or resistance to European laboratory findings. See: Phyllis Allen Richmond, "American Attitudes toward the Germ Theory of Disease (1860–1880)," *Journal of the History of Medicine and Allied Sciences* 9, no. 4 (1954): 428–54; Haller, *American Medicine in Transition, 1840–1910;* Rothstein, *American Physicians in the 19th Century—From Sects to Science;* and Warner, *The Therapeutic Perspective: Medical Practice, Knowledge, and Identity in America, 1820–1885;* Charles G. Lord, Lee Ross, and Mark R. Lepper, "Biased Assimilation and Attitude Polarization: The Effects of Prior Theories on Subsequently Considered Evidence," *Journal of Personality and Social Psychology* 37, no. 11 (1979): 2098–109; L. Rosenbaum, "Resisting the Suppression of Science," *N Engl J Med* 376, no. 17 (2017): 1607–9.
14. Alfred Stillé, *Therapeutics and Materia Medica,* 2 vols., vol. 1 (Philadelphia, PA: Henry C. Lea, 1874), 780; Austin Flint, *A Treatise on the Principles and Practice of Medicine; Designed for the Use of Practitioners and Students of Medicine* (Philadelphia, PA: Henry C. Lea, 1873).
15. Nelson Chesman, ed. *Rowell's American Newspaper Directory* (New York, NY: Geo. P. Rowell & Co., 1873), 249–250; Yandell, Lunsford P. Report of the Committee on Medical Literature: Association, *The Transactions of the American Medical Association.* 123–134.
16. For evidence of Reeves' abandonment of professional organizations see: Virginia, *Transactions of the Medical Society of the State of West Virginia; Transactions of the Medical Society of the State of West Virginia* (Wheeling, WV: Medical Society of West Virginia, 1875); American Medical Association,

The Transactions of the American Medical Association, vol. 25 (Philadelphia, PA: American Medical Association, 1874); The Transactions of the American Medical Association, vol. 26 (Philadelphia, PA: American Medical Association, 1875); in 1875 Reeves attended the APHA's annual meeting in Baltimore, where his parents lived, but he did not make a presentation: American Public Health Association, Public Health Reports and Papers, vol. 2 (New York, NY: Hurd and Houghton, 1876); For his new printing business see: Supplies: "River News," The Wheeling Daily Intelligencer, Wheeling, WV, February 16, 1874, 4, printing press: James Edmund Reeves (editor), The West Virginia Medical Student (Wheeling: The West Virginia Medical Student, 1875–1876), 404.

17. "We Are in Receipt," The Wheeling Daily Intelligencer, Wheeling, WV, July 5, 1875, 1; Landon B. Edwards (editor), "Bad Health: Its Physical and Moral Causes in American Women," The Virginia Medical Monthly 2, no. 5 (1875): 378.

18. James Edmund Reeves (editor), "Salutatory," The West Virginia Medical Student 1, no. 1 (1875): 23–25. 25, 23.

19. M.S. Hall (Letter), "To the Editor of the Medical Student," ibid., no. 2: 65; information on Hall: Atkinson, Physicians and Surgeons of the United States. 470; Editor, "Reviews and Notices—The West Virginia Medical Student," The Cincinnati Lancet and Observer 18, no. 12 (1875): 768; James Edmund Reeves (editor), "Credit to Whom Credit Is Due," The West Virginia Medical Student 1, no. 12 (1876): 404.

20. S. L. Jepson, "The Origin and Propagation of Typhoid Fever," ibid., no. 5: 149–58; William Budd, Typhoid Fever—Its Nature, Mode of Spreading, and Prevention (London, UK: Longmans, Green, and Company, 1873); For a discussion of the mechanism of water-borne infection, see Cabell, J.L. in: American Medical Association, The Transactions of the American Medical Association, vol. 29 (Philadelphia, PA: American Medical Association, 1878), 562.

21. Some historians have presented regulars of the time as bitterly opposed to botanical therapies (e.g., James C. Mohr, Licensed to Practice—The Supreme Court Defines the American Medical Profession [Baltimore, MD: Johns Hopkins University Press, 2013]), but the situation was more complicated. One prominent example of regulars' appreciation of the use of botanicals is that AMA founder Nathan Davis appointed himself to make a report on indigenous medical botany at the organization's first meeting in 1848. This report included a discussion of Cimicifuga Racemosa: Association, "The Transactions of the American Medical Association," 1848 341–357; Starling Loving, "Remarks on the Therapeutic Application of Cimicifuga Racemosa," The West Virginia Medical Student 1, no. 3 (1876): 77–87, 77; Cathi E. Dennehy and Candy Tsourounis, "Dietary Supplements & Herbal Medications," in Basic and Clinical Pharmacology, ed. Bertram G. Katzung and Anthony J. Trevor (New York, NY: McGraw-Hill Medical, 2015); P.R. Reamey, "Hydrochlorate of Ammonia—Introductory Remarks on Cimicifuga Racemosa," The West Virginia Medical Student 1, no. 7 (1876): 218–25.

22. Editor, "Memoranda," The Detroit Review of Medicine and Pharmacy 10, no. 12 (1875): 760–62. 760. Also Reeves (editor), The West Virginia Medical Student. 106.

23. "Personal Advertising," The West Virginia Medical Student 1, no. 1 (1875): 28–29. 29; Ashhurst, Jr., Transactions of the International Medical Congress; Hupp also sent personal notices to the Wheeling papers recording his departure to and return from the Congress, as he did for virtually every other medical meeting he attended. None of the other Wheeling physicians were so assiduous in publicly announcing their medical travels: "Personals," The Wheeling Daily Intelligencer, Wheeling, WV, August 31, 1876, 4, "Personals."

24. James Edmund Reeves (editor), "Reviews, Books, and Pamphlet Notices," The West Virginia Medical Student 1, no. 2 (1875): 70–74. 70, 73.

25. "Meeting of the State Medical Society," The West Virginia Medical Student 1, no. 7 (1876): 239–41. 239, 241.

26. West Virginians wrote only ten of the thirty-three Original Communications Reeves published in Volume 1 of the Medical Student.

27. Jepson, "The Healing Arts in the Pan-Handle."

28. S. L. Jepson, "Editorial. Here We Are.," The West Virginia Medical Journal 1, no. 1 (1906): 26–27. 27.

29. The Journal's Lactopeptine ads avoided the major problems of claiming unique status and offering lengthy testimonials. However, the product was still a branded, proprietary formulation: The Boston Medical and Surgical Journal. vol. 90 (Boston, MA: David Clapp & Son, 1874); by the AMA standards of the times, Lactopeptine had several problems. Firstly it was a proprietary preparation featuring a brand name; secondly it claimed uniquely effective status; and thirdly it featured endorsements by numerous physicians in their official organizational capacity. All of these would have been cause for reprobation in a lay publication and serious concern in a medical journal: Editor, "Advertisements," Journal of the American Medical Association I, no. 3 (1883): 89–90. The compound was also completely ineffective, but this was not known at the time. It was still marketed in 1922, but recognized by then to be worthless as a digestive aid: J. Deas, "Elixir Lactopeptine," Can Med Assoc J 12, no. 1 (1922): 44.

30. Association, "The Transactions of the American Medical Association," 1848. 284; for a contemporary discussion of this ethical inconsistency, see AMA President Sims' 1876 address: The Transactions of the American Medical Association, 98; James Harvey Young, The Toadstool Millionaires—A Social History of Patent Medicines in America before Federal Regulation (Princeton: Princeton University Press, 1961); The Medical Messiahs—A Social History of Health Quackery in Twentieth-Century America (Princeton: Princeton University Press, 1967); Eric W. Boyle, Quack Medicine—A History of Combating Health Fraud in Twentieth-Century America (Santa Barbara: Praeger, 2013); Morris Fishbein, "History of the American Medical Association: 1890–1894," JAMA 133, no. 6 (1947): 383–92.

31. Much of the biographical information on Lawrence was written after his business success and is sparse and sometimes conflicting on early details: Howard L. Conard, Encyclopedia of the History of Missouri, 6 vols., vol. 4 (New York: The Southern History Company, 1901), Hugh Buckner Johnston, "Lawrence, Joseph Joshua," in Dictionary of North Carolina Biography, ed. William S. Powell (Chapel Hill, NC: University of North Carolina Press, 1991), 30–31; Advertisement, "Rosadalis," The Daily Dis-

patch, Richmond, VA March 16, 1868, 2; "Koskoo!," *The Hillsborough Recorder*, Hillsborough, NC September 8, 1869, 3; the last advertisement I could find for these products was from February 1872: "Dr. Lawrence's Celebrated Medicines," *The Charlotte Democrat*, Charlotte, NC February 6, 1872, 4.

32. Joseph J. Lawrence (editor), "Will Be Enlarged to 50 Pages," *The Medical Brief* 1, no. 3 (1873): 1.

33. Chesman, *Rowell's American Newspaper Directory.*

34. Joseph J. Lawrence (editor), "Enlarged," *The Medical Brief* 1, no. 4 (1873): 1.

35. "The Wilson Plaindealer Says," *Wilmington Journal*, Wilmington, NC, October 24, 1873, 4; The new eclectic medical school that hired Lawrence was the American Medical College. It was a reputable institution for the time but could be confused by later readers with the American Eclectic Medical College of Cincinnati, the fraudulent institution that supplied Frank Dent's diploma in 1881: John M. Rauch (Secretary), *Fifth Annual Report of the State Board of Health of Illinois* (Springfield, IL: H.W. Rokker, 1883); Chesman, *Rowell's American Newspaper Directory.*

36. There appear to be no extant copies of issues #1 and #2 of volume 1. The motto is present on issue #3, volume 1, and subsequent issues: Lawrence (editor), "Will Be Enlarged to 50 Pages."

37. This therapeutic convergence has been well-described, but two examples illustrate the point: when asked to define eclecticism in 1872, the Iowa State Eclectic Medical Association asserted that it only differed from regular medicine in its refusal to use bleeding and metallic compounds, such as antimony salts, to which a regular medical journal editor replied that his profession did not use such treatments either: Editor, "What Is Eclecticism?," *Philadelphia Medical Times* 3, no. 1 (1872): 43–44. Likewise, a New York *Times* editorial observed in 1873: "In most important respects there is little real difference between the practice of an accomplished regular physician and that of the intelligent homeopathist who has abandoned the use of infinitesimal remedies." "Medical Union," *The New York Times*, New York, NY, February 7, 1873, 4.

38. Joseph J. Lawrence (editor), *The Medical Brief* (St Louis: The Medical Brief, 1876). Quotation p. 329.

39. *The Medical Brief* (St Louis: The Medical Brief, 1877). 33; *The Medical Brief* (St Louis: The Medical Brief, 1880), 552, 553.

Chapter 13

1. Medical Society of West Virginia, *Transactions of the Medical Society of the State of West Virginia* (Wheeling, WV: Medical Society of West Virginia, 1876); Reeves (editor), "Meeting of the State Medical Society," 240.

2. There was no mention of Reeves in the APHA's 1876 minutes American Public Health Association, *Public Health Reports and Papers*, vol. 3 (New York, NY: Hurd and Houghton, 1877) nor did he cover the event in the *Medical Student,* as he did for the 1875 meeting that he attended Reeves (editor), *The West Virginia Medical Student*; Association, *The Transactions of the American Medical Association*; "Personals"; Ashhurst, Jr., *Transactions of the International Medical Congress.*

3. *Transactions of the International Medical Congress.* xxxv, 1–20.

4. *Transactions of the International Medical Congress.* 254, 260; Samuel D. Gross, *Autobiography of Samuel D. Gross, M.D.*, vol. II (Philadelphia: George Barrie, 1887), 156.

5. Reeves (editor), "Meeting of the State Medical Society," 381. Note several pages are misnumbered in the original as 181–184.

6. Gibson L Cranmer, "Upper Ohio Valley," in *History of the Upper Ohio Valley*, ed. Gibson L Cranmer (Madison, WI: Brant & Fuller, 1890); Editor, "Mr. Sweeney's Position," *The Daily Intelligencer*, Wheeling, WV, February 1, 1861, 2; James Morton Callahan, *History of West Virginia Old and New and West Virginia Biography*, 3 vols., vol. 2 (Chicago, IL: The American Historical Society, Inc., 1923), 26–27.

7. "Barbour County"; In 1884 Woods was a member of the West Virginia Supreme Court and *The Intelligencer* bitterly opposed him, primarily by citing his Civil War allegiances Editor, "Judge Woods in Another Role," *ibid.*, August 20, 1884, 2.

8. "The Sixth Ward Democratic Club," *Wheeling Register*, Wheeling, WV, September 30, 1876, 4.

9. Newton, Nichols, and Sprankle, *History of the Pan-Handle; Being Historical Collections of the Counties of Ohio, Brooke, Marshall and Hancock, West Virginia*, 190.

10. "The Primaries," *The Wheeling Daily Intelligencer*, Wheeling, WV, January 8, 1877, 4; "Democratic City Convention," *The Wheeling Daily Intelligencer*, Wheeling, WV, January 9, 1877, 4.

11. John J. Coniff, ed. *Laws and Ordinances for the Government of the City of Wheeling, West Virginia* (Wheeling, WV: Intelligencer Publishing Co., 1901); "Full Returns," *The Wheeling Daily Intelligencer*, Wheeling, WV, January 27, 1877, 4.

12. "Full Returns"; "Second Branch," *The Wheeling Daily Intelligencer*, Wheeling, WV, January 31, 1877, 4.

13. Woods, "Our Gallery—James Edmund Reeves, M.D. of Wheeling W. Va," 482. The *Register* delighted in describing the beard-pulling confrontation while the *Intelligencer* did not mention it. "An Exciting Scene," *The Wheeling Daily Register*, Wheeling, WV, May 21, 1879, 4, "City Solons in Session," *The Wheeling Daily Intelligencer*, Wheeling, WV, May 21, 1879, 4.

14. "Section Book No. 2," *The Wheeling Daily Intelligencer*, Wheeling, WV, July 12, 1879, 4; "The Proposed Increase in the Police Force-an Interview with Dr. Reeves," *The Wheeling Daily Intelligencer*, Wheeling, WV, June 3, 1879, 1.

15. "City Council," *The Wheeling Daily Intelligencer*, Wheeling, WV, January 9, 1878, 4; estimate of meetings attended from the Wheeling *Intelligencer.* This number includes meetings where Reeves did not answer the roll call, but arrived later and offered a comment or resolution. Data from "Chronicling America Home Page," in *Chronicling America.*

16. "City Council—Second Branch," *The Wheeling Daily Intelligencer*, Wheeling, WV, June 16, 1877, 4; "Health Committee," *The Wheeling Daily Intelligencer*, Wheeling, WV, September 9, 1879, 4; "Official Returns," *The Wheeling Daily Intelligencer*, Wheeling, WV, January 25, 1879, 4; "Complete Council Tickets," *The Wheeling Daily Intelligencer*, Wheeling, WV, January 24, 1881, 4; Anonymous, "A Correspondent's Views," *The Wheeling Daily Register*, Wheeling, WV, January 9, 1882, 4.

17. "Personal Points," *The Wheeling Daily Intelligencer*, Wheeling, WV, March 25, 1878, 4; "Personalities," *The Wheeling Daily Register*, Wheeling, WV, March 25, 1878, 4; "City Chips," *The Wheeling Daily Register*, Wheeling, WV, April 22, 1878, 4; "Personal Points."

18. "We Are Indebted to Dr. Reeves...," *The Wheeling Daily Intelligencer*, Wheeling, WV, May 28, 1878, 2; Advertisements, "Advertisements," *ibid.*, 3.

19. Anonymous; Association, *The Transactions of the American Medical Association*; "Personal Points."

20. Anonymous.

21. "The City Medical Society," *The Wheeling Daily Register*, Wheeling, WV, April 5, 1879, 4.

22. For Brock: Kelly and Burrage, *American Medical Biographies*. 146; at age 30 Wilson returned to Wheeling in 1876 was elected County Health Officer. He was a generation younger than the Medical Society's old guard and soon showed his support for Reeves at the Wheeling and Ohio County Medical Society. Wilson authored Reeves' glowing memorial in 1896 Wilson, "James Edmund Reeves, M.D." For biographical information on Wilson, see S. L. Jepson, "In Memorium—Dr. Louis D. Wilson," *The West Virginia Medical Journal* 16, no. 3 (1921): 118–20; "Personal Mention," *The Wheeling Daily Intelligencer*, Wheeling, WV, April 4, 1879, 4.

23. Virginia, *Transactions of the Medical Society of West Virginia—Minutes of the First Annual Meeting*

24. *Transactions of the Medical Society of the State of West Virginia* (Wheeling, WV: Medical Society of West Virginia, 1878), 450, 452.

25. Frissell.

26. "Election of Officers," *The Wheeling Daily Intelligencer*, Wheeling, WV, October 4, 1879, 4; Medical Society member numbers from "Local Medical Society," *The Wheeling Daily Intelligencer*, Wheeling, WV, October 6, 1877, 4; American Medical Association, *The Transactions of the American Medical Association*, vol. 31 (Philadelphia, PA: American Medical Association, 1880).

27. *The Transactions of the American Medical Association*. 413.

28. Medical Society of West Virginia, *Transactions of the Medical Society of the State of West Virginia* (Wheeling, WV: Medical Society of West Virginia, 1880); 1880 president William Dent was the father of Frank Dent, the plaintiff in *Dent v. West Virginia*, but there is no evidence that Reeves had poor relationships with William. They were both founders of the Medical Society and, unlike Reeves' quarrel with Hupp, there was never any public friction. In the contentious 1879 state society meeting, Dent consistently voted with Reeves against Hupp *Transactions of the Medical Society of the State of West Virginia* (Wheeling, WV: Medical Society of West Virginia, 1879).

29. "West Virginia Medical Society," *The Wheeling Daily Intelligencer*, Wheeling, WV, June 28, 1880, 1; "Medical Matters," *The Wheeling Daily Register*, Wheeling, WV, June 29, 1880, 4.

30. Hupp died in 1908 and his official biographies are generally silent on his professional activities after 1880 Kelly and Burrage, *Dictionary of American Medical Biography*, Newspaper articles document him providing care until at least 1888 "A Serious Accident," *The Wheeling Daily Intelligencer*, Wheeling, WV, September 27, 1888, 4; Medical Society of West Virginia, *Transactions of the Medical Society of the State of West Virginia* (Wheeling, WV: Medical Society of West Virginia, 1882), pp. 837–840.

31. Association, *The Transactions of the American Medical Association*. 96.

32. Atkinson, *Physicians and Surgeons of the United States*; Victor Robinson (editor), "American Medical Biography," *Medical Review of Reviews* 24, no. 1 (1918): 1–15.

33. Atkinson, *A Biographical Dictionary of Contemporary American Physicians and Surgeons*.

34. Atkinson, *Physicians and Surgeons of the United States*. 8.

35. *Physicians and Surgeons of the United States*. 3.

36. James F. Baldwin (editor), "The Physicians and Surgeons of the United States," *The Ohio Medical Recorder* 3, no. 5 (1878): 213–17; George W. Paulson, *James Fairchild Baldwin, M.D.—An Extraordinary Surgeon* (Columbus, OH: Medical Heritage Center, 2005).

Chapter 14

1. Association, *The Transactions of the American Medical Association*. 398; H.G. Pickering, "Appendix IV—Digest of American Sanitary Law," in *Public Hygiene in America: Centennial Discourse on Public Hygiene and State Preventive Medicine*, ed. Henry I. Bowditch (Boston, MA: Little, Brown, and Company, 1876), 299–440; Association, *The Transactions of the American Medical Association*, 315. Louisiana technically had the first state board of health in 1855, but its jurisdiction was confined to New Orleans Duffy, *The Sanitarians—A History of American Public Health*.

2. Association, *Public Health Reports and Papers*. 526–528.

3. A. B. Stuart, "State Medicine and Public Hygiene," *The Sanitarian* 1, no. 10 (1874): 470–75; Association, *The Transactions of the American Medical Association*. 330.

4. *The Transactions of the American Medical Association*. 100–101; *The Transactions of the American Medical Association*, vol. 28 (Philadelphia, PA: American Medical Association, 1877), 42; *The Transactions of the American Medical Association*. 324–355; Pickering, "Appendix IV—Digest of American Sanitary Law."

5. Association, *The Transactions of the American Medical Association*, 401–402.

6. *The Transactions of the American Medical Association*, 324–355.

7. Stepen Rogers, "Correspondence. The New Medical Law of the State of New York " *New York Medical Journal* 20, no. 1 (1874): 64–72.

8. Medical Society of the State of New York, *Transactions of the Medical Society of the State of New York for the Year 1872* (Albany, NY: Medical Society of the State of New York, 1873), 49.

9. It is tempting to see the AMA's hand in health board and medical licensure development because the AMA and its surrogates took later ownership of the regulatory apparatus that arose Ronald Hamowy, "The Early Development of Medical Licensing Laws in the United States, 1875–1900," *Journal of Libertarian Studies* 3, no. 1 (1979): 73–119, Gregory Dolin, "Licensing Health Care Professionals: Has the United States Outlived the Need for Medical Licensure?," *The Georgetown Journal of Law and Public Policy* 2, no. 2

(2004): 315–36, Mohr, *Licensed to Practice—The Supreme Court Defines the American Medical Profession*, Stevens, *American Medicine and the Public Interest*, Starr, 1982), J. M. Harris, Jr., "It Is Time to Cancel Medicine's Social Contract Metaphor," *Acad Med* 92, no. 9 (2017): 1236–40.

10. Virginia, *Transactions of the Medical Society of the State of West Virginia*. 339, 341.

11. West Virginia Legislature, Charleston, WV, "Journal of the House of Delegates of the State of West Virginia for the Eleventh Session, 1872-'3," 1873; Virginia, *Transactions of the Medical Society of the State of West Virginia*. 543; Mohr states that another West Virginia physician, Silas Warrick Hall, was Medical Society President in 1874 Mohr, *Licensed to Practice—the Supreme Court Defines the American Medical Profession*. 42. His source was likely: Norma S. Hogshead, *Past Presidents of the West Virginia State Medical Association: 1867–1942* (Charleston, WV: Auxiliary to the West Virginia State Medical Association, 1942). Multiple issues of The Medical Society *Transactions* show that Moses Smith Hall was a member from 1870 and president in 1874, with no mention of Silas W. Hall: Virginia, *Transactions of the Medical Society of the State of West Virginia*. The distinction is important because of M. S. Hall's public respect for Reeves and his membership in the West Virginia House of Delegates; See Matthew Campbell's comments, *Transactions of the Medical Society of the State of West Virginia*. 31.

12. *Transactions of the Medical Society of the State of West Virginia*.

13. Reeves (editor), *The West Virginia Medical Student*. 28; Supplement to Issue 1, *The West Virginia Medical Student*; *The West Virginia Medical Student*. 64.

14. Samuel Jepson, "Editorial—A Bit of History," *The West Virginia Medical Journal* 10 (1915): 172–73; Virginia, *Transactions of the Medical Society of the State of West Virginia*. 341–352; West Virginia Legislature, Wheeling, WV, "Journal of the Senate of the State of West Virginia for the Fourteenth Session, 1877," 1877. 24, 29.

15. "To the Senate and House of Delegates of the State of West Virginia, Now in Legislative Session Assembled," *The Wheeling Daily Intelligencer*, Wheeling, WV, January 13, 1877, 2.

16. Association, *The Transactions of the American Medical Association*.

17. Wheeling, WV, "Journal of the Senate of the State of West Virginia for the Fourteenth Session, 1877," 81.

18. Virginia, *Transactions of the Medical Society of the State of West Virginia*. 350.

19. State numbers are based on an attempt to reconcile conflicting data: Samuel L. Baker, "Physician Licensure Laws in the United States, 1865–1915," *Journal of the History of Medicine* 39 (1984): 173–97; Association, *The Transactions of the American Medical Association*. 324–355; *The Transactions of the American Medical Association*. 101.

20. Walter L. Fleming, *Civil War and Reconstruction in Alabama* (New York: Columbia University Press,, 1905); Atkinson, *A Biographical Dictionary of Contemporary American Physicians and Surgeons*. 228; J.N. Baker, "Alabama's Contribution to Public Health," *The American Journal of Public Health* 30, no. 8 (1940): 859–65.

21. Medical Association of the State of Alabama, *Transactions of the Medical Association of the State of Alabama* (Montgomery, AL: Medical Association of the State of Alabama, 1875), 28.

22. Baker, "Alabama's Contribution to Public Health"; Cochran, 1893); Association, *The Transactions of the American Medical Association*. 325–326.

23. Baker, "Alabama's Contribution to Public Health"; Allen Johnston Going, *Bourbon Democracy in Alabama, 1874–1890* (Tuscaloosa, AL: University Alabama Press, 1992); Richard IV Hughes, Korisha Ramdhanie, Travis Wasserman et al., "State Boards of Health: Governance and Politics," *Journal of Law, Medicine, and Ethics* 39, no. Supplement (Spring) (2011): 37–41; in 1877, perhaps inspired by Alabama, the North Carolina legislature made the state medical society the state health board, without licensure authority or funding. The board was changed to a more traditional regulatory structure in 1879, but remained underfunded: Benjamin E. Washburn, *History of the North Carolina State Board of Health, 1877–1925* (Raleigh, NC: North Carolina State Board of Health, 1966).

24. Hamowy, "The Early Development of Medical Licensing Laws in the United States, 1875–1900"; Baker, "Alabama's Contribution to Public Health"; 500 members of an estimated physician population of 1,134 in 1873 (80 percent of census figures) Association, *The Transactions of the American Medical Association*, "Ninth Census of the United States, 1870"; Jerome Cochran, "The Medical Profession," in *Memorial Record of Alabama—A Concise Account of the State's Political, Military, Professional and Industrial Progress, Together with the Personal Memoirs of Many of Its People*, ed. Unknown (Madison, WI: Brant & Fuller, 1893), 107–40.

25. "Eighth Census of the United States, 1860," "Ninth Census of the United States, 1870." Property values based on true value. Literacy rates based on percent of population over age 10 able to read.

26. "Ninth Census of the United States, 1870." These data include all persons who self-identified as physicians. The total number for Alabama was 1,418, three of whom were women. For Illinois it was 4,801, 24 of whom were women (Table XXX). Missouri was even more crowded than Illinois, with 484 residents per physician; Illinois State Medical Society, *Transactions of the Illinois State Medical Society*, vol. 27 (Chicago, IL: The Illinois State Medical Society, 1877).

27. Board of Health of the City of Chicago, Chicago, IL, "Report of the Board of Health of the City of Chicago for 1867, 1868, 1869—And a Sanitary History of Chicago; from 1833 to 1870," 1870. 24–26; Chicago, IL, "Report of the Board of Health of the City of Chicago for 1870, 1871, 1872, and 1873," 1874; Atkinson, *A Biographical Dictionary of Contemporary American Physicians and Surgeons*; Reynolds, "Three Chicago and Illinois Public Health Officers: John H. Rauch, Oscar C. De Wolf, and Frank W. Reilly"; Duffy, *The Sanitarians—A History of American Public Health*; John B. Hamilton, "The Epidemics of Chicago," *Bulletin of the Society of Medical History of Chicago* 1, no. 1 (1911): 73–86.

28. For example, neither paid their dues in 1876 or attended that year's annual meeting: Illinois State Medical Society, *Transactions of the Illinois State Medical Society*, vol. 26 (Chicago, IL: The Illinois State Medical Society, 1876); Danforth, *The Life of Nathan Smith Davis*.

29. Society, *Transactions of the Illinois State Medical Society*. 27.

30. In 1872, with Davis' leadership, the AMA reaffirmed its constitutional prohibition on admitting any delegates, male or female, from women's medical colleges or women's hospitals (Association, *The Transactions of the American Medical Association*, p. 54). At this meeting, President Yandell confessed that women physicians might succeed, but told the delegates, "I hope they will never embarrass us by a personal application for seats in this Association. I could never vote for that" (*The Transactions of the American Medical Association*, p. 103). The practical problem the AMA faced, however, was that it had no constitutional prohibition on admitting women delegates. According to the Constitution and bylaws, any organized regular medical college or hospital could send delegates (*The Transactions of the American Medical Association*, pp:663–676). Davis soon moved to remedy the oversight. The following year, 1873, Davis proposed to amend the AMA's Constitution (Plan of Organization) by stipulating that only state medical societies, local societies in good standing within the state, and branches of the military could send delegates. The AMA would no longer seat delegates from medical colleges, hospitals, or any other non-medical society organizations, thus resolving any challenge from women's colleges and hospitals, as well other threats from medical colleges in general (*The Transactions of the American Medical Association*, p. 44). In 1874 the delegates adopted Davis' proposed change "by a large majority." *The Transactions of the American Medical Association*. Quotation p. 34.

31. Stanford Chaillé surveyed thirty-seven state medical societies in 1879 and found eleven that explicitly admitted doctresses *The Transactions of the American Medical Association*. 299–355; Society, *Transactions of the Illinois State Medical Society*. 203–222; *Transactions of the Illinois State Medical Society*. 27–28; like many women physicians of the time, Dr. Stevenson was well-qualified, having spent several years studying in Europe. She was later the first woman named to the Illinois State Board of Health. F.M. Sperry, *A Group of Distinguished Physicians and Surgeons of Chicago* (Chicago, IL: J.H. Beers & Co., 1904), 145–148.

32. State of Illinois, Springfield, IL, "Journal of the House of Representatives of the Thirtieth General Assembly of the State of Illinois," 1877; Springfield, IL, "Journal of the Senate of the Thirtieth General Assembly of the State of Illinois," 1877.

33. "Gov. Cullom," *Chicago Daily Tribune*, Chicago, IL, July 3, 1877, 4; "The Late Assembly," *Chicago Daily Tribune*, Chicago, IL, May 30, 1877, 8; "The Doctors—What They Think of the Bill Introduced by Senator Joslyn," *The Chicago Daily Tribune*, Chicago, IL, March 2, 1877, 7; Society, *Transactions of the Illinois State Medical Society*; "The Doctors—What They Think of the Bill Introduced by Senator Joslyn"; S.S. (Letter), "Doctors' Doings—Demand for a State Board of Medical Examiners to Stop the Slaughter," *ibid.*, March 15, 1877.

34. State Board of Health of Illinois, *Annual Report of the State Board of Health of Illinois Made to the Governor 1878* (Springfield, IL: Weber, Magie & Co.,, 1879), 12–15.

35. "Gov. Cullom"; *Annual Report of the State Board of Health of Illinois Made to the Governor 1878*;

Davenport, "John Henry Rauch and Public Health in Illinois 1877–1891."

36. General Assembly of Illinois, Springfield, IL, "Reports to the General Assembly of Illinois," 1879. 16.

37. Illinois, *Annual Report of the State Board of Health of Illinois Made to the Governor 1878*. 12.

38. Clinton Sandvick, "Enforcing Medical Licensing in Illinois: 1877–1890," *Yale Journal of Biology and Medicine* 82 (2009): 67–74; Starr, *The Social Transformation of American Medicine- the Rise of a Sovereign Profession and the Making of a Vast Industry*. 99. Eclecticism was more prominent in the Midwest than elsewhere, thus the percentage of regulars in Illinois could have been less than 80 percent: Rothstein, *American Physicians in the 19th Century—From Sects to Science*, but the overall impression from the data is that Illinois sectarians received licenses at about the same rate as they existed in the population; Illinois, *Annual Report of the State Board of Health of Illinois Made to the Governor 1878*.

39. Society, *Transactions of the Illinois State Medical Society*. Bone-setter reference 186. 196.

40. "Illinois State Board of Health," *Chicago Daily Tribune*, Chicago, IL December 9, 1877, 7.

41. Illinois, *Annual Report of the State Board of Health of Illinois Made to the Governor 1878*; John M. Rauch (Secretary), *Second Annual Report of the State Board of Health of Illinois* (Springfield, IL: H.W. Rokker, 1881), 16.

42. *Third Annual Report of the State Board of Health of Illinois* (Springfield, IL: H.W. Rokker, 1881); *Fourth Annual Report of the State Board of Health of Illinois* (Springfield, IL: H.W. Rokker, 1882); *Fifth Annual Report of the State Board of Health of Illinois*.

43. *Third Annual Report of the State Board of Health of Illinois*; *Eighth Annual Report of the State Board of Health of Illinois* (Springfield, IL: H.W. Rokker, 1886); Abraham Flexner, "Medical Education in the United States and Canada" (New York, NY: 1910); Shyrock, *Medical Licensing in America, 1650–1965*; Stevens, *American Medicine and the Public Interest*; Thomas Neville Bonner, *Iconoclast: Abraham Flexner and a Life in Learning* (Baltimore, MD: The Johns Hopkins University Press, 2002).

44. Isaac D. Rawlings, *The Rise and Fall of Disease in Illinois* (Springfield, IL: The State Department of Public Health, 1927); Sandvick, "Enforcing Medical Licensing in Illinois: 1877–1890"; Reynolds, "Three Chicago and Illinois Public Health Officers: John H. Rauch, Oscar C. De Wolf, and Frank W. Reilly."

45. John M. Rauch (Secretary), *Annual Reports of the State Board of Health of Illinois, for the Years Ending 1889, 1890, 1891* (Springfield, IL: H.W. Rokker, 1893), LXXXIX.

46. Council on Medical Education of the American Medical Association, "Second Annual Conference of the Council on Medical Education of the American Medical Association—Held in Chicago May 12, 1906," in *Annual Conference of the Council on Medical Education of the American Medical Association: 1905–1907* (Chicago, IL: American Medical Association, 1906), 11.

47. Barbara Gutmann Rosenkrantz, "Cart before Horse: Theory, Practice and Professional Image in American Public Health,1870–1920," *Journal of the History of Medicine and Allied Sciences* 29, no. 1 (1974): 55–73; Keith M. Macdonald, *The Sociology of the Professions* (London, UK: Sage Publications, 1999).

Chapter 15

1. Atkinson, *Bench and Bar of West Virginia*; For Daniel Webster comparison see: "House Happenings," *The Wheeling Daily Intelligencer*, Wheeling, WV, January 14, 1881, 2 and "Editorial Correspondence—Judge James H. Ferguson," *The Weekly Register*, Point Pleasant, WV, February 22, 1882, 2; Kenneth R. Bailey, *Alleged Evil Genius—The Life and Times of Judge James H. Ferguson* (Charleston, WV: Quarrier Press, 2006), 70.

2. Jepson, "Editorial—A Bit of History"; William W. Golden, "The Evolution of Medical Legislation in West Virginia," *ibid.* 12, no. 10 (1918): 361–70; Bailey, *Alleged Evil Genius—The Life and Times of Judge James H. Ferguson*; "Bills and Petitions Introduced," *The Wheeling Daily Intelligencer*, Wheeling, WV, January 20, 1881, 3; Atkinson and Gibbens, *Prominent Men of West Virginia*. 707–708.

3. Medical Society of West Virginia, *Transactions of the Medical Society of the State of West Virginia* (Wheeling, WV: Medical Society of West Virginia, 1881), 667; "Banquet to the Members of the Legislature," *The Wheeling Daily Intelligencer*, Wheeling, WV, February 11, 1881, 4.

4. "State Health Board," *Wheeling Register*, Wheeling, WV, January 27, 1881, 4; Editor, "Senate Bill No. 35," *The Wheeling Daily Intelligencer*, Wheeling, WV, January 31, 1881, 2.

5. James E. Reeves, "Annual Address by the President of the Medical Society of the State of West Virginia," ed. Medical Society of West Virginia (Wheeling, WV: Medical Society of West Virginia, 1882); "The Establishment of a State Board of Health," *The Wheeling Register*, Wheeling, WV, March 10, 1881, 2; "Physicians Parley," *The Wheeling Daily Intelligencer*, Wheeling, WV, February 3, 1881, 4; "Both the Bill...," *Wheeling Register*, Wheeling, WV, February 10, 1881, 2; "From Another Correspondent—Wheeling W. Va. Feb 2d, 1881," *The Weekly Register*, Point Pleasant, WV, February 9, 1881, 2; Doctor (Letter), "The Practice of Medicine in West Virginia—Remarks on the Proposed Legislation in Relation Thereto," *The Wheeling Daily Intelligencer*, Wheeling, WV, February 23, 1881, 3.

6. West Virginia Legislature, Wheeling, WV, *Acts of the Legislature of West Virginia at Its Fifteenth Session*," 1881. 327.

7. American Medical Association, *The Transactions of the American Medical Association*, vol. 33 (Philadelphia, PA: American Medical Association, 1882), 396.

8. "Board of Health to Be Commissioned by the Governor," *Wheeling Register*, Wheeling, WV, June 7, 1881, 4; "State Board of Health," *The Wheeling Daily Intelligencer*, Wheeling, WV June 22, 1881, 4; "Important Meeting," *The Wheeling Daily Intelligencer*, Wheeling, WV, June 25, 1881, 4.

9. *The Transactions of the American Medical Association*, vol. 32 (Philadelphia, PA: American Medical Association, 1881), 394–395, 582; The AMA created the Section on State Medicine from two existing sections on medical jurisprudence, chemistry, and psychology, and state medicine and public hygiene in 1879. *The Transactions of the American Medical Association*, 27.

10. *The Transactions of the American Medical Association*, 293–295.

11. Virginia, *Transactions of the Medical Society of the State of West Virginia*, 681.

12. Hogshead, *Past Presidents of the West Virginia State Medical Association: 1867–1942*; Virginia, *Transactions of the Medical Society of the State of West Virginia*, 681.

13. *Transactions of the Medical Society of the State of West Virginia*, 679.

14. The Wheeling Register reported this, naming Reeves as "Dr. J.E. Reed": "The Ohio Saw-Bones," *Wheeling Register*, Wheeling, WV, June 16, 1881, 1. The published *Transactions of the Ohio State Medical Society*, which are otherwise consistent with the *Register's* report, do not mention Reeves or Reed: Ohio State Medical Society, *Transactions of the Thirty-Sixth Annual Meeting of the Ohio State Medical Society* (Columbus, OH: Ohio State Medical Society, 1882).

15. Paulson, *James Fairchild Baldwin, M.D.—An Extraordinary Surgeon*.

16. *James Fairchild Baldwin, M.D.—An Extraordinary Surgeon*, 69.

17. Emilius O. Randall and Daniel J. Ryan, eds., *History of Ohio—The Rise and Progress of an American State*, 5 vols., vol. 5 (New York, NY: The Century History Company, 1912); James E. Reeves, "West Virginia Department," *The Ohio Medical Journal* 1, no. 1 (1881): 24–29, 28.

18. "Doctors Disagreeing," *Wheeling Register*, Wheeling, WV, August 1, 1881, 4; Advertisement, "M.J. Rhees, M.D.," *The Wheeling Daily Intelligencer*, Wheeling, WV, April 23, 1876, 3; M.J. (Letter) Rhees, "That Medical Commission," *ibid.*, August 1, 1881.

19. "Doctors Disagreeing"; James Edmund Reeves (Secretary), "First, Second, and Third Annual Reports: Years Ending December 31st, 1881, 1882, 1883," (Wheeling: Chas H. Taney, State Printer, 1883), 30; "Dr. Hopkins Again," *The Wheeling Daily Intelligencer*, Wheeling, WV, August 3, 1881, 4; Hopkins was litigious. He got in a strenuous and losing legal fight in 1881 with a stable owner over a horse that he had boarded, but refused to pay for: "A Lively Law Suit," *The Wheeling Daily Intelligencer*, Wheeling, WV, September 10, 1881, 4; it is not clear what happened to S.M. Hopkins after this episode. He disappeared from the Wheeling newspapers and Mohr states that after being drummed out of town by Reeves he moved to DeMossville Kentucky where Seymour (or Seymor) Marion Hopkins had a long and successful medical career: Mohr, *Licensed to Practice—The Supreme Court Defines the American Medical Profession*. This S.M. Hopkins was born in Kentucky in 1857 and died in Ohio in 1926. According to the AMA, he graduated from the Medical College of Ohio: Cincinnati Medical College, in 1885 and practiced in Kentucky his entire life: "Directory of Deceased American Physicians: 1804–1929," Ancestry.com, http://www.ancestry.com/. Census records show 23 year-old Seymour Hopkins living in Pendleton County Kentucky in 1880 and working as a laborer: U.S. Census, "Tenth Census of the United States, 1880," 1880; thus it is unlikely that Wheeling's combative S.M. Hopkins was also the respected Kentucky physician Seymour Marion Hopkins.

20. Reeves (Secretary), "First, Second, and Third Annual Reports: Years Ending December 31st, 1881, 1882, 1883," 1883. 32; Reeves did not report the year-end exam success rate in his annual report, but in an

October 1881 interview he cited 109 applicants and 20 failures. Clearly, most applicants passed the examination: "State Board of Health," *The Wheeling Register*, Wheeling, WV, October 10, 1881, 4.

21. "Tenth Census of the United States, 1880."

22. "Our Board of Health...," *The Weekly Register*, Point Pleasant, WV, September 14, 1881, 3; "We Don't Know...," *The Weekly Register*, Point Pleasant, WV, November 23, 1881, 3; Editor, "Is Not the Alarming Spread..." *Spirit of Jefferson*, Charles Town, WV, December 6, 1881, 2; "A Specimen Case of Quackery," *The Wheeling Daily Intelligencer*, Wheeling, WV, November 10, 1881, 1.

23. American Public Health Association, *Public Health Papers and Reports—Volume VII Presented at the Ninth Annual Meeting of the American Public Health Association—Savannah, Ga. Nov. 28–Dec. 3, 1881* (Boston: American Public Health Association, 1883); Jerrold M. Michael, "The National Board of Health: 1879–1883," *Public Health Reports* 126, no. January/February (2011): 123–29.

24. James E. Reeves, Circular Letter, December 24, 1881, 1881; "Operations of Our State Board of Health," *Wheeling Register*, Wheeling, WV, December 27, 1881, 2.

25. Fourth Street Record: Full Membership Approximately 1870–1920; Mary Paul Taylor, email from 7/28/2015 and written church records from 1882 and 1883 copied on 5/26/2016, 2016.

26. The records from St. Matthews show Reeves baptized as a Methodist and Frances baptized in the Episcopal Church; Wigger, *Taking Heaven by Storm—Methodism and the Rise of Popular Christianity in America*; Ahlstrom, *A Religious History of the American People*; Douglas M. Strong, "American Methodism in the Nineteenth Century: Expansion and Fragmentation," in *The Cambridge Companion to American Methodism*, ed. Jason E. Vickers (Cambridge, UK: Cambridge University Press 2013), 63–96; "Bishop Kain," *The Chattanooga Times*, Chattanooga, TN, April 20, 1891.

27. "Governor's Message," *The Wheeling Daily Intelligencer*, Wheeling, WV, January 12, 1882, 3; "Little Locals/Smallpox," *The Wheeling Daily Intelligencer*, Wheeling, WV, January 19, 1882, 4.

28. "Little Locals/Smallpox"; "Quarantine," *The Wheeling Daily Intelligencer*, Wheeling, WV, January 20, 1882, 4; "Individual Items," *Wheeling Register*, Wheeling, WV, January 25, 1882, 4.

29. West Virginia Legislature, Wheeling, WV, "Acts of the Legislature of West Virginia at Its Adjourned Session, Commencing January 11, 1882," 1882; Reeves (Secretary), "First, Second, and Third Annual Reports: Years Ending December 31st, 1881, 1882, 1883," 1883.

30. Callahan, *Genealogical and Personal History of the Upper Monongahela Valley—West Virginia*. 1309–1312; Rick Dent and Don Norman, "Descendants of Captain John Dent," Hacker's Creek Pioneer Descendants, Inc., https://hackerscreek.com/norman/DENT.htm; Wiley, *History of Preston County (West Virginia)*, 463; Virginia, *Transactions of the Medical Society of West Virginia—Including Proceedings of the Medical Convention Held at Fairmont April 10, 1867*; James Edmund Reeves (Secretary), Wheeling, WV, "The Fourth Annual Report of the Secretary of the State Board of Health of West Virginia for the Year Ending December 31, 1884," 1884; "Insane Asylum,"

The Weekly Register, Point Pleasant, WV, April 13, 1881, 2.

31. Reeves, "Annual Address by the President of the Medical Society of the State of West Virginia," 1882.

32. Paulson, *James Fairchild Baldwin, M.D.—An Extraordinary Surgeon*; James F. Baldwin (Editor), "The Columbus Medical College Imbroglio—Our Vindication," *The Columbus Medical Journal* 1, no. 5 (1882): Suppl 1–8.

33. The Columbus Medical College Imbroglio—Our Vindication"; W. C. Wile (editor), "Higher Medical Education," *New England Medical Monthly* 1, no. August (1882): 531–32. 531; "High Appreciation of a Wheeling Man," *The Wheeling Daily Intelligencer*, Wheeling, WV, August 26, 1882, 4.

34. Reeves, "Annual Address by the President of the Medical Society of the State of West Virginia," 1882; James F. Baldwin (editor), "Columbus Medical College," *The Ohio Medical Journal* 1 (1882): 417–18. 417–418.

35. "West Virginia State Medical Society," *The Columbus Medical Journal* 1 (1882): 30–31. 1; "Columbus Medical College Imbroglio," *The Wheeling Daily Intelligencer*, Wheeling, WV, September 6, 1882, 2; "The August Supplement," *The Columbus Medical Journal* 1 (1882): 139–40.

36. Announcement, "Dr. A.M. Dent Has Located," *The Weston Democrat*, Weston, WV, August 10, 1874, 3; Virginia, *Transactions of the Medical Society of the State of West Virginia*; *Transactions of the Medical Society of West Virginia—Minutes of the First Annual Meeting*.

37. "A 'Whitewash' After All," *The Wheeling Intelligencer*, Wheeling, WV, March 15, 1882, 4; "Temperance Mass Meeting," *The Wheeling Daily Intelligencer*, Wheeling, WV, February 11, 1881, 4.

38. Reeves (Secretary), "First, Second, and Third Annual Reports: Years Ending December 31st, 1881, 1882, 1883," 1883.

39. "Mrs. John G. Stewart," *The Coshocton Age*, Coshocton, OH, January 19, 1884, 1; "Tenderly Laid Away," *The Coshocton Age*, Coshocton, OH, April 13, 1900, 15.

40. Wheeling, WV, "The Fourth Annual Report of the Secretary of the State Board of Health of West Virginia for the Year Ending December 31, 1884"

41. Callahan, *Genealogical and Personal History of the Upper Monongahela Valley—West Virginia*; "Twelfth Census of the United States, 1900"; Wheeling, WV, "The Fourth Annual Report of the Secretary of the State Board of Health of West Virginia for the Year Ending December 31, 1884."

42. Wheeling, WV, "The Fourth Annual Report of the Secretary of the State Board of Health of West Virginia for the Year Ending December 31, 1884."

43. U.S. Supreme Court, Washington, D.C., "Transcript of Record: Supreme Court of the United States—October Term 1887 Vo. 119: Frank M. Dent Plaintiff in Error, Vs. The State of West Virginia," 1888; "Indictments," *Preston County Journal*, Kingwood, WV, December 7, 1882; "The Editor of the Journal...," *Preston County Journal*, Kingwood, WV, December 14, 1882, 2.

44. Wiley, *History of Preston County (West Virginia)*; Curry, *A House Divided—A Study of Statehood Politics and the Copperhead Movement in West Virginia*; "Insane Asylum"; John Phillip Reid, *An Ameri-*

can Judge—Marmaduke Dent of West Virginia (New York, NY: New York University Press, 1968); There is confusion about the relationship between Arthur M. and Marmaduke H. Dent. Arthur does not appear in a current Dent Family Genealogy: Dent and Norman, "Descendants of Captain John Dent." Early census records show that Marshall Dent and his first wife Carrie raised Arthur and Marmaduke, with Arthur born in 1848 and Marmaduke born in 1849: "Seventh Census of the United States, 1850," "Eighth Census of the United States, 1860." However, later census records, along with Arthur's 1892 application to the Sons of the American Revolution, show that Arthur was born in Illinois in December 1848 and Marmaduke was born in West Virginia in April 1849: "Tenth Census of the United States, 1880," "Twelfth Census of the United States, 1900," "U.S., Sons of the American Revolution Membership Applications, 1889–1970," (Provo, UT: Ancestry.com., 2011). Arthur was possibly adopted and certainly born to a different mother, but the two boys grew up as brothers.

45. Reid, *An American Judge—Marmaduke Dent of West Virginia*. 207.

46. "The Wind up—of the Democratic Circus," *The Wheeling Daily Intelligencer*, Wheeling, WV, August 14, 1882, 1.

47. "Hon. Samuel Woods—the New Supreme Judge of West Virginia," *Wheeling Register*, Wheeling, WV, January 2, 1883, 1; "Dr Frank Dent...," *The Wheeling Daily Intelligencer*, Wheeling, WV, May 26, 1883, 4; Alfred Caldwell, Charleston, WV, Attorney General, "Reports of Cases Argued and Determined in the Supreme Court of Appeals of West Virginia," 1885; Washington, D.C., "Transcript of Record: Supreme Court of the United States—October Term 1887 Vo. 119: Frank M. Dent Plaintiff in Error, Vs. The State of West Virginia."

48. Mohr argued that regulars such as Reeves fought to suppress all forms of irregular medicine and that Frank Dent was a pawn in this struggle. Mohr, *Licensed to Practice—The Supreme Court Defines the American Medical Profession*.

49. Evidence against the legitimacy of Dent's diploma in: Rauch (Secretary), *Fifth Annual Report of the State Board of Health of Illinois*, Reeves (Secretary), "First, Second, and Third Annual Reports: Years Ending December 31st, 1881, 1882, 1883," 1883, "A Doctor's Diploma," *The Wheeling Intelligencer*, Wheeling, WV, December 31, 1884, 4, and The American Medical Association, *American Medical Directory*, vol. 1 (Chicago, IL: American Medical Association, 1907), 707–708; data on acceptance of sectarian physicians in WV: Reeves (Secretary), "First, Second, and Third Annual Reports: Years Ending December 31st, 1881, 1882, 1883," 1883. 90.

50. Wheeling, WV, "The Fourth Annual Report of the Secretary of the State Board of Health of West Virginia for the Year Ending December 31, 1884." 22.

51. Charleston, WV, "Reports of Cases Argued and Determined in the Supreme Court of Appeals of West Virginia." 6; M.H. Dent, *Transcript of Argument in Behalf of Appellant at __, State V. Dent, 25 W.Va. 1 (1884)*, ed. Supreme Court of Appeals State of West Virginia, vol. 1—Fall Special Term 1884, Supreme Court Records & Briefs (Charleston, WV: Supreme Court of Appeals State of West Virginia, 1884).

52. Clerk of the Court, Charleston, WV, West Virginia Supreme Court of Appeals, "Court Records,"

1884; Charleston, WV, "Reports of Cases Argued and Determined in the Supreme Court of Appeals of West Virginia."

53. Charleston, WV, "Court Records"; Washington, D.C., "Transcript of Record: Supreme Court of the United States—October Term 1887 Vo. 119: Frank M. Dent Plaintiff in Error, Vs. The State of West Virginia"; Stephen K. Williams, ed. *United States Supreme Court Reports: Cases Argued and Decided in the Supreme Court of the United States in the October Terms 1887, 1889*, vol. 32, United States Supreme Court Reports (Rochester, NY: The Lawyers' Cooperative Publishing Company, 1889); *Dent V. West Virginia* (1889); the growing case backlog, which was several years in the 1880s, led to the creation of the United States circuit courts of appeals in 1891.

54. Wheeling, WV, "The Fourth Annual Report of the Secretary of the State Board of Health of West Virginia for the Year Ending December 31, 1884." 39.

55. "A Doctor's Diploma."

56. Sue Hersman, Letters, 10/9/2013, 2013; Dent's gravestone named him as "Dr. F.M. Dent." Tipton, "Find a Grave Search Form."

57. "Another Quack," *The Wheeling Daily Intelligencer*, Wheeling, WV, September 13, 1883, 1; Wheeling, WV, "The Fourth Annual Report of the Secretary of the State Board of Health of West Virginia for the Year Ending December 31, 1884."

58. Rauch (Secretary), *Fourth Annual Report of the State Board of Health of Illinois*. ix. Reynolds, "Three Chicago and Illinois Public Health Officers: John H. Rauch, Oscar C. De Wolf, and Frank W. Reilly."

59. Advertisement, "Dr. J.E. Smith," *The Wheeling Daily Intelligencer*, Wheeling, WV, February 6, 1883, 3.

60. "The State Board of Health," *Wheeling Register*, Wheeling, WV, July 15, 1882, 2; Reeves (Secretary), "First, Second, and Third Annual Reports: Years Ending December 31st, 1881, 1882, 1883," 1883; "Death Overrules Indictment against Dr. B.H. Stillyard," *The Wheeling Intelligencer*, Wheeling, WV, July 17, 1916, 10.

61. Perry H. Millard, "The Propriety and Necessity of State Regulation of Medical Practice," *JAMA* 9, no. 16 (1887): 491–93. 491.

62. "The Propriety and Necessity of State Regulation of Medical Practice," 493.

63. "The Small-Pox Scare," *The Wheeling Daily Intelligencer*, Wheeling, WV, May 23, 1883, 4; "Important and Interesting Meetings for to-Day," *Wheeling Register*, Wheeling, WV, January 12, 1883, 3

64. "Brief Locals—Dr. Reeves Yesterday...," *The Wheeling Daily Intelligencer*, Wheeling, WV, August 12, 1882, 4; Reeves (Secretary), "First, Second, and Third Annual Reports: Years Ending December 31st, 1881, 1882, 1883," 1883. 119–120, 171; Wheeling, WV, "The Fourth Annual Report of the Secretary of the State Board of Health of West Virginia for the Year Ending December 31, 1884"; "The Hog Cholera," *The Wheeling Daily Intelligencer*, Wheeling, WV, December 12, 1884, 4.

65. "First, Second, and Third Annual Reports: Years Ending December 31st, 1881, 1882, 1883," 1883. 26.

66. Reeves; "Operations of Our State Board of Health"; Association, *Public Health Papers and Reports—Volume VIII Presented at the Tenth Annual Meeting of the American Public Health Association—Indianapolis, Ind. Oct 17–20, 1882*. 234; A.N. Bell

(editor), "Editorial—The National and State Boards of Health," *The Sanitarian* 11, no. 1 (1883): 12–15.

Chapter 16

1. "The Water of Wheeling," *Wheeling Register*, Wheeling, WV, September 1, 1882, 4.
2. Robert Philip, "An Address on Koch's Discovery of the Tubercle Bacillus—Some of Its Implications and Results," *BMJ* 3, no. 3730 (1932): 1–5; Alex Sakula, "Robert Koch: Centenary of the Discovery of the Tubercle Bacillus, 1882," *Thorax* 37, no. 4 (1982): 246–51; Bunyan's quote is from his 1680 companion to *Pilgrim's Progress, The Life and Death of Mr. Badman*, Chapter XVIII. William Osler famously quoted this phrase in 1901 at the opening of the British Congress on Tuberculosis in London: Malcolm Morris, "Transactions" (paper presented at the British Congress on Tuberculosis for the Prevention of Consumption, London, UK, 1902), 12.
3. "Tuberculosis: Robert Koch and Tuberculosis: Koch's Famous Lecture," Nobel Media AB, https://www.nobelprize.org/educational/medicine/tuberculosis/readmore.html; Koch did not devise his stepwise approach, one that eventually claimed the term "Koch's postulates," rather he followed the philosophy of parasitic causation developed by his teacher, Jakob Henle. Koch suspected that not every organism associated with human disease would meet all of Henle's criteria. But the tuberculosis bacillus did: Alfred S. Evans, "Causation and Disease: The Henle-Koch Postulates Revisited," *Yale J Biol Med* 49, no. 2 (1976): 175–95.
4. Sakula, "Robert Koch: Centenary of the Discovery of the Tubercle Bacillus, 1882."
5. Philip, "An Address on Koch's Discovery of the Tubercle Bacillus—Some of Its Implications and Results," 2; "Supplying a Last Link," *New York Times*, New York, NY, May 3, 1882, 2; "An Important Discovery," *The Wheeling Daily Intelligencer*, Wheeling, WV, May 6, 1882, 3.
6. Austin Flint, *A Treatise on the Principles and Practice of Medicine*, fifth ed. (Philadelphia, PA: Henry C. Lea's Son & Co., 1881), 95.
7. *A Treatise on the Principles and Practice of Medicine—With an Appendix on the Researches of Koch and Their Bearing on the Etiology, Pathology, Diagnosis, Prognosis, and Treatment of Pulmonary Phthisis*, fifth ed. (Philadelphia, PA: Henry C. Lea's Son & Co., 1884); Bartlett, *Essay on the Philosophy of Medical Science*. 292–293.
8. Frederick P. Gorham, "The History of Bacteriology and Its Contribution to Public Health Work," in *A Half Century of Public Health*, ed. Mazÿck Ravenel (New York, NY: American Public Health Association, 1921), 66–93; Rosen, *A History of Public Health—Expanded Edition*; Harold M. Malkin, "The Trials and Tribulations of George Miller Sternberg: (1838–1915)—America's First Bacteriologist," *Perspectives in Biology and Medicine* 36, no. 4 (1993): 666–78.
9. For overviews of the adoption of the germ theory by American physicians see: Richmond, "American Attitudes toward the Germ Theory of Disease (1860–1880)"; Haller, *American Medicine in Transition, 1840–1910*; Rothstein, *American Physicians in the 19th Century—From Sects to Science*; Burnham,

Health Care in America: A History; Warner, *The Therapeutic Perspective: Medical Practice, Knowledge, and Identity in America, 1820–1885*.
10. Reeves, "Annual Address by the President of the Medical Society of the State of West Virginia," 1882, 6.
11. Association, *The Transactions of the American Medical Association*, 307.
12. Association, *Public Health Papers and Reports—Volume VIII Presented at the Tenth Annual Meeting of the American Public Health Association—Indianapolis, Ind. Oct 17–20, 1882*. Quotation p. 233; For evidence of the APHA's two-tier organizational structure, see the list of Active (almost entirely M.D.) and Associate (non–M.D.) members elected the following year *Public Health Papers and Reports*, ed. Irving A. Watson, vol. 10, Public Health Papers and Reports (Concord, NH: Republican Press Association, 1885), 533–536.
13. "Guarding the Public Welfare," *The Detroit Free Press*, Detroit, MI, November 15, 1883, 3; "Health Association," *The Wheeling Daily Intelligencer*, Wheeling, WV, November 15, 1883, 1, 3; James Edmund Reeves, "The Eminent Domain of Sanitary Science, and the Usefulness of State Boards of Health in Guarding the Public Welfare," *Public Health Papers and Reports* (1883): 171–84; "The Eminent Domain of Sanitary Science, and the Usefulness of State Boards of Health in Guarding the Public Welfare," *JAMA* 1, no. 21 (1883): 612–18; "The Eminent Domain of Sanitary Science, and the Usefulness of State Boards of Health in Guarding the Public Welfare," *The New York Medical Journal* 38 (1883): 538–44; Article Ii. The Eminent Domain of Sanitary Science, and the Usefulness of State Boards of Health in Guarding the Public Welfare," *Gaillard's Medical Journal* 36, no. 6 (1883): 604–14; "The Eminent Domain of Sanitary Science, and the Usefulness of State Boards of Health in Guarding the Public Welfare," *The Columbus Medical Journal* 2, no. 6 (1883): 250–64; "The Eminent Domain of Sanitary Science, and the Usefulness of State Boards of Health in Guarding the Public Welfare," *New England Medical Monthly* 3, no. March (1884): 256–67.
14. "The Eminent Domain of Sanitary Science, and the Usefulness of State Boards of Health in Guarding the Public Welfare," 171, 173, 181, 183–184; for changes in lifespan during the period, see: Hacker, "Decennial Life Tables for the White Population of the United States, 1790–1900"; Rosen, *A History of Public Health—Expanded Edition*.
15. Reeves, "The Eminent Domain of Sanitary Science, and the Usefulness of State Boards of Health in Guarding the Public Welfare," 181, 183–184; J. M. Harris, Jr., "James Edmund Reeves. 1883," *Am J Public Health* 104, no. 3 (2014): 417.
16. "State Medical Meeting," *The Wheeling Daily Intelligencer*, Wheeling, WV, May 25, 1882, 4.
17. "Personal Mention," *The Wheeling Daily Intelligencer*, Wheeling, WV, June 4, 1883, 4; Medical Society of West Virginia, *Transactions of the Medical Society of the State of West Virginia* (Wheeling, WV: Medical Society of West Virginia, 1883).
18. Association, *Public Health Papers and Reports*. 69–78, 79–85, 86–95; James E. Reeves, "Pollution of the Upper Ohio, and the Water-Supply of the Cities and Chief Towns Within the First Hundred Miles of Its Course," *JAMA* 3, no. 19 (1884): 512–17.

19. Association, *Public Health Papers and Reports.* 440; "West Virginia Honored by the Presidency of the American Public Health Association," *Wheeling Register,* Wheeling, WV, October 19, 1884, 4.

20. Reeves was elected to the AMA's Nominating Committee in 1881: Association, *The Transactions of the American Medical Association* and the Judicial Council in 1882: *The Transactions of the American Medical Association.* In 1884, AMA President Austin Flint named Reeves a member of the committee that selected trustees for the organization's newly-launched *Journal of the American Medical Association:* N.S. Davis (editor), "American Medical Association—Thirty-Fifth Annual Meeting," *JAMA* 2, no. 21 (1884): 561–80; "State Boards of Medical Examiners," *JAMA* 3, no. 18 (1884): 493–94; 499–501; James E. Reeves, *ibid.,* no. 21: 587–88.

21. N.S. Davis (editor), *ibid.,* 581–82.

22. "Personal Mention," *The Wheeling Daily Intelligencer,* Wheeling, WV, April 17, 1884, 4; "Capital Gossip," *The Wheeling Daily Intelligencer,* May 6, 1884, 1; Medical Society of West Virginia, *Transactions of the Medical Society of the State of West Virginia* (Wheeling, WV: Medical Society of West Virginia, 1884); Wheeling, WV, "The Fourth Annual Report of the Secretary of the State Board of Health of West Virginia for the Year Ending December 31, 1884"; Association, *Public Health Papers and Reports.*

23. "About People," *The Wheeling Daily Intelligencer,* Wheeling, WV, August 6, 1885, 4; James F. Baldwin (editor), "Resignation of Dr. James E. Reeves," *The Columbus Medical Journal* 3, no. 10 (1885): 474–75; "Dr. Reeves—Resigns the Secretaryship of the State Board of Health," *Wheeling Register,* Wheeling, WV, February 24, 1885, 4; for contemporary information on his illness (acute rheumatism): Flint, *A Treatise on the Principles and Practice of Medicine—With an Appendix on the Researches of Koch and Their Bearing on the Etiology, Pathology, Diagnosis, Prognosis, and Treatment of Pulmonary Phthisis;* for current information on hepatitis B: Mark Feldman, Lawrence S. Friedman, and Lawrence J. Brandt, eds., *Sleisenger and Fordtran's Gastrointestinal and Liver Disease,* tenth ed. (Philadelphia, PA: Saunders, 2016); also: L. S. Y. Tang, E. Covert, E. Wilson et al., "Chronic Hepatitis B Infection: A Review," *JAMA* 319, no. 17 (2018): 1802–13. Other diagnoses could be considered, particularly rheumatic fever: Stanford T. Shulman and Alan L. Bisno, "Nonsuppurative Post-streptococcal Sequelae: Rheumatic Fever and Glomerulonephritis," in *Mandell, Douglas, and Bennett's Principles and Practice of Infectious Diseases, Updated Edition,* ed. John E. Bennett, Raphael Dolin, and Martin J. Blaser (Philadelphia, PA: Saunders, 2015), but his wife's illness with similar symptoms several months later, his risk factors, and his subsequent liver cancer suggest a unifying diagnosis of hepatitis B.

24. "Dr. Reeves Resigns—His Place on Board of Health," *The Wheeling Daily Intelligencer,* Wheeling, WV, February 24, 1885, 4; "Dr. Reeves—Resigns the Secretaryship of the State Board of Health."

25. Baldwin (editor), "Resignation of Dr. James E. Reeves"; Editor, "Resignation of the Secretary of the State Board of Health of West Virginia," *Maryland Medical Journal* 12, no. February 28, 1885 (1885): 345; "Editor's Table," *The Sanitarian* 14, no. 184 (1885): 262–63.

26. Woods, "Our Gallery—James Edmund Reeves, M.D. of Wheeling W. Va." Quotation p. 483. The biography was penned over the pseudonym, "UET," and acknowledged by woods in an 1885 letter to Reeves.

27. Frances' illness: "About People"; Association, *Public Health Papers and Reports.*

28. "The Public Health—The Coming Meeting of an Important National Organization," *The Wheeling Daily Intelligencer,* Wheeling, WV, November 24, 1885, 4; "The Public Health," *The Wheeling Daily Intelligencer,* Wheeling, WV, November 3, 1885, 4.

29. "The Satitary [sic] Congress; Meeting of the American Public Health Association," *The Evening Star,* Washington, D.C. December 8, 1885, 8; *Public Health Papers and Reports,* ed. Irving A. Watson, vol. 11, Public Health Papers and Reports (Concord, NH: Republican Press Association, 1886).

30. Address of Dr. James E. Reeves, of Wheeling," *The Wheeling Daily Intelligencer,* Wheeling, WV, December 9, 1885, 2; Davis also reprinted the talk for the AMA: James E. Reeves, "Original Lectures—Annual Address Before the American Public Health Association," *JAMA* 5, no. 24 (1885): 645–49.

31. Irving A. Watson, ed. *Public Health—the Lomb Prize Essays* (Concord, NH: Republican Press Association, 1886); Association, *Public Health Papers and Reports;* Watson, *Public Health—The Lomb Prize Essays.*

32. Association, *Public Health Papers and Reports.* 384–390.

33. *Public Health Papers and Reports.* 330, 342–343.

34. *Public Health Papers and Reports.* 383; "Local Brevities," *The Wheeling Daily Intelligencer,* Wheeling, WV, December 14, 1885, 4.

35. *Public Health Papers and Reports,* ed. Irving A. Watson, vol. 14, Public Health Papers and Reports (Concord, NH: Republican Press Association, 1889), 264–265; *Public Health Papers and Reports,* ed. Irving A. Watson, vol. 12, Public Health Papers and Reports (Concord, NH: Republican Press Association, 1887); John Duffy, "The American Medical Profession and Public Health: From Support to Ambivalence," *Bulletin of the History of Medicine* 53, no. 1 (1979): 1–22; Committee for the Study of the Future of Public Health, *The Future of Public Health* (Washington, D.C.: National Academy Press, 1988); American Public Health Association, *Public Health Papers and Reports,* ed. Irving A. Watson, vol. 15, Public Health Papers and Reports (Concord, NH: Republican Press Association, 1890).

36. AMA Vice President Millard used the citadel metaphor in 1887, seconds before Reeves admonished him to exercise judgment in enforcing educational standards. He called for state legislatures to create: " such regulations of the practice of our profession as will place the standard thereof upon a citadel of greater strength and power." Millard, "The Propriety and Necessity of State Regulation of Medical Practice," 493.

37. Association, *Public Health Papers and Reports.* 17.

38. Nathan Allen, "The Relations Between Sanitary Science and the Medical Profession," *ibid.* 12 (1886): 85–98; D.N. Patterson, "Life and Character of Nathan Allen, M.D., Ll.D.," *Contributions of the Old Residents' Historical Association, Lowell, Mass.* 4, no. 2 (1889): 151–63.

39. Rice, *West Virginia: A History*; See Reeves' remarks at the 1885 APHA meeting, Association, *Public Health Papers and Reports* 343; The Governor and the State Board of Health," *The Wheeling Daily Intelligencer*, Wheeling, WV, July 18, 1887, 2; Medical Society of West Virginia, *Transactions of the Medical Society of the State of West Virginia* (Wheeling, WV: Medical Society of West Virginia, 1887). See p. 359.

40. "Governor Wilson—He Takes Notice of the Action of the State Board of Health," *Wheeling Register*, Wheeling, WV, August 18, 1887, 4; Golden, "The Evolution of Medical Legislation in West Virginia."

41. Duffy, *The Sanitarians—A History of American Public Health*; Jonathan Liebenau, *Medical Science and Medical Industry: The Formation of the American Pharmaceutical Industry* (Baltimore, MD: The Johns Hopkins University Press, 1987); Burnham, *Health Care in America: A History*; Golden, "The Evolution of Medical Legislation in West Virginia"; Hamowy, "The Early Development of Medical Licensing Laws in the United States, 1875–1900"; Clinton Matthew Sandvick, "Enforcing Medical Regulation in the United States 1875 to 1915" (University of Oregon, 2008).

Chapter 17

1. "About People," *The Wheeling Daily Intelligencer*, Wheeling, WV, May 11, 1886, 4; Association, *Public Health Papers and Reports*; *Public Health Papers and Reports*, ed. Irving A. Watson, vol. 13, Public Health Papers and Reports (Concord, NH: Republican Press Association, 1888); "Dr. Reeves Home," *The Wheeling Daily Intelligencer*, Wheeling, WV, November 14, 1887, 4.

2. Virginia, *Transactions of the Medical Society of the State of West Virginia*. Quotations p. 6.

3. James E. Reeves, *How to Work with the Bausch & Lomb Optical Company's Microtome and a Method of Demonstrating the Tubercle-Bacillus* (Rochester, NY: Bausch & Lomb Optical Company, 1886); Editor, "Book Reviews—How to Work with the Bausch and Lomb Co.'S Microtome," *The Microscope* 7, no. 3 (1887): 93–94; Simon Henry Gage, "Microscopy in America (1830–1945)," *Transactions of the American Microscopical Society* 83, no. 4 (Supplement) (1964): 1–125; Wilson, "James Edmund Reeves, M.D."

4. "Dr. Reeves at Chautauqua," *The Wheeling Daily Intelligencer*, Wheeling, WV, August 16, 1886, 4; "Creditable Work: Dr. Jas. E. Reeves' Contributions to Microscopy," *Wheeling Register*, Wheeling, WV, August 16, 1886, 4; American Society of Microscopists, *Proceedings of the American Society of Microscopists—Ninth Annual Meeting* (Buffalo, NY: Printing and Publishing House of Bigelow Brothers, 1886); *Proceedings of the American Society of Microscopists—Tenth Annual Meeting* (Peoria, IL: J.W. Franks and Sons, Printers and Binders, 1888).

5. Association of American Physicians, *Transactions of the Association of American Physicians*, vol. 1 (Philadelphia, PA: Wm. J. Dornan, Printer, 1886), 1; Esmond R. Long, *A History of American Pathology* (Springfield, IL: Charles C Thomas, 1962); for a record of the Association's antagonism to the AMA: King, *Transformations in American Medicine*.

6. Association of American Physicians, *Transactions of the Association of American Physicians*, vol. 2 (Philadelphia, PA: Wm. J. Dornan, Printer, 1887); Reeves attended in 1887, 1888, 1890, 1891, 1894. See Association *Transactions*.

7. James F. Baldwin (editor), "Editorial: Microscopical Work," *The Columbus Medical Journal* 6 (1887): 42–43; James E. Reeves, "Lupus and the Bacillus Tuberculosis," *The Medical News* 50, no. 26 (1887): 701–3; "Those Blood Spots," *The Wheeling Daily Intelligencer*, Wheeling, WV, July 30, 1887, 1.

8. "Local Brevities," *The Wheeling Daily Intelligencer*, Wheeling, WV, March 26, 1886, 4; "Dr. Reeves Not Ill," *Wheeling Register*, Wheeling, WV, October 12, 1887, 4; "About People," *The Wheeling Daily Intelligencer*, Wheeling, WV, October 12, 1887, 4; "Dr. Ford's Death," *The Wheeling Daily Intelligencer*, Wheeling, WV, September 22, 1887, 4; "Local Brevities," *The Wheeling Daily Intelligencer*, Wheeling, WV, November 9, 1887, 4; For an account of the social environment facing practitioners of the time: Steven J. Peitzman, "'I Am Their Physician': Dr. Owen J. Wister of Germantown and His Too Many Patients," *Bulletin of the History of Medicine* 83, no. 2 (2009): 245–70.

9. "Going South," *Wheeling Register*, Wheeling, WV, January 3, 1888, 4.

10. "Points on People," *Wheeling Register*, Wheeling, WV, November 17, 1887, 4; "In a Small Way—Reeves Disposes of His Residence," *Wheeling Register*, November 17, 1887, 4; Editor, "Medical News and Miscellany," *New Orleans Medical and Surgical Journal* 15, no. December (1887): 494; "Notes," *North Carolina Medical Journal* 20, no. 6 (1887): 371.

11. "Deed Book #80," Ohio County Recorder's Office, 1888; "Deed Book #83," Ohio County Recorder's Office, 1889; "Deed Book #61," Hamilton County Recorder's Office, 1889; Ann Jenks, Listing of real estate conveyances, 1888–1895 with either James E. or Frances M. Reeves as grantee, July 13, 2016, 2016.

12. U.S. Census, "Eleventh Census of the United States, 1890," 1890; the Chattanooga Chamber of Commerce painted a far rosier picture than the Census, claiming 50,000 people in 1889: John C Griffiss, W.R. Hall, and C.C. Murray, "Report of the Chamber of Commerce," (Chattanooga, TN: Chattanooga Chamber of Commerce, 1890); Day Otis Kellogg (editor), *New American Supplement to the Latest Edition of the Encyclopaedia Britannica* (New York: The Werner Company, 1898), 760–761; David Eichenthal and Tracy Windeknecht, "Chattanooga Tennessee," in *Restoring Prosperity* (Washington, D.C.: The Brookings Institution, 2008); James E. Reeves, "Health and Wealth of the City of Chattanooga," *Chattanooga Daily Times*, Chattanooga, TN, December 8, 1892, 46, *The Health and Wealth of the City of Wheeling—Including Its Physical and Medical Topography; Also General Remarks on the Natural Resources of West Virginia.*

13. "Wheeling Men in the South," *The Wheeling Daily Intelligencer*, Wheeling, WV, February 21, 1888, 1; "A Hint to the Immigration Society," *Wheeling Register*, Wheeling, WV, March 17, 1888, 4; "Dr. Reeves on the Colored Population of the South," *Wheeling Register*, Wheeling, WV, April 26, 1888, 2; for information on the *Southern Hub*: Charles D. McGuffey (editor), *Standard History of Chattanooga Tennessee* (Knoxville: Crew and Dorey, 1911), 252; Lester C. Lamon, *Blacks in Tennessee: 1791–1970* (Knoxville, TN: University of Tennessee Press, 1981); Chat-

tanooga's population was 43 percent "colored" while Wheeling's was 3 percent. "Eleventh Census of the United States, 1890."

14. Editor, "The Pathological and Histological Slides," *North Carolina Medical Journal* 21, no. 2 (1888): 115; none of Grant Medical College's faculty were paid: James W. Livingood, "Chattanooga's Medical Schools," in *Centennial History—Chattanooga and Hamilton County Medical Society: The Profession and Its Community* (Chattanooga, TN: Chattanooga and Hamilton County Medical Society, Inc., 1983), 45–51; Letters to his sister and niece were on professional stationary showing his prices. Jarvis, "Anna Jarvis Papers (1864–1948)," various years.

15. Margaret C. Fairlie, "The Yellow Fever Epidemic of 1888 in Jacksonville," *The Florida Historical Quarterly* 19, no. 2 (1940): 95–108.

16. Khaled Bloom, *The Mississippi Valley's Great Yellow Fever Epidemic of 1878* (Baton Rouge, LA: Louisiana State University Press, 1993); J. Berrien Lindsley (Secretary), "Yellow Fever Outlook," *State Board of Health Bulletin* 4, no. 1 (1888): 2–3 2.

17. "An Agent Down South," *The Daily American*, Nashville, TN, September 1, 1888, 3.

18. Examples of Reeves' reports: "Dr. Reeves Satisfied," *The Daily American*, Nashville September 5, 1888, 5 "Yellow Fever Scare," *The Daily American*, Nashville, TN, September 6, 1888, 5; Daily Reports of Inspectors," *State Board of Health Bulletin* 4, no. 2 (1888): 18–31; Fairlie, "The Yellow Fever Epidemic of 1888 in Jacksonville."

19. Association of American Physicians, *Transactions of the Association of American Physicians*, vol. 3 (Philadelphia, PA: Wm. J. Dornan, Printer, 1888).

20. Malkin, "The Trials and Tribulations of George Miller Sternberg: (1838–1915)—America's First Bacteriologist"; Physicians, *Transactions of the Association of American Physicians* 329; "Yellow Fever Germs," *The Wheeling Daily Intelligencer*, Wheeling, WV, December 24, 1888, 2.

21. American Society of Microscopists, *Proceedings of the American Society of Microscopists—Eleventh Annual Meeting* (Peoria, IL: J.W. Franks and Sons, Printers and Binders, 1888); Greg Cima, "Legends: Teacher, Researcher, and Inventor—Heinrich J. Detmers, 1833–1906," *JAVMA News*, no. June 1 (2013), https://www.avma.org/News/JAVMANews/Pages/130601g.aspx.

22. The *Tribune* misspelled Detmer's name as "Delmero" "He Has Found a Yellow Fever Germ," *Chicago Tribune*, Chicago, IL December 21, 1888, 1; also: "The Yellow Fever Germ," *The Memphis Appeal*, Memphis, TN, December 21, 1888, 1; "Fever Germs Photographed," *The New York Times*, New York, NY, December 23, 1888; "Some Science," *Daily Nebraska State Journal*, Lincoln, NE, January 4, 1889, 8; "Frank Seaver Billings," in *Biographical History of Massachusetts*, ed. Samuel Atkins Eliot (Boston, MA: Massachusetts Biographical Society, 1914).

23. Sternberg was one of the winners of the APHA's 1885 Lomb Prize: Watson, *Public Health—the Lomb Prize Essays*; he was also APHA president two years after Reeves: Association, *Public Health Papers and Reports*; Reeves took title to a property owned by R.M. Barton to secure notes from Barton to Sternberg: Jenks Deed Book 63–173.

24. Editor, "Medical Progress—Yellow Fever Germ," *JAMA* 12, no. 4 (1889): 124–25.

25. The viral cause of yellow fever was not discovered until 1927: Charles S. Bryan, "Discovery of the Yellow Fever Virus," *International Journal of Infectious Diseases* 2, no. 1 (1997): 52–54; in 1900, as Army Surgeon General, Sternberg organized Major Walter Reed's commission to Cuba, which definitively demonstrated the mosquito transmission of yellow fever: Malkin, "The Trials and Tribulations of George Miller Sternberg: (1838–1915)—America's First Bacteriologist"; also: Alan N. Clements and Ralph E. Harbach, "History of the Discovery of the Mode of Transmission of Yellow Fever Virus," *Journal of Vector Ecology* 42, no. 2 (2017): 208–22; W.W. Dawson, "Address—the President's Address," *JAMA* 13, no. 1 (1889): 1–10 5.

26. Washington, D.C., "Transcript of Record: Supreme Court of the United States—October Term 1887 Vo. 119: Frank M. Dent Plaintiff in Error, Vs. The State of West Virginia"; Williams, *United States Supreme Court Reports: Cases Argued and Decided in the Supreme Court of the United States in the October Terms 1887, 1889.*

27. Washington, D.C., "Transcript of Record: Supreme Court of the United States—October Term 1887 Vo. 119: Frank M. Dent Plaintiff in Error, Vs. The State of West Virginia."

28. David P. Currie, "The Constitution in the Supreme Court: The Protection of Economic Interests, 1889–1910," *The University of Chicago Law Review* 52, no. 2 (1985): 324–88; Mohr, *Licensed to Practice—The Supreme Court Defines the American Medical Profession* 147–149 FN 7–13; *Slaughterhouse Cases*, 83 U.S. (16 Wall) 36 (1872).

29. *Dent V. West Virginia*, 129 U.S. 114 (1889).

30. "The West Virginia Law," *The Wheeling Daily Intelligencer*, Wheeling, WV, January 15, 1889, 1; examples of minimal coverage: "Supreme Court Opinions," *New York Times*, New York, NY, January 15, 1889, 2; "National Supreme Court," *The Philadelphia Inquirer*, Philadelphia, PA, January 15, 1889, 7; Editor, "States May Regulate Medical Practice," *The Medical News* 54, no. January 26 (1889): 104–6.

31. Irenaeus D. Foulon, "Who Are Physicians before the Law?," *The Clinical Reporter* 2, no. 2 (1889): 29–34; for information on Foulon and his journal, see Thomas Lindsley Bradford, *Homoeopathic Bibliography of the United States—From the Year 1825 to the Year 1891, Inclusive* (Philadelphia, PA: Boericke & Tafel, 1892); John M. Rauch (Secretary), *Eleventh Annual Report of the State Board of Health of Illinois* (Springfield, IL: H.W. Rokker, 1892).

32. Albert Horton, Chief Justice of the Kansas Supreme Court, made the public's point to the APHA shortly after *Dent*: American Public Health Association, *Public Health Papers and Reports*, ed. Irving A. Watson, vol. 17, Public Health Papers and Reports (Concord, NH: Republican Press Association, 1892) 24–33; for the medical profession's perspective: Perry H. Millard, "The Legal Restriction of Medical Practice in the United States," *JAMA* 13, no. 14 (1889): 470–75 471, 472; for the persisting issues: Ruth Horowitz, *In the Public Interest—Medical Licensing and the Disciplinary Process* (New Brunswick, NJ: Rutgers University Press, 2013).

33. Reeves, "On All Sides a Learned Doctor" 595; examples of local contributions: Fred B. Stapp, "Chattanooga Medical Society," *Virginia Medical Monthly* 17, no. 8 (1890): 649; "Chattanooga Medical Society," *Virginia Medical Monthly* 19, no. 1 (1892): 146–47;

Uncle Jimmy: "Doctor's Memory Honored by Group," *Chattanooga Times*, Chattanooga, TN, June 14, 1936, 3.

34. Landon B. Edwards (editor), "Tri-State Medical Association of Alabama, Georgia, and Tennessee," *Virginia Medical Monthly* 16, no. 8 (1889): 666–78; Fred B. Stapp, "Chattanooga Medical Society," *ibid.* 17 (1890): 649; Osler reference: James E. Reeves, "Some Points on the Natural History of Enteric or Typhoid Fever," in *Transactions of the Association of American Physicians*, ed. Henry Hun (Philadelphia, PA: Association of American Physicians, 1890), 1–20 20.

35. "Bishop Kain"; "Return from Mexico," *Wheeling Register*, Wheeling, WV, December 20, 1892, 8; a letter from Reeves stated that he planned to meet Anna's train on September 16, 1891: Personal letter, courtesy of International Mother's Day Shrine, Grafton, WV, August 27, 1891; Anna also stated that she moved to Philadelphia from Chattanooga: Jarvis, "Anna Jarvis Papers (1864–1948)," various years; also: Katharine Lane Antolini, "Memorializing Motherhood: Anna Jarvis and the Struggle for Control of Mother's Day" (University of West Virginia, 2009).

36. "Health and Wealth of the City of Chattanooga."

Chapter 18

1. Volume 7, Manufactures, Table 1 "Twelfth Census of the United States, 1900"; There are no 1880 data for the value of druggists' preparations, but this category also increased dramatically, from $6.7 million in 1890 to $23.2 million in 1900. See: Volume 7, Manufactures, Table 1 "Twelfth Census of the United States, 1900."

2. Enrique Ravina, *The Evolution of Drug Discovery* (Weinheim, FRG: Wiley-VCH, 2011); Warner, *The Therapeutic Perspective: Medical Practice, Knowledge, and Identity in America, 1820–1885*; Harry M. Marks, *The Progress of Experiment: Science and Therapeutic Reform in the United States, 1900–1990* (Cambridge: Cambridge University Press, 1997); Alan Wayne Jones, "Early Drug Discovery and the Rise of Pharmaceutical Chemistry," *Drug Testing and Analysis* 3 (2011): 337–44; Ravina, *The Evolution of Drug Discovery*; M. J. R. Desborough and D. M. Keeling, "The Aspirin Story—from Willow to Wonder Drug," *Br J Haematol* 177, no. 5 (2017): 674–83; one way to estimate major changes in pharmaceutical therapies is to compare versions of the U.S. Pharmacopoeia, noting when drugs later found to be important entered. Between 1880 and 1900 the *U.S. Pharmacopoeia* added 205 new preparations and removed 241. Many all of these were adjustments to existing items. For instance, codeine sulphate was added to codeine and *petrolatum* and *aloe* replaced similar terms. Over the period, the major additions were acetanilide, cocaine, and physostigmine in 1890 and phenazone (antipyrine), acetphenetidinum (phenacetin), colchicine, adrenal and thyroid extracts, and diphtheria antitoxin in 1900: The United States Pharmacopœial Convention Inc., *The Pharmacopeia of the United States of America*, Seventh ed. (Philadelphia, PA: J.B. Lippincott Company, 1893), *The Pharmacopeia of the United States of America*, Seventh ed. (Philadelphia, PA: P. Blakiston's Son and Company, 1905).

3. Benjamin Ward Richardson, *The Asclepiad*, 11

vols., vol. 2 (London, UK: Longmans, Green, and Company, 1885), 352. This work was also published in Boston and Philadelphia.

4. Victor Mataja, "The Economic Value of Advertising," *The International Quarterly* 8, no. December–March (1904): 379–98; Sidney Sherman, "Advertising in the United States," *Publications of the American Statistical Association* 7, no. 52 (1900): 1–44; Liebenau, *Medical Science and Medical Industry: The Formation of the American Pharmaceutical Industry*; Albert N. Blodgett, "The Influence of Proprietary Pharmacy Upon the Practice of Medicine " *The Boston Medical and Surgical Journal* 120, no. 1 (1889): 11–15; Solomon Solis-Cohen, "Shall Physicians Become Sales-Agents for Patent Medicines?," *Proceedings of the Philadelphia County Medical Society* 13 (1892): 213–16; Samuel Hopkins Adams, *The Great American Fraud—Reprinted from Collier's Weekly* (New York, NY: P.F. Collier & Son, 1905); Frank Billings, "The Medical Profession and the Medical Journals in Relation to Nostrums," *The Boston Medical and Surgical Journal* 154, no. 9 (1906): 231–35.

5. Association, *The Transactions of the American Medical Association*. 134; N.S. Davis, "Association Journal—Report of the Board of Trustees on the Establishment of the Journal of the American Medical Association," *JAMA* 1, no. 1 (1883): 4–7.

6. The *Journal's* advertising income in 1898 was less than $10,000. In 1946 it was $1,750,000: Morris Fishbein, "History of the American Medical Association: 1902–1904," *ibid.* 133, no. 9 (1947): 605–13; N.S. Davis (editor), "Journal of the American Medical Association—Financial Progress," *ibid.* 4, no. 12 (1885): 323–24; AMA revenue estimates are based on data that the *Journal's* trustees and AMA treasurer Dunglison reported: Board of Trustees, "Report of the Board of Trustees for the Publication of the Journal of the American Medical Association," *ibid.* 14, no. 22 (1890): 799 Richard J. Dunglison, "Treasurer's Report," *ibid.*, no. 24: 878.

7. Lawrence (editor), *The Medical Brief*. 553; *The Medical Brief*, vol. 9 (St Louis: The Medical Brief, 1881). The subscription price increase came in 1882: *The Medical Brief*, vol. 10 (St Louis: The Medical Brief, 1882).

8. *The Medical Brief*. 365, 388; further information on ingredient names and known properties at the time: John S. Wright, ed. *A Guide to the Organic Drugs of the United States Pharmacopoeia 1890* (Indianapolis, IN: Eli Lilly & Company, 1895); the development of Listerine is unclear. Many sources quote the Warner Lambert Company's assertion that Lawrence developed and began manufacturing Listerine in 1879: Leon Morgenstern, "Gargling with Lister," *Journal of the American College of Surgeons* 204, no. 3 (2007): 495–97; "From Surgery Antiseptic to Modern Mouthwash," Johnson and Johnson Consumer, Inc., https://www.listerine.com/about; the Smithsonian's National Museum of American History states that Listerine was co-invented by Lawrence and Jordan Lambert in 1879: Kenneth E. Behring Center National Museum of American History, "Listerine," The National Museum of American History, http://americanhistory.si.edu/collections/search/object/nmah_1170944; Lambert's alma mater, Randolph-Macon College named part of its campus after Lambert and the town (Ashland, VA) museum claims that he invented Listerine: "Jordan Wheat Lambert 1851–

1889," Ashland Museum, http://americanhistory.si. edu/collections/search/object/nmah_1170944 as does a relatively contemporary biography: "Lambert, Jordan W.," in *Encyclopedia of the History of St. Louis*, ed. William Hyde and Howard L. Conard (New York, NY: The Southern History Company, 1899), 1214–15; given the men's training, Lawrence as an eclectic physician and Lambert as an accountant with an interest in chemistry, the product's original developer was almost certainly Lawrence. There is no mention of Listerine in Lawrence's journal or anywhere else before 1881, which is also the year the trademark was filed. The AMA measured Listerine's alcohol content in 1931 as 26.08 percent: P.N. Leech, "Listerine—Report of Chemical and Bacteriologic Investigations," *JAMA* 96, no. 16 (1931): 1303–6.

9. Lawrence (editor), *The Medical Brief.* 360.

10. For example of laboratory studies: *The Medical Brief*, 309–310; example of other journals: Lunsford P. Yandell and Louis McMurtry, eds., *The Louisville Medical News—A Weekly Journal of Medicine and Surgery*, vol. 13 (Louisville, KY: The Louisville Medical News, 1881); Lawrence (editor), *The Medical Brief.* April 1882, Advertisements p. 22; tuberculosis: *The Medical Brief.* 391, 474.

11. Leech, "Listerine—Report of Chemical and Bacteriologic Investigations"; A. Emil Hiss, *Thesaurus of Proprietary Preparations and Pharmaceutical Specialties* (Chicago, IL: G.P. Engelhard & Company, 1898).

12. Solis-Cohen, "Shall Physicians Become Sales-Agents for Patent Medicines?"

13. Leech, "Listerine—Report of Chemical and Bacteriologic Investigations."

14. "Lambert, Jordan W.," 1899 1214–15; *Warner-Lambert Pharm. Co. V. John J. Reynolds, Et Al.* (1959); Johnston, "Lawrence, Joseph Joshua," 1991 30–31, "End Trust in Estate of Originator of Listerine," *Joplin (Missouri) Globe*, July 20, 1929.

15. William R. Amick, "Diseases of the Eye," *The Cincinnati Lancet and Observe* 21, no. 2 (1878): 175–82; "Catarrhal Deafness," *The Cincinnati Medical News* (1879): 742–46; "Aural Polypi," *The Cincinnati Medical News* (1879): 1–5; "Objective Snapping Noises in the Ear," *Cincinnati Medical News* (1879): 586–90; "The Effects of Sanitation on the Organs of Vision," *JAMA* (1884): 287–91; "Wealthy Doctors—Some of the Solid Men in the Profession," *Cincinnati Enquirer*, June 22, 1891, 8.

16. Sakula, "Robert Koch: Centenary of the Discovery of the Tubercle Bacillus, 1882."

17. Editor, "Koch's Treatment of Tuberculosis—Official Prussian Report," *The Boston Medical and Surgical Journal* 124, no. March 26 (1891): 318–20; "Further Experience with Tuberculin in New York Hospitals," *Boston Medical and Surgical Journal* 124, no. May 14 (1891): 492.

18. Sakula, "Robert Koch: Centenary of the Discovery of the Tubercle Bacillus, 1882"; Philip, "An Address on Koch's Discovery of the Tubercle Bacillus—Some of Its Implications and Results"; "Lymph Called a Failure," *The New York Times*, New York, NY, July 28, 1891.

19. Barry Smith, "Gullible's Travails: Tuberculosis and Quackery 1890–1930," *Journal of Contemporary History* 20, no. 4 (1985): 733–56; Katherine Ott, *Fevered Lives: Tuberculosis in American Culture since 1870* (Cambridge, MA: Harvard University Press, 1996); William Osler, *The Principles and Practice of Medicine—Designed for the Use of Practitioners and Students of Medicine* (New York: D. Appleton and Company, 1892); Adams, *The Great American Fraud—Reprinted from Collier's Weekly.* 11.

20. The most recent innocuous article was: William R. Amick, "Drunkenness," *The Cincinnati Lancet-Clinic* 28 (1892): 174–76; "A Chemical Cure for Consumption and Asthma," *The Cincinnati Lancet-Clinic* (1892): 297–308.

21. Osler, *The Principles and Practice of Medicine—Designed for the Use of Practitioners and Students of Medicine.* 184.

22. Amick, "A Chemical Cure for Consumption and Asthma," 299.

23. "A Chemical Cure for Consumption and Asthma."

24. The editorial was unsigned and Richardson's name did not appear on the *Lancet-Clinic* masthead in 1892, which it did in 1891. However, Richardson was named by Amick in his article and referenced in the local press as a *Lancet-Clinic* editor. Given the editorial's mention of the newspaper article, its author had to Richardson: Editor, "A Question of Ethics and Equity," *The Cincinnati Lancet Clinic* (1892): 348–49. 348–9.

25. The public's gullibility was (is) understandable. That many, probably most, physicians were poor scientists and did not stay current with the medical literature was also well recognized. For a discussion of the period, see: Duffy, *The Sanitarians—a History of American Public Health*; Warner, *The Therapeutic Perspective: Medical Practice, Knowledge, and Identity in America, 1820–1885*. For a discussion of the problem today, see: Richard Smith, *The Trouble with Medical Journals* (London: Royal Society of Medicine Press Ltd., 2006); M. Jiwa, "Doctors and Medical Science," *Australas Med J* 5, no. 8 (2012): 462–7; Milton Packer to Revolution and Revelation, March 28, 2018, https://www.medpagetoday.com/blogs/revolution andrevelation/72029.

26. George Edward Stevens, "A History of the Cincinnati Post" (University of Minnesota, 1969); the *Post* claimed that its weekday circulation in Ohio, Kentucky, West Virginia, and Tennessee was 20,000 more than any other Ohio newspaper: "This Paper Guarantees to Every Advertiser/ Honest Circulation," *The Cincinnati Post*, March 15, 1892, 2; Gerald J. Baldasty, *E.W. Scripps and the Business of Newspapers* (Urbana and Chicago, IL: University of Illinois Press, 1999).

27. "I've Found It—Triumphantly Exclaims Dr. Amick of Cincinnati," *Cincinnati Post*, March 5, 1892, 8; for evidence that Amick authored his own press reports, see testimony in: Editor, "W.R. Amick Vs J.C. Culbertson," *The Cincinnati Lancet-Clinic* (1894): 386–94; *W.R. Amick vs. James E. Reeves—Action for Libel* (1895).

28. "Sure Cure. Has Dr. Amick Discovered One for Consumption? Local Physicians Inclined to Believe It," *Cincinnati Post*, March 7, 1892, 1.

29. "Phthisis Pulmonalis—Its Terrors Dispelled by Dr. Amick," *St Louis Republic*, St Louis, MO 1892, 13.

30. "Here You Are—Dr. Amick Will Treat a Test Case to Prove the Value of His Cure.," *Cincinnati Post*, March 9, 1892, 1.

31. "Square Deal," *The Cincinnati Post*, Cincinnati, OH, March 11, 1892, 1; "The Great Test," *The Cincin-*

nati Post, Cincinnati, OH, March 15, 1892, 2; "Asthma Departs—Mrs. Madison Draws a Free Breath Again," *The Cincinnati Post*, March 29, 1892, 2; "A Modern Joshua—He Turns Back Life's Fast Setting Sun," *The Cincinnati Post*, Cincinnati, OH, March 26, 1892, 1.

32. "Secret Remedies," *The Cincinnati Lancet-Clinic* (1892): 402–3; "Editorial Notes," *The Cincinnati Lancet-Clinic* (editorial) (1892): 633–34.

33. Antikamnia was the prototypical secret nostrum used by the profession. It contained varying amounts of caffeine, sodium bicarbonate, and acetanilide, the latter a dangerous, but mildly effective and non-addicting analgesic that was listed in the U.S. Pharmacopoeia and sold by itself as Antifebrin. Pharmacologists easily discovered the ingredients, although many physicians never bothered to understand the implications and often prescribed several branded compounds containing acetanilide at the same time: Hiss, *Thesaurus of Proprietary Preparations and Pharmaceutical Specialties*; Robert A. Hatcher and Martin I. Wilbert, *The Pharmacopeia and the Physician* (Chicago, IL: American Medical Association Press, 1906); William J. Robinson, "The Composition of Some So-Called Synthetics and "Ethical" Nostrums," *JAMA* 42, no. 16 (1904): 1016–20; Adams, *The Great American Fraud—Reprinted from Collier's Weekly*.

34. Editor, "The Medical Practice Act," *The Cincinnati Lancet-Clinic* 27 (1891): 831–32. 832.

35. The Cincinnati *Post* reported William Amick's departure from the college as a matter of principle: "Amick Resigns from the Cincinnati College of Medicine," *The Cincinnati Post*, May 16, 1892, 3; A later lawsuit provided ample uncontested physician testimony that he was a medical pariah: "W.R. Amick vs J.C. Culbertson"; Marion's resignation was mentioned in his biography: Charles Theodore Greve, *Centennial History of Cincinnati and Representative Citizens*, vol. II (Chicago: Biographical Publishing Company, 1904).

36. "Amick's Triumph—Mrs Madison Walks into the Post's Office—Palatial New Institute Opened Wednesday by Amick," *The Cincinnati Post*, May 4, 1892, 4; Amick was covered in the *Post* on: 4/4, 4/8, 4/23, 4/29, 5/4, 5/5, 5/16, 5/28, 6/14, 7/9, 10/27. A searchable archive of The Cincinnati Post is available at: "Genealogy Bank," (Naples, FL: NewsBank, Inc., 2018).

37. "Medical Science," *The Cincinnati Post*, Cincinnati, OH, April 23, 1892, 8.

38. "Test Cases—May Be Treated by Dr. Irvine K. Mott," *The Cincinnati Post*, Cincinnati, OH, July 30, 1894, 3.

39. "Harvard Helps—in the Selection of the Post's Test Patients," *The Cincinnati Post*, Cincinnati, OH, August 27, 1894, 4; one of these drug names, brucin, referred to a known toxin, brucine, that is related to strychnine and had no therapeutic use: United States Pharmacopœial Convention Inc., *The Pharmacopeia of the United States of America*; Harvard Concurs—by a Verdict of Unqualified Success," *The Cincinnati Post*, Cincinnati, OH, October 27, 1894, 8; The *Post* reported fourteen times on Mott's accomplishment in 1894, but only twice in the following five years; There are numerous examples of Mott's later ads, all of which were similar and based on the *Post* articles. See Advertisement, "Cures the Kidneys—Dr. Mott of Cincinnati Has Found the Exact Remedies," *Chicago*

Daily News, Chicago, IL, November 6, 1897, 7; "Bright's Disease and Diabetes Cured," *Pearson's Magazine*, 1901.

40. Norman Hapgood, "Editorial Talks—Uncle Sam's Efficiency," *Collier's—The National Weekly*, August 12, 1905, 22; "Bright's Disease and Diabetes," *San Francisco Chronicle*, San Francisco, CA April 4, 1915, 37; Mott died in 1920: "Deaths," *JAMA* 74, no. 10 (1920): 689.

41. Background on the Amick Chemical Company from: "Asthma Too—The Post Will Present Dr. Amick a Case—A Sanitarium to Be Established Here—Abundant Capital Will Furnish the Facilities," *The Cincinnati Post*, March 10, 1892, 3; "New Enterprises," *The Cincinnati Enquirer*, Cincinnati, OH, August 16, 1892, 5; "Home Page," *Companies Ohio*, http://www.companies-ohio.com/; Editor, "W.R. Amick vs J.C. Culbertson"; "Dr. Amick's Chemical Treatment for Consumption, Asthma, Chronic Bronchitis, Catarrh, Hay Fever and All Kindred Diseases. (Second Annual Report of the Amick Chemical Company)," (Cincinnati, OH: Amick Chemical Company, 1894).

42. "Death's Doors Were Swung Back by Dr. Amick—S.G. Sea, the Chicago Herald's Business Manager Lauds a Cincinnati Physician's Cure for Consumption," *The Cincinnati Post*, October 7, 1892, 5; Sea's association was never publicly announced. In 1894, Marion Amick Described Mr. See (*sic*) as one of the four principals.

43. "Exit Prof. Amick," *The St Louis Medical and Surgical Journal* 62, no. 6 (1892): 361.

44. Joseph J. Lawrence (editor), "A Seasonable Word," *The Medical Brief* 20, no. 12 (1892): 1457; *The Medical Brief*, vol. 20 (St Louis: The Medical Brief, 1892).

45. *The Medical Brief*. 878, 1123–1138, 1275, 1507. Quotation 1124.

46. Advertisement, "Dr. Amick's Chemical Cure for Consumption," *The Medical Summary* 14, no. 9 (1892): xxi–xxxvi.

47. "All America Applauds the Investigation," *New York Recorder*, New York, NY, December 25, 1892, 24.

48. There is little scholarly information on The New York *Recorder* and its archives are not yet digitized. This information is from an unpublished Master's thesis: Lorna Watson, "The New York Recorder as a Woman's Newspaper 1891–1894," (Madison: University of Wisconsin, 1939) and the *Recorder's* announcements: "The Recorder—Its History and Its Home," *New York Recorder*, New York, NY, February 19, 1893, 47. See also: Doris Faber, *Printer's Devil to Publisher: Adolph S. Ochs of the New York Times* (Hensonville, NY: Black Dome Press, 1996), 81, and Kenneth Whyte, *The Uncrowned King*, vol. Toronto, Canada (Random House Canada, 2008).

49. "From Far and near—Eminent Physicians on the Recorder's Consumption Investigation," *New York Recorder*, New York, NY, December 28, 1892, 7; "Has Koch a Rival? An Eminent Cincinnati Physician's Interesting Theory," *The New York Recorder*, New York, NY, December 29, 1892, Unknown page (torn); "The Investigation—A Western Newspaper Confirms the Recorder Correspondence Regarding Dr. Amick's Discovery," *New York Recorder*, New York, NY, December 30, 1892, 7.

50. "Amick Is Willing—His Discoveries Indorsed by the Public, Physicians, and Medical Journals of the West," *New York Recorder*, New York, NY, January 31,

1892, 9; presumably the *Medical Brief* article referenced by the *Recorder* was Amick's September one; otherwise the statement was a complete falsehood, as there were no comparable articles on consumption published in either the December 1892 or January 1893 issues of *The Medical Brief.*

51. "Koch and Virchow to Be Interviewed—Dr. Amick's Discovery to Be Tested," *New York Recorder*, New York, NY, January 1, 1893, 10; If Sternberg was not in New York in December 1892, he was not far away: "National Control Urged," *New York Times*, New York, NY, December 14, 1892, 9, 10.

52. "Koch and Amick—a Chance to Compare the Merits of Their Methods," *New York Recorder*, New York, NY January 12, 1893, 9.

53. The *Recorder* is currently not stored digitally. The count of articles is based on a manual review of issues in microfilm format between December 1, 1892, and May 23, 1893. Citations are (1893): 1/7, 1/8, 1/9, 1/11, 1/12, 1/13, 1/14, 1/15, 1/17, 1/22, 1/24, 1/29, 2/1, 2/3, 2/5, 2/6, 2/12, 2/15, 2/17, 2/19, 2/21, 2/26, 3/6, 3/12, 3/19, 4/16; "The Award Is Made—the Recorder Presents Dr. Amick with One Thousand Dollars," *New York Recorder*, New York, NY, April 23, 1893, 30–31.

54. "A Great Newspaper's Achievement," *Phillipsburg Herald*, March 9, 1893, 7; "Consumption Cured," *The Buffalo Sunday Morning News*, Buffalo, NY, April 23, 1893, 1.; "Curing Them All—the Recorder's Discovery Now Generally Recognized by Physicians and Newspapers Everywhere," *New York Recorder*, New York, NY, May 14, 1893, 38.

55. "Dr. Amick's Chemical Treatment for Consumption, Asthma, Chronic Bronchitis, Catarrh, Hay Fever and All Kindred Diseases. (Second Annual Report of the Amick Chemical Company)," 1894; Classified Ad, "Consumption and Catarrh Treated," *Los Angeles Herald*, Los Angeles, CA, July 9, 1893, 6.

56. The *Enquirer* published one of Amick's Chattanooga dispatches on July 26, 1893, but was otherwise silent until Reeves' arrest on August 26, 1893: Digital records for the *Enquirer*: "Newspapers.Com," (Ancestry.com); Manual search of the *Times-Star* for March 5–June 30, 1892, showed no mentions of Amick: Linda Dietrich, June 30, 2018.

57. "Timesmachine," in *New York Times* (New York, NY: New York Times); Searchable database for *Herald, World,* and *Tribune*: "Newspaperarchive.com" (Wilmington, DE: Heritage World Archives SEZC).

58. "A Medium for Cheats—How Frauds Are Worked Through the Mails," *Cincinnati Enquirer*, Cincinnati, OH, May 7, 1892, 14; example of consumption ad: Advertisement, "Fifty Years Settles It—Consumption Can Be Cured," *ibid.,* December 19, 8.

59. Adams, *The Great American Fraud—Reprinted from Collier's Weekly.* 5.

60. It is hard to know if New York physicians were completely silent, but there was no mention of Amick or his miraculous cure in the largest New York medical journal or the state medical society meetings: Frank P. Foster (editor), *The New York Medical Journal*, vol. 57 (Jan–June) (New York: D. Appleton and Company, 1893); *The New York Medical Journal*, vol. 58 (July–Dec) (New York: D. Appleton and Company, 1893); *Transactions of the Medical Society of the State of New York for the Year 1893*, (Albany, NY: The Medical Society of the State of New York 1893); *Transac-

tions of the Medical Society of the State of New York for the Year 1894*, (Albany, NY: The Medical Society of the State of New York 1894).

61. George N. Aronoff, "The Doctrine of Libel Per Se in Ohio," *Case Western Reserve Law Review* 9, no. 1 (1957): 43–55; Douglas R. Matthews, "American Defamation Law: From Sullivan, through Greenmoss, and Beyond," *Ohio State Law Journal* 48, no. 2 (1987): 513–32.

62. "The Truth. Can Consumption Be Cured?," *The Cincinnati Post*, Cincinnati, OH, April 14, 1893, 4.

63. Editor, "Radam's Libel Suit," *The Druggists Circular and Chemical Gazette* 37, no. 6 (1893): 121–22.

64. "Radam's Microbe Killer in Court—Oral Testimony Before the New York Supreme Bench—Evidence of Its Phenomenal Curative Virtues Decided to Be Absolutely Conclusive," *The Chicago Tribune*, Chicago, IL, June 24, 1893, 3; Young, *The Toadstool Millionaires—A Social History of Patent Medicines in America before Federal Regulation; The Medical Messiahs—A Social History of Health Quackery in Twentieth-Century America.*

65. Faber, *Printer's Devil to Publisher: Adolph S. Ochs of the New York Times.*

66. Connecticut Medical Society, *Secretary Letter*, Proceedings of the Connecticut Medical Society, 1893 (Bridgeport, CT: Connecticut Medical Society, 1893), 22; "News Items. The Pan-American Medical Congress," *The Medical News* 63, no. 7 (1893): 196; "Uncle Jimmy" reference: "Doctor's Memory Honored by Group."

Chapter 19

1. "That Bubbling Mercury," *The Daily Times*, Chattanooga, TN, July 8, 1893, 2; "Hanged—Then Burned!," *The Daily Times*, Chattanooga, TN, July 8, 1893, 2; "Going to Give It a Trial," *The Daily Times*, Chattanooga July 8, 1893, 5.

2. "Almost Miraculous," *The Sunday Times*, Chattanooga, TN, July 9, 1893, 1; for samples of similar articles in other papers see: "Newspapers.com," "Newspaperarchive.com,".

3. "Chattanooga's Tribute to the Merits of the Wonderful Amick Consumption Cure," *The Daily Times*, Chattanooga, TN, July 26, 1893, 2; "Mrs. Springfield's Life. The 'Squire Tells How It Was Despaired Of," *The Daily Times*, Chattanooga, TN, July 28, 1893, 8; "More Surprises Daily—At the Hands of the Chattanooga Doctors," *The Daily Times*, Chattanooga, July 30, 1893, 10.

4. Andrew Porwancher, "Objectivity's Prophet: Adolph S. Ochs and the *New York Times*, 1896–1935," *Journalism History* 36, no. 4 (2011): 186–95.

5. "The Amick Cure—Dr. James E. Reeves Doesn't Believe in Its Virtues," *The Daily Times*, Chattanooga, TN, August 3, 1893, 8.

6. "Free and Full Tests—to Be Held by a Committee of Physicians," *The Daily Times*, Chattanooga, TN, August 8, 1893, 2; "Two Liberal Doctors—Six Consumptives Will Be Benefitted Through Their Skill," *The Daily Times*, August 9, 1893, 5; "Discussing the Amick," *The Daily Times*, Chattanooga, TN, August 7, 1893, 2; Editor, "The Amick Treatment for Consumption," *North Carolina Medical Journal* 32, no. 2 (1893): 105.

7. "A Postal Card Written by Dr. James E. Reeves

Gets Him into Trouble," *The Chattanooga News*, Chattanooga, TN, August 26, 1893, 1.

8. "A Postal Card Written by Dr. James E. Reeves Gets Him into Trouble"; "Their Biggest Ad—Dr. Amick Causes the Arrest of Dr. Jas. E. Reeves," *The Sunday Times*, Chattanooga, TN, August 27, 1893, 5; "Fixed at $1,000," *The Daily Times*, Chattanooga, TN, August 29, 1893, 6; For information on Gosdorfer: *W.R. Amick vs. James E. Reeves—Action for Libel*. Note that Gosdorfer's name was spelled at least three ways in the *Times* article and the court records, including "Grosdorfer" and "Gosdoffer." Twenty-two year-old Milton *Gosdorfer* from Cincinnati showed up in an unrelated libel suit in 1894: Samuel A. Blatchford, New York, NY, United States Circuit Court of Appeals for the Second Circuit, "United States Court of Appeals Report," 1896. 169–170.

9. "Their Biggest Ad—Dr. Amick Causes the Arrest of Dr. Jas. E. Reeves"; "Amick Gets Back," *The Cincinnati Post*, Cincinnati, OH, August 26, 1893, 1.

10. James F. Baldwin, "Prosecuted on Account of a Postal Card," *The Columbus Medical Journal* 12, no. 3 (1893): 142; George M Gould (editor), "Dr. Reeves and the "Amick Cure" (1)," *The Medical News* 63 (1893): 357.

11. "Dr. Reeves Is Sued—The Amick Company Wants $25,000 Damages from Him," *The Daily Times*, Chattanooga, TN, September 7, 1893, 2.

12. Howard F. Hansell, "George Milbry Gould, A.M., M.D.," *Transactions of the American Ophthalmological Society* 21 (1923): 14–20; James E. Reeves, Letter to William Pepper, Jr., September 15, 1893.

13. "Dr. Amick—Is Recognized by the World—Paris Physicians Couple His Name with Pasteur's," *The Cincinnati Post*, Cincinnati, OH, September 7, 1893, 4; "It Is a Success," *The St. Joseph Sunday Herald*, St. Joseph, MO, October 1, 1893, 1. Numerous papers carried this dispatch.

14. "Dr. Reeves Wins," *The Daily Times*, Chattanooga, TN, October 10, 1893, 8.

15. George M Gould (editor), "Dr. Reeves and the 'Amick Cure' (2)," *The Medical News* 63 (1893): 467–68; Editor, "Dr. Reeves and the 'Amick Cure,'" *The St. Louis Medical and Surgical Journal* 65, no. 5 (1893): 325–26; George M Gould (editor), "Editorial Comments—The Philadelphia County Medical Society and Nostrums," *The Medical News* 63, no. 18 (1893): 498; James F. Baldwin (editor), "Dr. Reeves and the Amick," *The Columbus Medical Journal* 12, no. 4 (1893): 183–84; Editor, "Miscellany—Dr. Reeves and the Amick Cure," *The Boston Medical and Surgical Journal* 129, no. 17 (1893): 428–29; "The Amick Treatment," *North Carolina Medical Journal* 32, no. 5 (1893): 246–47; George F. Shrady (editor), "The Philadelphia Medical Society and Nostrums," *Medical Record* 44, no. 19 (1893): 595.

16. For biographical information on Culbertson see: "Culbertson, James Coe," in *The National Cyclopaedia of American Biography* (New York, NY: James T. White & Company, 1904), 47; see also: Kelly and Burrage, *Dictionary of American Medical Biography*; J. C. Culbertson (editor), "Druggist and Physician," *JAMA* 29, no. 25 (1892): 732.

17. "Editorial—Our Politics: The Amick Consumption Cure," *The Cincinnati Lancet Clinic* 31 (1893): 486–88; "Dr. Amick Enters Suit against Dr. Culbertson for Libel," *The Cincinnati Post*, Cincinnati, OH, November 6, 1893, 1. This article also mentions

a prior suit against the *Lancet-Clinic*, but I could find no record of one. It may have been a mistaken reference to the April 1893 suit Amick filed against the Ohio Medical College. To further confuse matters, Culbertson stated in December 1893 that the suit was for $100,000: "Incompatibles," *The Cincinnati Lancet-Clinic* 31 (1893): 739–40.

18. Editor, "Editorial Opinions on the Latest Quack," *The St Louis Clinique* 6, no. 11 (1893): 505–7; "Called Him a Quack," *St. Louis Post-Dispatch*, St. Louis, MO, December 7, 1893, 9.

19. J. C. Culbertson (editor), "Editorial—at It Again," *The Cincinnati Lancet-Clinic* 31 (1893): 710.

20. "Philadelphia—The Quack Aspects of American Life," *British Medical Journal* 2 (1893): 1350–51.

21. "Judgment Rendered," *The Cincinnati Post*, Cincinnati, OH February 28, 1894, 2; for example of wire reports: "Judgment Rendered," *Trenton Evening Times*, Trenton, NJ, March 5, 1894, 8; "Amick's Suit Settled," *St. Louis Post-Dispatch*, St. Louis, MO, February 28, 1894, 11.

22. "Criminal Libel," *The Cincinnati Post*, Cincinnati, OH, February 27, 1894, 1; for details on Ohio law see: Florien Giauque, ed. *The Revised Statutes of the State of Ohio*, 6th ed., vol. 2 (Cincinnati, OH: Robert Clarke & Co., 1894); Editor, "W.R. Amick Vs J.C. Culbertson"; J.C. Culbertson (editor), "The Amick Quack Combination," *The Cincinnati Lancet-Clinic* 33, no. July 14 (1894): 38–39.

23. *Cincinnati Medical Journal* cited in: "Philadelphia," *British Medical Journal* 1 (1894): 770; Advertisement, "Doctors Disagree," *The Medical Brief* 22, no. 8 (1894): 989; "It Cures Consumption," *Columbus Daily Enquirer*, Columbus, GA, October 19, 1894, 1.

24. W.R. Amick, "One and One Are Two," *The Medical Journal* 10, no. 6 (1895): 404–10; among many examples of Amick's anti–isolation activities: "The Consumption Panic," *The Boston Daily Globe*, Boston, MA, February 20, 1895, 7.

25. Samuel M. Taylor, Columbus, OH, Secretary of State, "Annual Report of the Secretary of State," 1896. 510.

26. J.M. Hays, "A Plea for the More General Use of the Microscope in Every Day Practice," *North Carolina Medical Journal* 32, no. 2 (1893): 76–83.

27. John Harley Warner, "'Exploring the Inner Labyrinths of Creation': Popular Microscopy in Nineteenth-Century America," *Journal of the History of Medicine and Allied Sciences* 37, no. 1 (1982): 7–33; Lester S. King, "XIX. Medical Education: The Decade of Massive Change," *JAMA* 251, no. 2 (1984): 219–24; Joseph G. Richardson, *A Handbook of Medical Microscopy* (Philadelphia, PA: J.B. Lippincott & Co., 1871).

28. "Book Reviews—Medical Microscopy. A Guide to the Use of the Microscope in Medical Practice," *JAMA* 29, no. 25 (1892): 734.

29. James E. Reeves, *Hand-Book of Medical Microscopy* (Philadelphia, PA: P. Blakiston, Son & Co., 1894).

30. "Book Notices—a Handbook of Medical Microscopy," *JAMA* 23, no. 13 (1894): 516–17; J. C. Culbertson (editor), "Bibliography—A Hand-Book of Medical Microscopy," *The Cincinnati Lancet-Clinic* 33 (1894): 132; H.C.F., "Book Reviews—A Hand-Book of Medical Microscopy," *Columbus Medical Journal* 13, no. 8 (1894): 430–31; Editor, "Book Notices—

Hand-Book of Medical Microscopy," *Virginia Medical Monthly* 21, no. 8 (1894): 786.

31. James E. Reeves, Personal letter, courtesy of Mrs. Joan Webb, March 30, 1895.

32. Details of trial: *W.R. Amick vs. James E. Reeves—Action for Libel.* 8; "Peculiar Libel Suit—Twenty-Five Thousand Dollars the Damages Claimed," *The Daily Times*, Chattanooga, TN, April 11, 1895, 5; "Dr. Reeves Acquitted," *The Daily Times*, Chattanooga, TN, April 12, 1895, 6.

33. *W.R. Amick vs. James E. Reeves—Action for Libel.* 19.

34. "Dr. Reeves Acquitted"; *W.R. Amick vs. James E. Reeves—Action for Libel.*

35. "Dr. Reeves Vindicated," *The Wheeling Daily Intelligencer*, Wheeling, WV, April 13, 1895, 7.

36. George M Gould (editor), "A Defeat for Quackery," *The Medical News* 66 (1895): 469.

37. "Should Physicians Deal Honorably and Courteously with One Another," *The Medical News* 66, no. 17 (1895): 465–66. 466. This editorial reads like a synopsis of Cronin's 1938 English novel, *The Citadel.* In 1892, the Philadelphia Medical Society, led by Solomon Solis-Cohen from the Polyclinic, began a campaign to remove secret nostrum advertisements from the *Journal of the American Medical Association* (See Solis-Cohen, "Shall Physicians Become Sales-Agents for Patent Medicines?"). In 1895, Solis-Cohen achieved victory: "Association News—American Medical Association," *JAMA* 24, no. 20 (1895): 755–67.

38. James F. Baldwin (editor), "Dr. George M. Gould," *Columbus Medical Journal* 15, no. 1 (1895): 44; George M. Gould, "Professional Indifference to Professional Enemies," *The Medical News*, June 29, 1895, 735–36; John B. Hamilton (editor), "'Medicine and Cricket," *JAMA* 25, no. 2 (1895): 78.

39. George M Gould (editor), "Editorial Comments—The James E. Reeves Fund," *The Medical News* 67, no. 10 (1895): 274–75.

40. J. C. Culbertson (editor), "Lost!," *The Cincinnati Lancet-Clinic* 34 (1895): 440; "Dr. Reeves Vindicated," *The Cincinnati Lancet-Clinic* 34 (1895): 440; "A Quack Consumption Cure," *The Cincinnati Lancet-Clinic* 36 (1896): 221. Culbertson reprinted this editorial in the *Indiana Medical Journal*, which he also owned: Editor, "Lung-Savior Edson," *Indiana Medical Journal* 14, no. 9 (1896): 328–29.

41. "Scipio—Dr. W.R. Amick Has Returned from Cincinnati," *Columbus (IN) Daily Herald*, September 4, 1895; for Marion: Amerious V. Williams (editor), *Williams Cincinnati Business Directory* (Cincinnati: Cincinnati Directory Office, 1896); the *Indiana Medical Journal* reported Amick's consumption in 1896: Editor, "Lung-Savior Edson"; "Funeral of Dr. Amick," *Columbus (IN) Daily Times*, September 1, 1900, 4; Greve, *Centennial History of Cincinnati and Representative Citizens.* 393; "Dr. Amick Cannot Recover," *Abilene Daily Reflector*, Abilene, KS November 14, 1904, 4; "Deaths—Amick," *The Cincinnati Post*, Cincinnati, OH, November 17, 1904, 11.

42. For example of advertising: "A Son Saved from Certain Death," *Topeka State Journal*, Topeka, KS March 24, 1898, 9; the Amick Company timeline is based on listings in subsequent annual Cincinnati *Business Directories.* The Amick Chemical Company was relisted in 1897, showing three officers (Henry Roos, president) and a company physician. Similar

listings continued until 1903. After that, no officers were listed. Presumably, Roos *et al.* serviced existing clients until 1903–4 and then abandoned operations. Copies of the Williams Cincinnati Business Directory available at "Search Us City Directories," Ancestry. com, http://search.ancestry.com/search/db.aspx?dbid= 2469.

43. "Association News—American Medical Association," "Association News—American Medical Association"; "Dr. Reeves Dead"; "Dr. James E. Reeves"; for Sims: McGuffey (editor), *Standard History of Chattanooga Tennessee.*

44. "Dr. Reeves Dead." This report also mentions another individual, the "professor of surgery" of Johns Hopkins, presumably William Halstead. Other reports only mention Osler. A personal letter from Osler to Baldwin, written well after the malignant course of Reeves' disease was apparent, related that Osler first told Reeves he thought the liver tumor was a benign adenoma, as Reeves had hoped to hear: Osler; A second letter from Osler, after Reeves had died, mentioned the physical finding of liver nodules: Personal letter from William Osler to P.D. Sims. Owned by Barbara Boren., January 10, 1896; the gifts from Reeves to Osler had the same dedication: "To Dr. Wm Osler, with love, James E. Reeves, Chattanooga, Tenn. Oct. 17th, 1895: A.P.W. Philip, *A Treatise on Indigestion and Its Consequences*, Fourth ed. (New York, NY: Evert Duyckink and George Long, 1824); Sir Richard Blackmore, *Dissertations on a Dropsy, a Tympany, the Jaundice, the Stone, and a Diabetes* (London, UK: James and John Knapton, 1727) (Bibliotheca Osleriana #2049); John Cheyne, *An Essay on Cynanche Trachealis or Croup* (Philadelphia: Anthony Finley, 1813) (Bibliotheca Osleriana #2307); George M. Gould, Personal letter owned by Barbara Boren, October 15, 1895.

45. Gould; "Dr. Reeves Dead."

46. Personal letter from George Gould to James Reeves, owned by Barbara Boren, November 24, 1895; "Dr. James E. Reeves."

47. "Dr Reeves Dying"; For example of dispatches about Reeves' illness: "Dr. James Edmund Reeves Dying," *The Inter Ocean*, Chicago, IL December 27, 1895, 3.

48. "Dr. Reeves Dead."

49. "Dr. Reeves Dead"; "Funeral of Dr. Reeves."

50. "Death of Dr. Reeves," *Wheeling Register*, Wheeling, WV, January 5, 1896, 5; "Dr. James E. Reeves," *Wheeling Daily Intelligencer*, Wheeling, WV, January 6, 1896, 8; "Funeral of Dr. J.E. Reeves."

51. Examples of newspaper death notices: "Telegraphic Briefs," *Charlotte Observer*, Charlotte, NC, January 5, 1896, 1; a few papers ran lengthier pieces, noting Reeves' public health career: "Dr. Reeves Dead," *The Atlanta Constitution*, Atlanta, GA, January 5, 1896, 14; Watson, *Physicians and Surgeons of America: A Collection of Biographical Sketches of the Regular Medical Profession*; journal obituaries included: "Necrology. James Edmund Reeves," *JAMA* 26, no. 3 (1896): 141–42; Editor, "Obituary," *The Sanitarian* 36, no. March (1896): 277–78; "Medical Items—James Edmund Reeves," *New Orleans Medical and Surgical Journal* 23, no. 8 (1896): 501–2; J. Riddle Goffe (editor), "Obituary," *The Medical News* 68, no. 7 (1896): 196; The Association of American Physicians eulogy: A. Jacobi, "President's Address," *Boston Medical and Surgical Journal* 134, no. 19 (1896): 453–55.

Epilogue

1. Wilson, "James Edmund Reeves, M.D.," 1325.
2. Editor, "The Fairmont Meeting," *The West Virginia Medical Journal* 32, no. 5 (1936): 231; T.M. Hood, "Founders' Monument Address," *ibid.*, no. 8: 370–71; "Doctor's Memory Honored by Group."
3. It's difficult (impossible) to prove that something does not exist, but considerable digging finds very few 20th-century references to James Reeves. I've cited the few I located and some examples of pertinent negatives: James Morton Callahan, *History of West Virginia Old and New and West Virginia Biography*, 3 vols., vol. II–III (Chicago, IL: The American Historical Society, Inc., 1923); John Alexander Williams, *West Virginia: A History* (New York, NY: W.W. Norton and Company, Inc., 1976; repr., 1984); Otis K. Rice and Stephen W. Brown, *West Virginia: A History* (Lexington, KY: University Press of Kentucky, 1985); Reeves was mentioned in the 20th-century Mother's Day literature, not always accurately: Kendall, *Mothers Day—A History of Its Founding and Its Founder*; Wolfe, *Mothers Day and the Mothers Day Church*; Jepson, "Editorial—A Bit of History"; JE Rader, "Founding of the West Virginia State Medical Association—President's Address," *WV Med J* 12, no. 4 (1917): 161–68; Hood, "Founders' Monument Address"; Reeves was not mentioned in the first edition of Kelly's compendium of American physicians Kelly, *A Cyclopedia of American Medical Biography*, but the oversight was corrected in the second edition Howard A. Kelly and Burrage Walter L., *Dictionary of American Medical Biography* (New York, NY: D. Appleton and Company, 1928), 1024–1025; Citing only his own opinion, AMA historian Lester King described Reeves' 1894 *Hand-Book of Medical Microscopy* as a "stupendous failure." King, "XIX. Medical Education: The Decade of Massive Change," 220.
4. Mohr, *Licensed to Practice—The Supreme Court Defines the American Medical Profession*, 28, 79.
5. Everett Rogers' classic work on innovation diffusion seems surprisingly overlooked by medical historians: Everett M. Rogers, *Diffusion of Innovations* (New York, NY: Free Press, 2003); ABIM Foundation. American Board of Internal Medicine, ACP-ASIM Foundation. American College of Physicians-American Society of Internal Medicine, and Medicine European Federation of Internal, "Medical Professionalism in the New Millennium: A Physician Charter," *Ann Intern Med* 136, no. 3 (2002): 243–6.
6. T. L. Beauchamp, "Internal and External Standards for Medical Morality," *J Med Philos* 26, no. 6 (2001): 601–19; John M. Harris, Jr., "Medical Ethics, Methodism, and a Nineteenth Century West Virginian's Battles with Quackery," *West Virginia History* 9, no. Spring (2016): 27–44; John M. Harris, Jr., and Lynette Reid, "In Reply to Cruess Et Al.," *Acad Med* 92, no. 12 (2017): 1650–51.

Bibliography of
Selected Sources

Ackerknecht, Erwin. "Aspects of the History of Therapeutics." *Bulletin of the History of Medicine* 36, no. 5 (1962): 389–419.

Ackerknecht, Erwin. "Elisha Bartlett and the Philosophy of the Paris Clinical School." *Bulletin of the History of Medicine* 24, no. Jan (1950): 43–60.

Adams, George Worthington. *Doctors in Blue*. Dayton, OH: Morningside House, Inc., 1985.

Adams, Samuel Hopkins. *The Great American Fraud—Reprinted from Collier's Weekly*. New York, NY: P.F. Collier & Son, 1905.

Ahlstrom, Sydney E. *A Religious History of the American People*. Second ed. New Haven, CT: Yale University Press, 2004. 1972.

Allen, Nathan. "The Relations between Sanitary Science and the Medical Profession." *Public Health Papers and Reports* 12 (1886): 85–98.

Ambler, Charles Henry *Sectionalism in Virginia from 1776 to 1861*. Chicago: University of Chicago Press, 1910.

Ambler, Charles H., and Festus P. Summers. *West Virginia—The Mountain State*. Second ed. Englewood Cliffs, NJ: Prentice Hall, Inc., 1958.

Ambrose, Charles T. "The Secret Kappa Lamda Society of Hippocrates (and the Origin of the American Medical Association's Principles of Medical Ethics)." *Yale J Biol Med* 78, no. 1 (2005): 45–56.

Anbinder, Tyler G. *Nativism and Slavery: The Northern Know Nothings and the Politics of the 1850s*. Oxford, UK: Oxford University Press, 1992.

Antolini, Katharine Lane "Memorializing Motherhood: Anna Jarvis and the Struggle for Control of Mother's Day." University of West Virginia, 2009.

Aronoff, George N. "The Doctrine of Libel Per Se in Ohio." *Case Western Reserve Law Review* 9, no. 1 (1957): 43–55.

Atkinson, George W. *Bench and Bar of West Virginia*. Charleston, WV: Virginian Law Book Company, 1919.

Atkinson, George W., and Alvaro Franklin Gibbens. *Prominent Men of West Virginia*. Wheeling, WV: W. L. Callin, 1890.

Atkinson, William B. *A Biographical Dictionary of Contemporary American Physicians and Surgeons*. Philadelphia: D.G. Brinton, 1880.

Atkinson, William B. *Physicians and Surgeons of the United States*. Philadelphia: Charles Robson, 1878.

Bacon, Francis. *The Advancement of Learning*. Edited by Henry Morley. Project Gutenburg ed. London, UK: Cassell & Company, Limited 1893.

Bacon, Francis. *The Works of Francis Bacon—Containing Novum Organon Scientiarium*. Translated by Baron Verulam. Edited by Baron Verulam Vol. 4, London, UK: M. Jones, 1815.

Bacon, Francis. *The Works of Lord Bacon*. 2 vols. Vol. II, London, UK: Henry G. Bohn, 1854.

Bailey, Kenneth R. *Alleged Evil Genius—The Life and Times of Judge James H. Ferguson*. Charleston, WV: Quarrier Press, 2006.

Baker, J.N. "Alabama's Contribution to Public Health." *The American Journal of Public Health* 30, no. 8 (1940): 859–65.

Baker, Robert B. "The American Medical Ethics Revolution." In *The American Medical Ethics Revolution*, edited by Robert B. Baker, Arthur L. Caplan, Linda L. Emanuel and Stephen R. Latham, 17–51. Baltimore: The Johns Hopkins University Press, 1999.

Baker, Robert B. "A National Code of Medical Ethics." In *Before Bioethics: A History of American Medical Ethics from the Colonial Period to the Bioethics Revolution* Oxford: Oxford University Press, 2014. www.oxfordscholarship.com.

Baker, Samuel L. "Physician Licensure Laws in the United States, 1865–1915." *Journal of the History of Medicine* 39 (1984): 173–97.

Baldasty, Gerald J. *E.W. Scripps and the Business of Newspapers.* Urbana and Chicago, IL: University of Illinois Press, 1999.

Bartlett, Elisha. *Essay on the Philosophy of Medical Science.* Philadelphia, PA: Lea & Blanchard, 1844.

Bartlett, Elisha. *The History Diagnosis and Treatment of Typhoid and of Typhus Fever; with an Essay on the Diagnosis of Bilious Remittent and of Yellow Fever.* Philadelphia, PA: Lea and Blanchard, 1842.

Beauchamp, T. L. "Internal and External Standards for Medical Morality." *J Med Philos* 26, no. 6 (Dec 2001): 601–19.

Beecher, C. H. "The Management of Congestive Heart Failure." *New England Journal of Medicine* 209, no. 24 (1933): 1226–28.

Berlant, Jeffry. *Profession and Monopoly: A Study of Medicine in the United States and Great Britain.* Berkeley: University of California Press, 1975.

Bladek, John David "'Virginia Is Middle Ground': The Know Nothing Party and the Virginia Gubernatorial Election of 1855." *The Virginia Magazine of History and Biography* 106, no. 1 (1998): 35–70.

Blake, John B. "From Buchan to Fishbein: The Literature of Domestic Medicine." In *Medicine Without Doctors—Home Health Care in American History,* edited by Gunter B; Numbers Risse, Ronald L; Leavitt, Judith Walker, 11–30. New York, NY: Science History Publications, 1977.

Blane, Sir Gilbert. *Elements of Medical Logick.* Second ed. London, UK: Thomas and George Underwood, 1821.

Blanton, Wyndham B. *Medicine in Virginia in the Nineteenth Century.* Richmond: Garrett & Massie Inc., 1933.

Bledstein, Burton J. *The Culture of Professionalism—The Middle Class and the Development of Higher Education in America.* New York, NY: W.W. Norton & Company, 1978.

Bloom, Khaled. *The Mississippi Valley's Great Yellow Fever Epidemic of 1878.* Baton Rouge, LA: Louisiana State University Press, 1993.

Blustein, Bonnie Ellen. *Preserve Your Love for Science—Life of William A. Hammond, American Neurologist.* Cambridge History of Medicine. Edited by Charles Webster and Charles Rosenberg Cambridge, UK: Cambridge University Press, 2002. 1991.

Blustein, Bonnie Ellen. "'To Increase the Efficiency of the Medical Department': A New Approach to U.S. Civil War Medicine." *Civil War History* 33, no. 1 (1987): 22–41.

Bollet, Alfred Jay. *Civil War Medicine—Challenges and Triumphs.* Tucson, AZ: Galen Press, 2002.

Bonner, Thomas Neville. *Iconoclast: Abraham Flexner and a Life in Learning.* Baltimore, MD: The Johns Hopkins University Press, 2002.

Boss, J. "The Medical Philosophy of Francis Bacon (1561–1626)." *Med Hypotheses* 4, no. 3 (May–June 1978): 208–20.

Bowditch, Henry I. *Public Hygiene in America.* Boston, MA: Little, Brown and Company, 1877.

Boyle, Eric W. *Quack Medicine—A History of Combating Health Fraud in Twentieth-Century America.* Santa Barbara: Praeger, 2013.

Bradford, Thomas Lindsley. *Homoeopathic Bibliography of the United States—From the Year 1825 to the Year 1891, Inclusive.* Philadelphia, PA: Boericke & Tafel, 1892.

Bradford, Thomas Lindsley. *The Life and Letters of Dr. Samuel Hahnemann.* Philadelphia: Boerickle & Tafel, 1895.

Brieger, Gert H. "American Surgery and the Germ Theory of Disease." *Bulletin of the History of Medicine* 40, no. 2 (1966): 135–45.

Brieger, Gert H. "Sanitary Reform in New York City: Stephen Smith and the Passage of the Metropolitan Health Bill." *Bulletin of the History of Medicine* 40, no. 5 (1966): 407–29.

Brieger, Gert. "Therapeutic Conflicts and the American Medical Profession in the 1860's." *Bulletin of the History of Medicine* 41, no. 3 (1967): 215–22.

Broussolle, E, F Gobert, T Danaila, S Thobois, O Walusinski, and J Bogousslavsky. "History of Physical and 'Moral' Treatment of Hysteria." *Frontiers of Neurology and Neuroscience* 35 (2014): 181–97.

Bryan, Charles S. "Discovery of the Yellow Fever Virus." *International Journal of Infectious Diseases* 2, no. 1 (1997): 52–54.

Budd, William. *Typhoid Fever—Its Nature, Mode of Spreading, and Prevention.* London, UK: Longmans, Green, and Company, 1873.

Burnham, John C. *Health Care in America: A History.* Baltimore, MD: Johns Hopkins University Press, 2015.

Byford, Wm H. *A Treatise on the Theory and Practice of Obstetrics.* New York, NY: William Wood & Co, 1870.

Bynum, W. F. *Science and the Practice of Medicine in the Nineteenth Century.* Cambridge, UK: Cambridge University Press, 1994.

Callahan, James Morton. *Genealogical and Personal History of the Upper Monongahela Valley—West Virginia.* Edited by Bernard L. Butcher3 vols. New York, NY: Lewis Historical Publishing Company, 1912.

Callahan, James Morton. *History of West Virginia Old and New and West Virginia Biography.* 3 vols. Vol. II-III, Chicago, IL: The American Historical Society, Inc., 1923.

Callahan, James Morton. *History of West Virginia Old and New and West Virginia Biography.* 3 vols. Vol. 2, Chicago, IL: The American Historical Society, Inc., 1923.

Callahan, James Morton. *History of West Virginia—Old and New.* 3 vols. Vol. 1, Chicago and New York: The American Historical Society, Inc., 1923.

Callahan, James Morton. *Semi-Centennial History of West Virginia.* Charleston, WV: Semi-Centennial Commission of West Virginia, 1913.

Camden, Thomas Bland. *My Recollections and Experiences of the Civil War or a Citizen of Weston During the Late Unpleasantness.* Parsons, WV: The Friends of the Louis Bennett Public Library, 2000.

Cannon, M. Hamlin "The United States Christian Commission." *The Mississippi Valley Historical Review* 38, no. 1 (1951): 61–80.

Cassedy, James H. "Edwin Miller Snow: An Important American Public Health Pioneer." *Bulletin of the History of Medicine* 35, no. 1 (1961): 156–62.

Cassedy, James H. "The Microscope in American Medical Science, 1840–1860." *Isis* 67, no. March (1976): 76–97.

Chapin, Charles V. "The Evolution of Preventive Medicine." *JAMA* 76, no. January 22, 1921 (1921): 215–22.

Chapin, Charles V. "History of State and Municipal Control of Disease." In *A Half Century of Public Health*, edited by Mazÿck Ravenel, 133–60. New York, NY: American Public Health Association, 1921.

Chesley, L. C. "History and Epidemiology of Preeclampsia-Eclampsia." *Clin Obstet Gynecol* 27, no. 4 (Dec 1984): 801–20.

Churchill, Fleetwood. *On the Theory and Practice of Midwifery.* Fifth ed. London, UK: Henry Renshaw, 1866.

Churchill, Fleetwood. *On the Theory and Practice of Midwifery.* Second ed. London, UK: Henry Renshaw, 1850.

Clarke, Edward H., Henry J. Bigelow, Samuel D. Gross, T. Gaillard Thomas, and John S. Billings. *A Century of American Medicine: 1776–1876.* Philadelphia: Henry C. Lea, 1876.

Clements, Alan N., and Ralph E. Harbach. "History of the Discovery of the Mode of Transmission of Yellow Fever Virus." *Journal of Vector Ecology* 42, no. 2 (2017): 208–22.

Cochran, Jerome. "The Medical Profession." Chap. 8 In *Memorial Record of Alabama—A Concise Account of the State's Political, Military, Professional and Industrial Progress, Together with the Personal Memoirs of Many of Its People*, edited by Unknown, 107–40. Madison, WI: Brant & Fuller, 1893.

Conard, Howard L. *Encyclopedia of the History of Missouri.* 6 vols. Vol. 4, New York: The Southern History Company, 1901.

Coulter, Harris L. *Divided Legacy; The Conflict Between Homoeopathy and the American Medical Association.* Second ed. Berkeley, CA: North Atlantic Books, 1982. 1973.

Cranmer, Gibson L. *History of Wheeling City and Ohio County, West Virginia and Representative Citizens.* Chicago, IL: Biographical Pub. Co., 1902.

Cranmer, Gibson L. "Upper Ohio Valley." In *History of the Upper Ohio Valley*, edited by Gibson L Cranmer. Madison, WI: Brant & Fuller, 1890.

Cunningham, Horace Herndon. *Doctors in Gray—The Confederate Medical Service.* Gloucester, MA: Peter Smith, 1970. 1958.

Curran, Thomas J. *Xenophobia and Immigration, 1820–1930.* Woodbridge CT: Twayne Publishers, 1975.

Currie, David P. "The Constitution in the Supreme Court: The Protection of Economic Interests, 1889–1910." *The University of Chicago Law Review* 52, no. 2 (1985): 324–88.

Curry, Richard Orr. "Crisis Politics in West Virginia, 1861–1870." Chap. 3 In *Radicalism, Racism, and Party Alignment: The Border States During Reconstruction*, edited by Richard Orr Curry, 80–104. Baltimore, MD: The Johns Hopkins Press, 1969.

Curry, Richard Orr. *A House Divided—A Study of Statehood Politics and the Copperhead Movement in West Virginia.* Pittsburgh, PA: University of Pittsburgh Press, 1964.

Dabney, Virginius. *Virginia—The New Dominion: A History from 1607 to the Present.* Charlottesville, VA: University Press of Virginia, 1971.

Danforth, I.N. *The Life of Nathan Smith Davis.* Chicago, IL: Cleveland Press, 1907.

Darlington, Thomas. "The Present Status of the Midwife." *American Journal of Obstetrics and Diseases of Women and Children* 63, no. 5 (1911): 870–76.

Davenport, Charles B. "Biographical Memoir of Frederick Augustus Porter Barnard: 1809–1889." In *Biographical Memoirs of the National Academy of Sciences*, edited by Unknown Washington, D.C.: National Academy of Sciences, 1938. http://www.nasonline.org/publications/biographical-memoirs/.

Davenport, F. Garvin. "John Henry Rauch and Public Health in Illinois 1877–1891." *Journal of the Illinois State Historical Society* 50, no. 3 (1957): 277–94.

Davico, Rosalba, ed. *The Autobiography of Edward Jarvis (1803–1884)*, Medical History Supplement Number 12. London, UK: Wellcome Institute for the History of Medicine, 1992.

Davis, Nathan S. *History of the American Medical Association from Its Organization up to January, 1855.* Philadelphia: Lippincott, Grambo and Company, 1855.

Davis, N.S. *History of Medical Education and Institutions in the United States.* Chicago, IL: S.C. Griggs & Company, 1851.

Dayton, Ruth Woods. *Samuel Woods and His Family.* Charleston, WV: Hood-Heserman-Brodhag Company, 1939.

"Death of Carl Pfeiffer, Architect." *The American Architect and Building News* 23, no. 648 (May 26, 1888): 241.

Dennehy, Cathi E., and Candy Tsourounis. "Dietary Supplements & Herbal Medications." Chap. 64 In *Basic and Clinical Pharmacology,* edited by Bertram G. Katzung and Anthony J. Trevor. New York, NY: McGraw-Hill Medical, 2015.

Dent, M.H. *Transcript of Argument in Behalf of Appellant at __, State V. Dent, 25 W.Va. 1 (1884).* Supreme Court Records & Briefs. Edited by Supreme Court of Appeals State of West Virginia Vol. 1 - Fall Special Term 1884, Charleston, WV: Supreme Court of Appeals State of West Virginia, 1884.

Desborough, M. J. R., and D. M. Keeling. "The Aspirin Story—From Willow to Wonder Drug." *Br J Haematol* 177, no. 5 (Jun 2017): 674–83.

Devine, Shauna. *Learning from the Wounded—The Civil War and the Rise of American Medical Science* Civil War America. Edited by Gary W. Gallagher, Peter S. Carmichael, Caroline E. Janney and Sheehan-Dean Aaron Chapel Hill, NC: The University of North Carolina Press, 2014.

Dewees, William P. *A Compendious System of Midwifery.* 12th ed. Philadelphia, PA: Blanchard and Lea, 1853.

Dicke, Willemijn, and Martin Albrow. "Reconstituting the Public-Private Divide under Global Conditions." *Global Social Policy* 5, no. 2 (2011): 227–48.

Dolin, Gregory. "Licensing Health Care Professionals: Has the United States Outlived the Need for Medical Licensure?." *The Georgetown Journal of Law and Public Policy* 2, no. 2 (2004): 315–36.

Douglas, George H. *The Golden Age of the Newspaper.* Westport, CT: Greenwood Press, 1999.

Dudley, P.H. "The Inception and Progress of Railways." *Transactions of the New York Academy of Science* 5 (1886): 137–51.

Duffin, Jacalyn. *To See with a Better Eye: A Life of R. T. H. Laennec.* Princeton, NJ: Princeton University Press, 1998.

Duffin, Jacalyn, and Pierre Rene. "'Anti-Moine; Anti-Biotique': The Public Fortunes of the Secret Properties of Antimony Potassium Tartrate (Tartar Emetic)." *Journal of the History of Medicine and Allied Sciences* 46, no. 4 (1991): 440–56.

Duffy, John. "The American Medical Profession and Public Health: From Support to Ambivalence." *Bulletin of the History of Medicine* 53, no. 1 (1979): 1–22.

Duffy, John. *The Sanitarians—A History of American Public Health.* Urbana, IL: University of Illinois Press, 1992.

Dunglison, Robely. *Medical Lexicon: A New Dictionary of Medical Science, Containing a Concise Account of the Various Subjects and Terms.* Second ed. Philadelphia, PA: Lea and Blanchard, 1839.

Dunglison, Robely, ed. *The Cyclopaedia of Practical Medicine.* 4 vols. Vol. 1. Philadelphia, PA: Lea & Blanchard, 1845.

Dunnington, George A. *History and Progress of the County of Marion, West Virginia: From Its Earliest Settlement by the Whites Down to the Present, Together with Biographical Sketches of Its Most Prominent Citizens.* Fairmont, WV: George A. Dunnington, 1880.

Dyer, Frederick H. *A Compendium of the War of the Rebellion.* Des Moines, IA: Dyer Publishing Company, 1908.

Ernst, Edzard. *Homeopathy: The Undiluted Facts.* Basel, Switzerland: Springer, 2016.

Ethics, AMA Committee on Medical. *Code of Medical Ethics of the American Medical Association.* Chicago: American Medical Association Press, 1847.

Evans, Alfred S. "Causation and Disease: The Henle-Koch Postulates Revisited." *Yale J Biol Med* 49, no. 2 (1976): 175–95.

Faber, Doris. *Printer's Devil to Publisher: Adolph S. Ochs of the New York Times.* Hensonville, NY: Black Dome Press, 1996. 1963.

Fairlie, Margaret C. "The Yellow Fever Epidemic of 1888 in Jacksonville." *The Florida Historical Quarterly* 19, no. 2 (1940): 95–108.

Feldman, Mark, Lawrence S. Friedman, and Lawrence J. Brandt, eds. *Sleisenger and Fordtran's Gastrointestinal and Liver Disease.* Tenth ed. Philadelphia, PA: Saunders, 2016.

Felts, J. H. "Henry Ingersoll Bowditch and Oliver Wendell Holmes: Stethoscopists and Reformers." *Perspect Biol Med* 45, no. 4 (Fall 2002): 539–48.

Fleming, Walter L. *Civil War and Reconstruction in Alabama.* New York: Columbia University Press,, 1905.

Flint, Austin. *Clinical Reports on Continued Fever Based on Analyses of One Hundred and Sixty-Four Cases.* Philadelphia, PA: Lindsay & Blakiston, 1855.

Flint, Austin. *A Treatise on the Principles and Practice of Medicine.* Fifth ed. Philadelphia, PA: Henry C. Lea's Son & Co., 1881.

Flint, Austin. *A Treatise on the Principles and Practice of Medicine; Designed for the Use of Practitioners and Students of Medicine.* Philadelphia, PA: Henry C. Lea, 1873.

Flint, Austin. *A Treatise on the Principles and Practice of Medicine—With an Appendix on the Researches of Koch and Their Bearing on the Etiology, Pathology, Diagnosis, Prognosis, and Treatment of Pulmonary Phthisis.* Fifth ed. Philadelphia, PA: Henry C. Lea's Son & Co., 1884.

Foulon, Irenaeus D. "Who Are Physicians before the Law?." *The Clinical Reporter* 2, no. 2 (1889): 29–34.

Fox, Henry J., and W. B. Hoyt. *Fox and Hoyt's Quadrennial Register of the Methodist Episcopal Church and Universal Church Gazetteer: 1852–1856.* Hartford, CT: Case, Tiffany, & Co., 1852.

Fox, William L. *Regimental Losses in the American Civil War: 1861–1865.* Albany, NY: Albany Publishing Company, 1889.

Frampton, Sally. "Defining Difference: Competing Forms of Ovarian Surgery in the Nineteenth Century." Chap. 3 In *Technological Change in Modern Surgery: Historical Perspectives on Innovation,* edited by Thomas Schlich and Christopher Crenner, 51–70. Rochester, NY: University of Rochester Press, 2017.

Freemon, Frank R. "Lincoln Finds a Surgeon General: William A. Hammond and the Transformation of the Union Army Medical Bureau." *Civil War History* 33, no. 1 (1987): 5–21.

Gage, Simon Henry. "Microscopy in America (1830–1945)." *Transactions of the American Microscopical Society* 83, no. 4 (Supplement) (1964): 1–125.

Garceau, Oliver. *The Political Life of the American Medical Association.* Hamden, CT: Archon Books, 1961.

Gariepy, Thomas P. "The Introduction and Acceptance of Listerian Antisepsis in the United States." *Journal of the History of Medicine and Allied Sciences,* 49, no. 2 (1994): 167–206.

Gerhard, W.W. "On the Typhus Fever, Which Occurred at Philadelphia in the Spring and Summer of 1836; Illustrated by Clinical Observations at the Philadelphia Hospital; Showing the Distinction between This Form of Disease and Dothinenteritis or the Typhoid Fever with Alteration of the Follicles of the Small Intestine. Part 1." *The American Journal of the Medical Sciences* 38, no. February 1837 (1837): 289–322.

Goen, C.C. *Broken Churches, Broken Nation—Denominational Schisms and the Coming of the American Civil War.* Macon, GA: Mercer University Press, 1985.

Going, Allen Johnston. *Bourbon Democracy in Alabama, 1874–1890.* Tuscaloosa, AL: University Alabama Press, 1992. 1951.

Golden, William W "The Evolution of Medical Legislation in West Virginia." *The West Virginia Medical Journal* 12, no. 10 (1918): 361–70.

Gooden, Randall Scott. "The Completion of a Revolution: West Virginia from Statehood through Reconstruction." University of West Virginia, 1995.

Goodman, Louis S., and Alfred Gilman. *The Pharmacological Basis of Therapeutics.* New York, NY: The Macmillan Company, 1955.

Gorham, Frederick P. "The History of Bacteriology and Its Contribution to Public Health Work." In *A Half Century of Public Health,* edited by Mazÿck Ravenel, 66–93. New York, NY: American Public Health Association, 1921.

Grant, J. A. C. "The Gild Returns to America 1 & 2." *The Journal of Politics* 4, no. 3 & 4 (1942): 303–36, 458–77.

Greve, Charles Theodore. *Centennial History of Cincinnati and Representative Citizens.* Vol. II, Chicago: Biographical Publishing Company, 1904.

Gross, Samuel D. *Autobiography of Samuel D. Gross, M.D.* Vol. II, Philadelphia: George Barrie, 1887.

Hahnemann, Samuel. *Materia Medica Pura.* Translated by Charles Julius Hempel. First ed. New York, NY: William Radde, 1846. 1811.

Hahnemann, Samuel. *Organon Der Rationellen Heilkunde.* Dresden: Arnoldischen Buchandlung, 1810.

Hahnemann, Samuel. *Organon of the Rational Art of Healing—Translated from the First Edition.* Translated by C.E. Wheeler. Everyman's Library—Science. Edited by Ernest Rhys London, UK: J.M. Dent & Sons, Ltd., 1913.

Hall, Courtney R. "Jefferson on the Medical Theory and Practice of His Day." *Bulletin of the History of Medicine* 37, no. January 1, 1957 (1957): 235–45.

Haller, John S., Jr. *American Medicine in Transition, 1840–1910.* Urbana, IL: University of Illinois Press, 1981.

Haller, John S., Jr. *The History of American Homeopathy: The Academic Years, 1820–1935.* New York, NY: Pharmaceutical Products Press, 2005.

Haller, John S., Jr. *The People's Doctors—Samuel Thomson and the American Botanical Movement, 1790–1860.* Carbondale, IL: Southern Illinois University Press, 2000.

Hammond, William A. *A Treatise on Hygiene: With Special Reference to the Military Service.* Philadelphia, PA: J. B. Lippincott & Co., 1863.

Hamowy, Ronald. "The Early Development of Medical Licensing Laws in the United States, 1875–1900." *Journal of Libertarian Studies* 3, no. 1 (1979): 73–119.

Hansell, Howard F. "George Milbry Gould, A.M., M.D." *Transactions of the American Ophthalmological Society* 21 (1923): 14–20.

Harris, J. M., Jr. "It Is Time to Cancel Medicine's Social Contract Metaphor." *Acad Med* 92, no. 9 (2017): 1236–40.

Harris, J. M., Jr. "James Edmund Reeves. 1883." *Am J Public Health* 104, no. 3 (Mar 2014): 417.

Harris, John M. "James Edmund Reeves (1829–1896) and the Contentious 19th Century Battle for Medical Professionalism in the United States." *Journal of Medical Biography* (May 15, 2014).

Harris John M., Jr. "Medical Ethics, Methodism, and a Nineteenth Century West Virginian's Battles with Quackery." *West Virginia History* 9, no. Spring (2016): 27–44.

Harris John M., Jr., and Lynette Reid. "In Reply to Cruess Et Al." *Acad Med* 92, no. 12 (2017): 1650–51.

Hatcher, Robert A., and Martin I. Wilbert. *The Pharmacopeia and the Physician.* Chicago, IL: American Medical Association Press, 1906.

Health, Committee for the Study of the Future of Public. *The Future of Public Health.* Washington, D.C.: National Academy Press, 1988.

Heitzenrater, Richard P. *Wesley and the People Called Methodists.* Second ed. Nashville, TN: Abingdon Press. 1995.

Henry (Editor), Frederick P. *Standard History of the Medical Profession of Philadelphia.* Chicago, IL: Goodspeed Brothers, 1897.

Hirschhorn, Norbert, Robert G. Feldman, and Ian Greaves. "Abraham Lincoln's Blue Pills: Did Our 16th President Suffer from Mercury Poisoning?" *Perspectives in Biology and Medicine* 44, no. 3 (2001): 315–32.

Hiss, A. Emil. *Thesaurus of Proprietary Preparations and Pharmaceutical Specialties.* Chicago, IL: G.P. Engelhard & Company, 1898.

Hogshead, Norma S. *Past Presidents of the West Virginia State Medical Association: 1867–1942.* Charleston, WV: Auxiliary to the West Virginia State Medical Association, 1942.

Holt, Michael F. *The Rise and Fall of the American Whig Party: Jacksonian Politics and the Onset of the Civil War.* Oxford, UK: Oxford University Press, 1999.

Holzhey, Helmut, and Vilem Mudroch. *Historical Dictionary of Kant and Kantianism.* Historical Dictionaries of Religions Philosophies, and Movements. Vol. 60, Lanham, MD: Scarecrow Press, 2005.

Home, Everard, ed. *A Treatise on the Blood, Inflammation, and Gun-Shot Wounds by the Late John Hunter.* London, UK: John Richardson, 1794.

Horowitz, Ruth. *In the Public Interest—Medical Licensing and the Disciplinary Process.* New Brunswick, NJ: Rutgers University Press, 2013.

Hughes, Richard IV, Korisha Ramdhanie, Travis Wasserman, and Travis Moscettie. "State Boards of Health: Governance and Politics." *Journal of Law, Medicine, and Ethics* 39, no. Supplement (Spring) (2011): 37–41.

Humphreys, Margaret. *Marrow of Tragedy—The Health Crisis of the American Civil War.* Baltimore, MD: The Johns Hopkins University Press, 2013.

Hunt, Gaillard, ed. *The First Forty Years of Washington Society Portrayed by the Family Letters of Mrs. Samuel Harrison Smith.* New York, NY: Charles Scribner's Sons, 1906.

Huntington, Elisha. *An Address on the Life, Character, and Writings of Elisha Bartlett, M.D., M.M.S.S.* Lowell, MA: Middlesex North District Medical Society, 1856.

Illinois, State Board of Health of. *Annual Report of the State Board of Health of Illinois Made to the Governor 1878.* Springfield, IL: Weber, Magie & Co., 1879.

"Improved Rail-Road Cars." *Scientific American* 1, no. 1 (1845): 1.

Ioannidis, J. P. "Why Most Published Research Findings Are False." *PLoS Med* 2, no. 8 (Aug 2005): e124.

Jameson, Edwin M. *Clio Medica—Gynecology and Obstetrics.* New York, NY: Hafner Publishing Company, 1962. 1962. 1936.

Jenner, Edward. *An Inquiry into the Causes and Effects of the Variola Vaccine.* London, UK: Sampson Low, 1798.

Jepson, Samuel. "The Healing Arts in the Pan-Handle." Chap. 18 In *History of the Upper Ohio Valley,* edited by Gibson L Cranmer, 563–93. Madison, WI: Brant & Fuller, 1890.

Jiwa, M. "Doctors and Medical Science." *Australas Med J* 5, no. 8 (2012): 462–7.

Jobe, Abraham. *A Mountaineer in Motion—The Memoir of Dr. Abraham Jobe 1817–1906.* Edited by David C. Hsuing Knoxville, TN: The University of Tennessee Press, 2009.

Jones, Alan Wayne. "Early Drug Discovery and the Rise of Pharmaceutical Chemistry." *Drug Testing and Analysis* 3 (2011): 337–44.

Jones, Gordon. "Obstetrical Practice in Civil War Times." *JAMA* 184, no. 5 (1963): 254–61.

Jones, Russell M. "American Doctors and the Parisian Medical World, 1830–1840: Part 1." *Bulletin of the History of Medicine* 47, no. 1 (1973): 40–65.

Jones, Russell M. "American Doctors and the Parisian Medical World, 1830–1840: Part 2." *American Doctors and the Parisian Medical World, 1830–1840: Part 1* 47, no. 2 (1973): 177–204.

Jonsen, Albert R. *A Short History of Medical Ethics.* New York, NY: Oxford University Press, 2000.

Kelly, Howard A. *A Cyclopedia of American Medical Biography.* 2 vols. Vol. II, Philadelphia, PA: W. B. Saunders Co, 1912.

Kelly, Howard A., and Walter L. Burrage. *American Medical Biographies.* Baltimore, MD: The Norman, Remington Company, 1920.

Kelly, Howard A., and Walter L. Burrage. *Dictionary of American Medical Biography.* New York, NY: D. Appleton and Company, 1928.

Kendall, Norman F. *Mothers Day—A History of Its Founding and Its Founder.* Grafton, WV: D. Grant Smith, 1937.

King, Lester S. "Medical Logic." *Journal of the History of Medicine and Allied Sciences* 33, no. 3 (1978): 377–85.

King, Lester S. *Transformations in American Medicine.* Baltimore, MD: The Johns Hopkins University Press, 1991.

King, Lester S. "XIX. Medical Education: The Decade of Massive Change." *JAMA* 251, no. 2 (1984): 219–24.

Kramer, Howard D. "Effect of the Civil War on the Public Health Movement." *The Mississippi Valley Historical Review* 35, no. 3 (1948): 449–62.

Kuvandik, C., I. Karaoglan, M. Namiduru, and I. Baydar. "Predictive Value of Clinical and Laboratory Findings in the Diagnosis of the Enteric Fever." *New Microbiol* 32, no. 1 (Jan 2009): 25–30.

Laennec, René-Théophile-Hyacinthe. *A Treatise on the Diseases of the Chest.* Translated by John Forbes. London: T. and G. Underwood, 1821.

Lamon, Lester C. *Blacks in Tennessee: 1791–1970.* Knoxville, TN: The University of Tennessee Press, 1981.

Leake, C. D. "Theories of Ethics and Medical Practice." *JAMA* 208, no. 5 (May 5, 1969): 842–7.

Leech, P.N. "Listerine—Report of Chemical and Bacteriologic Investigations." *JAMA* 96, no. 16 (1931): 1303–6.

Lesser, W. Hunter. *Rebels at the Gate—Lee and McClellan on the Front Line of a Nation Divided.* Naperville, IL: Sourcebooks, Inc., 2004.

Lewis, Ronald L. *Transforming the Appalachian Countryside.* Chapel Hill, NC: The University of North Carolina Press, 1998.

Liebenau, Jonathan. *Medical Science and Medical Industry: The Formation of the American Pharmaceutical Industry.* Baltimore, MD: The Johns Hopkins University Press, 1987.

Lind, James. *A Treatise on the Scurvy.* Second ed. London, UK: A Millar, 1757.

Lister, Joseph. "Illustrations of the Antiseptic System of Treatment in Surgery." *The Lancet* 90, no. 2309 (November 30, 1867): 668–69.

Lister, Joseph. "On a New Method of Treating Compound Fracture, Abscesses, Etc.—With Observations on the Conditions of Suppuration." *The Lancet* 89, no. 2273 (March 23, 1867): 326–29.

Livingood, James W. "Chattanooga's Medical Schools." Chap. 8 in *Centennial History—Chattanooga and Hamilton County Medical Society: The Profession and Its Community,* 45–51. Chattanooga, TN: Chattanooga and Hamilton County Medical Society, Inc., 1983.

Long, Esmond R. *A History of American Pathology.* Springfield, IL: Charles C Thomas, 1962.

Lord, Charles G., Lee Ross, and Mark R. Lepper. "Biased Assimilation and Attitude Polarization: The Effects of Prior Theories on Subsequently Considered Evidence." *Journal of Personality and Social Psychology* 37, no. 11 (1979): 2098–109.

Louis, Pierre-Charles-Alexandre. *Anatomical, Pathological and Therapeutic Researches Upon the Disease Known Under the Name of Gastro-Enterite, Putrid, Adynamic, Ataxic, or Typhoid Fever, Etc.: Compared with the Most Common Acute Diseases.* Translated by Henry I. Bowditch. 2 vols. Boston, MA: Isaac R. Butts, Hilliard Gray & Co., 1836.

Louis, Pierre-Charles-Alexandre. *Researches on the Effects of Bloodletting in Some Inflammatory Diseases.* Translated by C.G. Putnam. Boston, MA: Hilliard, Gray, & Company, 1836.

Loving, David A. "The Development of American Public Health, 1850–1925." University of Oklahoma, 2008.

Ludlum, David M. *The Weather Factor.* Boston, MA: American Meteorological Society, 1989. 1984.

Macdonald, Keith M. *The Sociology of the Professions* London, UK: Sage Publications, 1999. 1995.

Malkin, Harold M. "The Trials and Tribulations of George Miller Sternberg: (1838–1915)—America's First Bacteriologist." *Perspectives in Biology and Medicine* 36, no. 4 (1993): 666–78.

Marks, Harry M. *The Progress of Experiment: Science and Therapeutic Reform in the United States, 1900–1990.* Cambridge: Cambridge University Press, 1997.

Mataja, Victor. "The Economic Value of Advertising." *The International Quarterly* 8, no. December–March (1904): 379–98.

Mattaliano, Jane K., and Lois G. Omonde. *Milestones: A Pictorial History of Philippi, West Virginia, 1844–1994*. Virginia Beach, VA: The Donning Company, 1994.

Matthews, Douglas R. "American Defamation Law: From Sullivan, Through Greenmoss, and Beyond." *Ohio State Law Journal* 48, no. 2 (1987): 513–32.

Maxwell, Hu. *The History of Barbour County, West Virginia*. Parsons, WV: McClain Printing Company, 1968. 1968. 1899.

McCullough, David. *The Greater Journey—Americans in Paris*. New York, NY: Simon & Schuster, 2011.

McGuffey (Editor), Charles D. *Standard History of Chattanooga Tennessee*. Knoxville: Crew and Dorey, 1911.

McPherson, James M. *Battle Cry of Freedom—The Civil War Era*. The Oxford History of the United States. Edited by C. Vann Woodward. 11+ vols. Vol. 6, Oxford, UK: Oxford University Press, 1988.

Medicine, ABIM Foundation. American Board of Internal, ACP-ASIM Foundation. American College of Physicians-American Society of Internal Medicine, and Medicine European Federation of Internal. "Medical Professionalism in the New Millennium: A Physician Charter." *Ann Intern Med* 136, no. 3 (Feb 5, 2002): 243–6.

Meigs, Charles D. *Obstetrics—The Science and the Art*. Second ed. Philadelphia, PA: Blanchard and Lea, 1852. 1849.

Meyer, Balthasar Henry ed. *History of Transportation in the United States Before 1860*. Washington, D.C.: Carnegie Institution of Washington, 1917.

Michael, Jerrold M. "The National Board of Health: 1879–1883." *Public Health Reports* 126, no. January/February (2011): 123–29.

Millard, Candice. *Destiny of the Republic*. New York: Doubleday, 2011.

Miller, Thomas Condit, and Hu Maxwell. *West Virginia and Its People*. 3 vols. Vol. 1, New York, NY: Lewis Historical Publishing Company, 1913.

Mohr, James C. *Doctors & the Law: Medical Jurisprudence in Nineteenth-Century America*. New York, NY: Oxford University Press, 1993.

Mohr, James C. *Licensed to Practice—The Supreme Court Defines the American Medical Profession*. Baltimore, MD: The Johns Hopkins University Press, 2013.

Mohr, James C. *The Radical Republicans and Reform in New York During Reconstruction*. Ithaca, NY: Cornell University Press, 1973.

Moore, Wendy. *The Knife Man: Blood, Body Snatching, and the Birth of Modern Surgery*. New York, NY: Broadway Books, 2005.

Morabia, A. "P. C. A. Louis and the Birth of Clinical Epidemiology." *J Clin Epidemiol* 49, no. 12 (Dec 1996): 1327–33.

Morgenstern, Leon. "Gargling with Lister." *Journal of the American College of Surgeons* 204, no. 3 (2007): 495–97.

Morris, Malcolm. "Transactions." British Congress on Tuberculosis for the Prevention of Consumption, London, UK, 1902.

Newton, J. H., G. G. Nichols, and A. G. Sprankle. *History of the Pan-Handle; Being Historical Collections of the Counties of Ohio, Brooke, Marshall and Hancock, West Virginia*. Wheeling: J.A. Caldwell, 1879.

Novak, William J. *The People's Welfare: Law and Regulation in Nineteenth-Century America*. Chapel Hill, NC: The University of North Carolina Press, 1996.

Novotny, Patrick. *The Press in American Politics, 1787–201*. Santa Barbara, CA: Praeger, 2014.

Numbers, Ronald L. "Do-It-Yourself the Sectarian Way." In *Medicine Without Doctors*, edited by Gunter B; Numbers Risse, Ronald L; Leavitt, Judith Walker, 49–72. New York, NY: Science History Publications, 1977.

O'Connor, Bob. *The Amazing Legacy of James E. Hanger, Civil War Soldier*. West Conshocken, PA: Infinity Publishing, 2014.

Ong, S. "Pre-Eclampsia: A Historical Perspective." In *Pre-Eclampsia : Current Perspectives on Management*, edited by Philip Baker and John Kingdom. Boca Raton, FL: CRC Press, 2004.

Osler, William. "Elisha Bartlett—A Rhode Island Philosopher." In *An Alabama Student and Other Biographical Essays*, 108–58. London: Oxford University Press, 1929. Reprint, 1929.

Osler, William. *The Evolution of Modern Medicine—A Series of Lectures Delivered at Yale University on the Silliman Foundation in April, 1913*. New Haven, CT: Yale University Press, 1921.

Osler, William. *The Principles and Practice of Medicine—Designed for the Use of Practitioners and Students of Medicine*. New York: D. Appleton and Company, 1892.

Osler, William. *The Problem of Typhoid Fever in the United States*. Baltimore, MD: John Murphy Company, 1899.

Otis, George A. *The Medical and Surgical History of the War of Rebellion—Surgical History*. The Medical and Surgical History of the War of Rebellion. Edited by Joseph K. Barnes 2 vols. Vol. 2—Part 1, Washington, D.C.: Government Printing Office, 1870.

Otis, George A. *The Medical and Surgical History of the War of Rebellion—Surgical History*. The Medical and Surgical History of the War of Rebellion. Edited by Joseph K. Barnes 2 vols. Vol. 2—Part 2, Washington, D.C.: Government Printing Office, 1877.

Otis, George A., and D.L. Huntington. *The Medical and Surgical History of the War of Rebellion—Surgical History.* The Medical and Surgical History of the War of Rebellion. Edited by Joseph K. Barnes2 vols. Vol. 2 - Part 3, Washington, D.C.: Government Printing Office, 1883.

Ott, Katherine. *Fevered Lives: Tuberculosis in American Culture since 1870.* Cambridge, MA: Harvard University Press, 1996.

Parker, Granville. *The Formation of the State of West Virginia and Other Incidents of the Late Civil War.* Wellsburg, WV: Glass & Son, Book and Job Printers, 1875.

Parry, C. M., T. T. Hien, G. Dougan, N. J. White, and J. J. Farrar. "Typhoid Fever." *N Engl J Med* 347, no. 22 (Nov 28, 2002): 1770–82.

Paulson, George W. *James Fairchild Baldwin, M.D.—An Extraordinary Surgeon.* Columbus, OH: Medical Heritage Center, 2005.

Peitzman, Steven J. "'I Am Their Physician': Dr. Owen J. Wister of Germantown and His Too Many Patients." *Bulletin of the History of Medicine* 83, no. 2 (2009): 245–70.

Percival, Thomas. *Medical Ethics or a Code of Institutes and Precepts, Adapted to the Professional Conduct of Physicians and Surgeons.* London: S. Johnson, St. Paul's Church Yard and R. Bickerstaff, 1803.

Peters, DeWitt Clinton. *The Life and Adventures of Kit Carson—The Nestor of the Rocky Mountains from Facts Narrated by Himself.* New York, NY: W. R. C. Clark & Co., 1858.

Philip, Robert. "An Address on Koch's Discovery of the Tubercle Bacillus—Some of Its Implications and Results." *BMJ* 3, no. 3730 (1932): 1–5.

Pickering, H.G. "Appendix IV - Digest of American Sanitary Law." In *Public Hygiene in America: Centennial Discourse on Public Hygiene and State Preventive Medicine,* edited by Henry I. Bowditch, 299–440. Boston, MA: Little, Brown, and Company, 1876.

Porter, Roy. *The Greatest Benefit to Mankind—A Medical History of Humanity.* NY, NY: W.W. Norton and Company, 1997.

Porwancher, Andrew. "Objectivity's Prophet: Adolph S. Ochs and the *New York Times*, 1896–1935." *Journalism History* 36, no. 4 (2011): 186–95.

Potter, David M. *The Impending Crisis : 1848–1861.* New York, NY: Harper & Row, 1976.

Quinn, Kate. "A Heinous Offence." *Upper Ohio Valley Historical Review* 30, no. 1 (2007): 3–8.

Ramsbotham, Francis H. *The Principles and Practice of Obstetric Medicine and Surgery.* London, UK: John Churchill, 1856.

Rankin, Stephen W. "Wesley and War: Guidance for Modern Day Heirs?" *Methodist Review* 3 (2011): 101–39.

Ratner, Lorman A., Paula T. Kaufman, and Dwight L. Teeter Jr. *Paradoxes of Prosperity: Wealth-Seeking Versus Christian Values in Pre-Civil War America.* Urbana, IL: University of Illinois Press, 2009.

Ravenel, Mazÿck. "The American Public Health Association: Past, Present, and Future." In *A Half Century of Public Health,* edited by Mazÿck Ravenel, 13–55. New York, NY: American Public Health Association, 1921.

Ravina, Enrique. *The Evolution of Drug Discovery.* Weinheim, FRG: Wiley-VCH, 2011.

Rawlings, Isaac D. *The Rise and Fall of Disease in Illinois.* Springfield, IL: The State Department of Public Health, 1927.

Redford, A.H. *History of the Organization of the Methodist Episcopal Church South.* Nashville, TN: Methodist Episcopal Church South, 1871.

Reeves, James E. *Hand-Book of Medical Microscopy.* Philadelphia, PA: P. Blakiston, Son & Co., 1894.

Reeves, James E. *The Health and Wealth of the City of Wheeling—Including Its Physical and Medical Topography; Also General Remarks on the Natural Resources of West Virginia.* Baltimore: The Sun Book and Job Office, 1871.

Reeves, James E. *How to Work with the Bausch & Lomb Optical Company's Microtome and a Method of Demonstrating the Tubercle-Bacillus.* Rochester, NY: Bausch & Lomb Optical Company, 1886.

Reeves, James E. *The Physical and Medical Topography, Including Vital, Manufacturing and Other Statistics of the City of Wheeling.* Wheeling: Daily Register Book and Job Office, 1870.

Reeves, James E. *A Practical Treatise on Enteric Fever; Its Diagnosis and Treatment: Being an Analysis of One Hundred and Thirty Consecutive Cases Derived from Private Practice and Embracing a Partial History of the Disease in Virginia.* Philadelphia, PA: J. B. Lippincott & Co., 1859.

Reeves, James Edmund. "The Eminent Domain of Sanitary Science, and the Usefulness of State Boards of Health in Guarding the Public Welfare." *JAMA* 1, no. 21 (1883): 612–18.

Reid, John Phillip. *An American Judge—Marmaduke Dent of West Virginia.* New York, NY: New York University Press, 1968.

Reid, Whitelaw. *Ohio in the War—Her Statesmen, Soldiers, and Generals.* 2 vols. Vol. 1, Columbus, OH: Eclectic Publishing Company, 1893.

Reynolds, Arthur R. "Three Chicago and Illinois Public Health Officers: John H. Rauch, Oscar C. De Wolf, and Frank W. Reilly." *Bulletin of the Society of Medical History of Chicago* 1, no. 2 (1911): 89–108.

Rice, Otis K. *West Virginia: A History.* Lexington, KY: The University Press of Kentucky, 1985.

Rice, Otis K., and Stephen W. Brown. *West Virginia: A History.* Lexington, KY: The University Press of Kentucky, 1985.

Rice, Philip Morrison "The Know-Nothing Party in Virginia, 1854–1856 (Concluded)." *The Virginia Magazine of History and Biography* 55, no. 2 (1947): 159–67.

Richmond, Phyllis A. "Glossary of Historical Fever Terminology." *Journal of the History of Medicine:* 16, no. 1 (1961): 76–77.

Richmond, Phyllis Allen. "American Attitudes toward the Germ Theory of Disease (1860–1880)." *Journal of the History of Medicine and Allied Sciences* 9, no. 4 (1954): 428–54.

Riley, James C. *Rising Life Expectancy: A Global History.* Cambridge, UK: Cambridge University Press, 2001.

Rogal, S. J. "Pills for the Poor: John Wesley's Primitive Physick." *Yale J Biol Med* 51, no. 1 (Jan–Feb 1978): 81–90.

Rogers, Everett M. *Diffusion of Innovations.* New York, NY: Free Press, 2003. 1962.

Rolleston, J. D. "F. J. V. Broussais (1772–1838): His Life and Doctrines: (Section of the History of Medicine)." *Proc R Soc Med* 32, no. 5 (Mar 1939): 405–13.

Rolt, L.T.C. *George & Robert Stephenson—The Railway Revolution.* Westport, CT: Greenwood Press, 1977. 1960.

Rosen, George. *Fees and Fee Bills: Some Economic Aspects of Medical Practice in Nineteenth Century America* Supplement 6 to the Bulletin of the History of Medicine. Edited by Henry E. Sigerist Baltimore: Johns Hopkins University Press, 1946.

Rosen, George. *A History of Public Health—Expanded Edition.* Second ed. Baltimore, MD: The Johns Hopkins University Press, 1993. 1958.

Rosenbaum, L. "Resisting the Suppression of Science." *N Engl J Med* 376, no. 17 (Apr 27 2017): 1607–9.

Rosenberg, Charles E. "The Therapeutic Revolution: Medicine, Meaning and Social Change in Nineteenth Century America." *Perspectives in Biology and Medicine* 20, no. 4 (1977): 485–506.

Rosenburg, Charles E. "'The Fielding H. Garrison Lecture': Medical Text and Social Context: Explaining William Buchan's *Domestic Medicine.*" *Bulletin of the History of Medicine* 57, no. Spring (1983): 22–42.

Rosenkrantz, Barbara Gutmann. "Cart before Horse: Theory, Practice and Professional Image in American Public Health,1870–1920." *Journal of the History of Medicine and Allied Sciences* 29, no. 1 (1974): 55–73.

Rothstein, William G. *American Physicians in the 19th Century—From Sects to Science.* Baltimore, MD: Johns Hopkins University Press, 1992.

Rush, Benjamin. *Medical Inquiries and Observations.* Vol. 4, Philadelphia: Thomas Dobson, 1796.

Rush, Benjamin. *Sixteen Introductory Lectures.* Philadelphia, PA: Bradford and Innskeep, 1811.

Sakula, Alex. "Robert Koch: Centenary of the Discovery of the Tubercle Bacillus, 1882." *Thorax* 37, no. 4 (1982): 246–51.

Sandvick, Clinton. "Enforcing Medical Licensing in Illinois: 1877–1890." *Yale Journal of Biology and Medicine* 82 (2009): 67–74.

Scheel, Eugene. *Culpeper—A Virginia County's History Through 1920.* Orange, VA: Green Publishers, Inc., 1982.

Schlesinger, Arthur M. *The Age of Jackson.* Old Saybrook, CT: Konecky & Konecky, 1971. 1971. 1945.

Schmidt, J. M. "200 Years Organon of Medicine—A Comparative Review of Its Six Editions (1810–1842)." *Homeopathy* 99, no. 4 (Oct 2010): 271–7.

Shaffer, John W. *Clash of Loyalties—A Border County in the Civil War.* Morgantown, WV: West Virginia University Press, 2003.

Shaffer, John W. *Union and Confederate Soldiers and Sympathizers of Barbour County, West Virginia.* Baltimore, MD: Genealogical Publishing Company, 2005.

Sheets, L. Wayne. *Mother's Day—The Legacy of Anna Jarvis.* Parsons, WV: McClain Printing Company, 2013.

Sherman, Sidney. "Advertising in the United States." *Publications of the American Statistical Association* 7, no. 52 (1900): 1–44.

Shulman, Stanford T., and Alan L. Bisno. "Nonsuppurative Poststreptococcal Sequelae: Rheumatic Fever and Glomerulonephritis." Chap. 200 In *Mandell, Douglas, and Bennett's Principles and Practice of Infectious Diseases, Updated Edition,* edited by John E. Bennett, Raphael Dolin and Martin J. Blaser. Philadelphia, PA: Saunders, 2015.

Shyrock, Richard Harrison. "The American Physician in 1846 and 1946—A Study in Professional Contrasts." *JAMA* 134, no. 5 (1947): 417–24.

Shyrock, Richard Harrison. *Medical Licensing in America, 1650–1965.* Baltimore: Johns Hopkins Press, 1967.

Shyrock, Richard Harrison. *Medicine and Society in America: 1660–1860.* New York, NY: New York University Press, 1960. 1963.

Sigerist, Henry E. *American Medicine.* Translated by Hildegard Nagel. New York: W.W. Norton & Company, Inc., 1934.

Smart, Charles. *The Medical and Surgical History of the War of Rebellion—Medical History Part 3.* 2 vols. Vol. 1, Washington, D.C.: Government Printing Office, 1888.

Smillie, Wilson G. *Public Health: Its Promise for the Future.* New York, NY: The Macmillan Company, 1955.

Smith, Barry. "Gullible's Travails: Tuberculosis and Quackery, 1890–1930." *Journal of Contemporary History* 20, no. 4 (1985): 733–56.

Smith, Richard. *The Trouble with Medical Journals* London: Royal Society of Medicine Press Ltd., 2006.

Smith, Roy C. *Adam Smith and the Origins of American Enterprise: How the Founding Fathers Turned to a Great Economist's Writings and Created the American Economy.* New York, NY: Truman Talley Books, 2002.

Smith, Stephen. *The City That Was.* New York, NY: Frank Allaben, 1911.

Smith, Stephen. "Historical Sketch of the American Public Health Association." *Public Health Papers and Reports* 5 (1880): xvii–liv.

Smith-Rosenberg, Carroll. "The Female Animal: Medical and Biological Views of Women." Chap. 2 In *No Other Gods: On Science and American Social Thought,* edited by Charles E. Rosenberg, 54–70. Baltimore, MD: The Johns Hopkins University Press, 1997.

Smith-Rosenberg, Carroll, and Charles Rosenberg. "The Female Animal: Medical and Biological Views of Woman and Her Role in Nineteenth-Century America." Chap. 1 In *Women and Health in America—Historical Readings,* edited by Judith Walzer Leavitt, 12–27. Madison, WI: The University of Wisconsin Press, 1984.

Snell, Mark A. *West Virginia and the Civil War.* Civil War Sesquicentennial Series. Edited by Doug Bostick Charleston, SC: The History Press, 2011.

Snyder, C. "Our Ophthalmic Heritage. Julius Homberger, M.D." *Arch Ophthalmol* 68 (Dec 1962): 875–8.

Solis-Cohen, Solomon. "Shall Physicians Become Sales-Agents for Patent Medicines?" *Proceedings of the Philadelphia County Medical Society* 13 (1892): 213–16.

Spencer, H. R. "The History of Ovariotomy: (Section of the History of Medicine)." *Proc R Soc Med* 27, no. 11 (Sep 1934): 1437–44.

Sperry, F.M. *A Group of Distinguished Physicians and Surgeons of Chicago.* Chicago, IL: J.H. Beers & Co., 1904.

Starr, Paul. *The Social Transformation of American Medicine—The Rise of a Sovereign Profession and the Making of a Vast Industry.* New York: Basic Books, 1982.

Stempsey, William E., ed. *Elisha Bartlett's Philosophy of Medicine.* Edited by H. Tristram Engelhardt, Jr., and S.F. Spicker Vol. 83, Philosophy and Medicine. Dordrecht, The Netherlands: Springer, 2005.

Stevens, George Edward. "A History of the Cincinnati Post." University of Minnesota, 1969.

Stevens, Rosemary. *American Medicine and the Public Interest.* New Haven, CT: Yale University Press, 1971.

Stevenson, Lloyd G. "Exemplary Disease: The Typhoid Pattern." *Journal of the History of Medicine* 37, no. 2 (1982): 159–81.

Stillé, Charles *History of the United States Sanitary Commission—Being the General Report of Its Work During the War of the Rebellion.* Philadelphia, PA: J.B. Lippincott & Co, 1866.

Stover, John F.. *History of the Baltimore and Ohio Railroad.* West Lafayette, IN: Purdue University Press, 1987.

Stowe, Steven M.. *Doctoring the South—Southern Physicians and Everyday Medicine in the Mid-Nineteenth Century.* Chapel Hill, NC: The University of North Carolina Press, 2004.

Strong, Douglas M. "American Methodism in the Nineteenth Century: Expansion and Fragmentation." Chap. 3 In *The Cambridge Companion to American Methodism,* edited by Jason E. Vickers, 63–96. Cambridge, UK: Cambridge University Press 2013.

Stuart, A. B. "State Medicine and Public Hygiene." *The Sanitarian* 1, no. 10 (1874): 470–75.

Studd, John. "Ovariotomy for Menstrual Madness and the Pre-Menstrual Syndrome—19th Century History and Lessons for Current Practice." *Gynecology and Endocrinology* 22 (2006): 411–15.

Sullivan, Robert B. "Sanguine Practices: A Historical and Historiographic Reconsideration of Heroic Therapy in the Age of Rush." *Bulletin of the History of Medicine* 68, no. Summer (1994): 211–34.

Summers, Festus P. *Johnson Newlon Camden—A Study in Individualism.* New York, NY: G.P. Putnam's Sons, 1937.

Summers, Mark Wahlgren. *The Ordeal of the Reunion—A New History of Reconstruction.* Chapel Hill, NC: The University of North Carolina Press, 2014.

Sweet, William W. *Religion on the American Frontier 1783–1840.* Vol. IV—The Methodists, Chicago: The University of Chicago Press, 1946.

Tang, L. S. Y., E. Covert, E. Wilson, and S. Kottilil. "Chronic Hepatitis B Infection: A Review." *JAMA* 319, no. 17 (May 1, 2018): 1802–13.

Thomas, William G. *The Iron Way—Railroads, the Civil War, and the Making of Modern America.* New Haven, CT: Yale University Press, 2011.

Thomson, Samuel. *New Guide to Health; or Botanic Family Physician.* Second ed. Boston, MA: E. G. House, 1825. 1822.

Torney, George H. "Surgery of the Battlefield." *New York State Journal of Medicine* 12, no. 9 (1912): 483–88.

Traylor, John H. "Relative Strength of the Two Armies." *Confederate Veteran* 12, no. 11 (1904): 534–36.

Uchimura, Kazuko. "Coal Operators and Market Competition: The Case of West Virginia's Smokeless Coalfields and the Fairmont Field, 1853–1933." *West Virginia History* 4, no. 2 (2010): 59–86.

Velpeau, Alfred-Armand-Louis-Marie. *Complete Treatise on Midwifery: Or Principles of Tokology and Embryology.* Translated by Charles D. Meigs. Fourth American ed. Philadelphia: Lindsay and Blakiston, 1852.

Velpeau, Alfred-Armand-Louis-Marie. *Elementary Treatise on Midwifery: Or Principles of Tokology and Embryology.* Translated by Charles D. Meigs. First American ed. Philadelphia: J. Grigg, 1831.

Velpeau, Alfred-Armand-Louis-Marie. *Elementary Treatise on Midwifery: Or Principles of Tokology and Embryology.* Translated by Charles D. Meigs. Second American ed. Philadelphia: Grigg & Elliot, 1838.

Virchow, Rudolph. *Collected Essays on Public Health and Epidemiology.* Translated by Anne Gismann. Resources in Medical History. Edited by L.J. Rather 2 vols. Vol. 2, Canton, MA: Science History Publications/U.S.A., 1985. 1879.

Waite, F. C. "American Sectarian Medical Colleges Before the Civil War." *Bull Hist Med* 19 (Feb 1946): 148–66.

Warner, John Harley. *Against the Spirit of System—The French Impulse in Nineteenth-Century American Medicine.* Princeton, NJ: Princeton University Press, 1998.

Warner, John Harley. "'Exploring the Inner Labyrinths of Creation': Popular Microscopy in Nineteenth-Century America." *Journal of the History of Medicine and Allied Sciences* 37, no. 1 (1982): 7–33.

Warner, John Harley. "The Idea of Southern Medical Distinctiveness: Medical Knowledge and Practice in the Old South." Chap. 9 In *Science and Medicine in the Old South,* edited by Ronald L. Numbers and Todd L. Savitt, 179–205. Baton Rouge, LA: Louisiana State University Press, 1989.

Warner, John Harley. "A Southern Medical Reform: The Meaning of the Antebellum Argument for Southern Medical Education." Chap. 10 In *Science and Medicine in the Old South,* edited by Ronald L. Numbers and Todd L. Savitt, 206–25. Baton Rouge, LA: Louisiana State University Press, 1989.

Warner, John Harley. *The Therapeutic Perspective: Medical Practice, Knowledge, and Identity in America, 1820–1885.* Princeton, NJ: Princeton University Press, 1997.

Warner, John Harley, and Janet A. Tighe, eds. *Major Problems in the History of American Medicine and Public Health,* Major Problems in American History. Boston, MA: Houghton Mifflin Company, 2001.

Washburn, Benjamin E. *History of the North Carolina State Board of Health, 1877–1925.* Raleigh, NC: North Carolina State Board of Health, 1966.

Watson, Irving A. *Physicians and Surgeons of America: A Collection of Biographical Sketches of the Regular Medical Profession.* Concord, NH: Republican Press Association, 1896.

Wayland, John W. *A History of Rockingham County, Virginia.* Dayton, VA: Ruebush-Elkins Company, 1912.

Wayland, John W. *A History of Shenandoah County, Virginia.* Baltimore. MD: Regional Publishing Company, 1980. 1927.

Weisz, George. *Divide and Conquer : A Comparative History of Medical Specialization.* Oxford, UK: Oxford University Press, 2006.

Wesley, John. *Notes on the Bible.* Grand Rapids, MI: Christian Classics Ethereal Library, 1754.

Wesley, John. *Thoughts Upon Slavery.* Second ed. London: R. Hawes, 1774.

White, John H. *The American Railroad Passenger Car.* 2 vols. Vol. 2, Baltimore: The Johns Hopkins University Press, 1985. 1978.

Whooley, Owen. *Knowledge in the Time of Cholera—The Struggle Over American Medicine in the Nineteenth Century.* Chicago, IL: The University of Chicago Press, 2013.

Whyte, Kenneth *The Uncrowned King.* Vol. Toronto, Canada: Random House Canada, 2008.

Wicker, E. R. "Railroad Investment before the Civil War." In *Trends in the American Economy in the Nineteenth Century,* edited by The Conference on Research in Income and Wealth, 503–46. Princeton, NJ: Princeton University Press, 1960.

Wigger, John H. *Taking Heaven by Storm—Methodism and the Rise of Popular Christianity in America.* Urbana and Chicago: University of Illinois Press, 2001.

Wiley, S. T. *History of Preston County (West Virginia).* Kingwood, WV: Journal Printing House, 1882.

Williams, John Alexander. "The New Dominion and the Old: Ante-Bellum and Statehood Politics as the Background of West Virginia's' Bourbon Democracy." *West Virginia History* 33, no. 4 (1972): 317–407.

Williams, John Alexander. *West Virginia: A History.* New York, NY: W.W. Norton and Company, Inc., 1976. 1984. 1976.

Williams, John Alexander. *West Virginia and the Captains of Industry.* Morgantown, WV: West Virginia University Press, 2003. 1976.

Wilsey, John D. *American Exceptionalism and Civil Religion: Reassessing the History of an Idea.* Downers Grove, IL: InterVarsity Press, 2015.

Wilson, Louis D. "James Edmund Reeves, M.D.." *Transactions of the Medical Society of the State of West Virginia* (1896): 1319–27.

Winkelstein Jr., Warren. "Austin Flint, Clinician Turned Epidemiologist." *Epidemiology* 18, no. 2 (2007): 279.

Wolfe, Howard H. *Mother's Day and the Mother's Day Church.* Kingsport, TN: Privately Printed, 1962.

Wood, George Bacon. *A Treatise on the Practice of Medicine.* 1 ed. 2 vols. Philadelphia, PA: Grigg, Elliot, and Co., 1847.

Wood, George Bacon. *A Treatise on the Practice of Medicine.* 5 ed. 2 vols. Philadelphia, PA: J.B. Lippincott and Co, 1858.

Wood, George Bacon. *A Treatise on the Practice of Medicine.* 6 ed. 2 vols. Philadelphia, PA: J.B. Lippincott and Co, 1866.

Woods, Samuel. "Our Gallery—James Edmund Reeves, M.D. Of Wheeling W. Va.." *New England Medical Monthly* 4 (1885): 480–83.

Woodward, J.J. *The Medical and Surgical History of the War of the Rebellion—Medical History Part 1.* Edited by Joseph K. Barnes 2 vols. Vol. 1, Washington, D.C.: Government Printing Office, 1870.

Woodward, J.J. *The Medical and Surgical History of the War of the Rebellion—Medical History Part 2.* Edited by Joseph K. Barnes 2 vols. Vol. 1, Washington, D.C.: Government Printing Office, 1879.

York, Council of Hygiene and Public Health of the Citizens' Association of New. *Report Upon the Sanitary Condition of the City.* New York, NY: D. Appleton and Company, 1865.

Young, James Harvey. *The Medical Messiahs—A Social History of Health Quackery in Twentieth-Century America.* Princeton: Princeton University Press, 1967.

Young, James Harvey. *The Toadstool Millionaires—A Social History of Patent Medicines in America Before Federal Regulation.* Princeton: Princeton University Press, 1961.

Zaunders, Bo. *The Great Bridge Building Contest.* New York, NY: Harry N. Abrams, 2004.

Zimring, David R. "'Secession in Favor of the Constitution': How West Virginia Justified Separate Statehood During the Civil War." *West Virginia History (New Series)* 3, no. 2 (2009): 23–51.

Index